A Clinician's Guide to Multiple Sclerosis

A Clinician's Guide to Multiple Sclerosis

Editor: Floyd Freemont

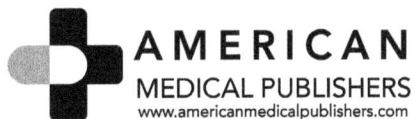

AMERICAN
MEDICAL PUBLISHERS
www.americanmedicalpublishers.com

AMERICAN
MEDICAL PUBLISHERS
www.americanmedicalpublishers.com

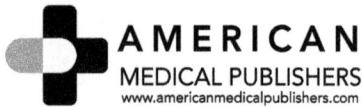

Cataloging-in-Publication Data

A clinician's guide to multiple sclerosis / edited by Floyd Freemont.
   p. cm.
Includes bibliographical references and index.
ISBN 978-1-63927-278-5
1. Multiple sclerosis. 2. Virus diseases. 3. Myelin sheath--Diseases. 4. Demyelination.
5. Neurology. I. Freemont, Floyd.
RC377 .C55 2022

616.834--dc23

American Medical Publishers,
41 Flatbush Avenue,
1st Floor, New York,
NY 11217, USA

ISBN 978-1-63927-278-5 (Hardback)

Contents

Permissions

List of Contributors

Index

Preface

This book has been an outcome of determined endeavour from a group of educationists in the field. The primary objective was to involve a broad spectrum of professionals from diverse cultural background involved in the field for developing new researches. The book not only targets students but also scholars pursuing higher research for further enhancement of the theoretical and practical applications of the subject.

Multiple sclerosis is a form of demyelinating disease. It is the disease of the nervous system in which the neuron's myelin sheath, a lipid-rich substance is damaged. The myelin is responsible for insulating axons to ensure the rapid flow of information from one nerve cell to another. This damage causes an inability in the parts of the nervous system to communicate. The signs and symptoms of the disease include mental, physical and psychiatric problems. Multiple sclerosis is the most common immune-mediated disorder that affects the central nervous system. The symptoms are determined by the locations of the lesions in the nervous system. This includes changes in sensation such as tingling, pins or numbness, muscle weakness and spasms, blurred vision or difficulty in moving. The person diagnosed with multiple sclerosis also experiences difficulties in coordination and balance, problems with speech or swallowing and chronic pain. This book includes some of the vital pieces of work being conducted across the world, on various topics related to multiple sclerosis. It consists of contributions made by international experts. It will provide comprehensive knowledge to the readers.

It was an honour to edit such a profound book and also a challenging task to compile and examine all the relevant data for accuracy and originality. I wish to acknowledge the efforts of the contributors for submitting such brilliant and diverse chapters in the field and for endlessly working for the completion of the book. Last, but not the least; I thank my family for being a constant source of support in all my research endeavours.

Editor

A cross-sectional and longitudinal study evaluating brain volumes, RNFL, and cognitive functions in MS patients and healthy controls

Jessica Frau[1*†], Giuseppe Fenu[1†], Alessio Signori[2], Giancarlo Coghe[1], Lorena Lorefice[1], Maria Antonietta Barracciu[3], Vincenzo Sechi[3], Federico Cabras[3], Mauro Badas[1], Maria Giovanna Marrosu[1] and Eleonora Cocco[1]

Abstract

Background: The principal biomarker of neurodegeneration in multiple sclerosis (MS) is believed to be brain volume, which is associated with cognitive functions and retinal nerve fibre layer (RNFL). A cross-sectional and longitudinal assessment of the relationship between RNFL, cognitive functions and brain volume.

Methods: At baseline, relapsing patients and healthy controls underwent 1.5 T MRI to estimate the normalized volume of brain (NBV), grey (NGV), white (NWV) and peripheral grey (pNGV) matter. Cognitive functions were evaluated by BICAMS, RNFL by Spectral-Domain OCT. Patients were re-evaluated after 12 months.

Results: Cognitive functions, brain volume, and RNFL differed between the group of 66 patients and that of 16 healthy controls. In the MS group, at baseline, an association was found between: p-NGV and symbol-digit (SDMT) ($p = 0.022$); temporal-RNFL and NBV ($p = 0.007$), NWV ($p = 0.012$), NGV ($p = 0.048$), and p-NGV ($p = 0.021$); papillo-macular bundle-RNFL and NBV ($p = 0.013$), NWV ($p = 0.02$), NGV ($p = 0.049$), and p-NGV ($p = 0.032$). Over the observational period, we found a reduction of brain volume ($p < 0.001$), average-RNFL ($p = 0.001$), temporal-RNFL ($p = 0.006$), and papillo-macular bundle-RNFL ($p = 0.009$). No association was found between OCT, MRI, and cognitive changes.

Conclusions: Brain volume, cognitive functions, and RNFL are continuous measures of different neurodegenerative aspects. BICAMS and OCT have low costs and can be easily used in clinical practice to monitor neurodegeneration.

Keywords: Multiple sclerosis, Brain volume, Retinal nerve Fiber layer thickness, Cognitive impairments, BICAMS

Background

Multiple Sclerosis (MS) is a chronic disease involving the central nervous system. The clinical course is generally relapsing at onset, and later progressive [1]. Both the inflammatory and neurodegenerative component is present from the early stages [1]. While the first aspect has been well documented and is monitored in clinical practice using conventional magnetic resonance imaging (MRI), the study of neurodegeneration is more

difficult [2]. At present, an important biomarker of the neurodegenerative aspect in MS is the evaluation of brain volume by non-conventional techniques of MRI [3]. Indeed, the loss of brain volume appears to be related to the progression of the disease and the permanent accumulation of disability [3, 4]. One of the most important symptoms related to brain atrophy is the deficit of cognitive functions [5]. This is associated with several MRI markers, in particular grey matter pathology, both in terms of focal lesions and volume loss [5]. Cognitive impairment, which has variable severity and has been identified at all stages of the disease and clinical courses, affects between 40 and 70% of MS patients [6]. It appears to be associated with age, disease

* Correspondence: jessicafrau@hotmail.it
†Equal contributors
[1]Multiple Sclerosis Center Binaghi Hospital, Department of Medical Sciences and Public Health, University of Cagliari, via Is Guadazzonis 2, 09126 Cagliari, Italy
Full list of author information is available at the end of the article

duration and disability [7]. Many diagnostic tools are able to explore cognitive functions in MS patients [8], although the majority of these are time consuming and require qualified personnel [8]. However, a recently developed neuropsychological assessment named "Brief International Cognitive Assessment for Multiple Sclerosis" (BICAMS) can be administered by non-specifically trained healthcare staff in around 15 min [8].

In the last decades, optic coherence tomography (OCT), a new instrument for evaluating the neurodegenerative aspect of MS, has been widely studied [9, 10]. OCT is able to evaluate the thickness of the retinal nerve fibre layer (RNFL), a defined marker of axonal loss. RNFL measurement could differentiate MS patients from healthy subjects, and it is clearly related to brain atrophy, disease duration, and disability [10–14]. The most involved RNFL region is the temporal quadrant [15]. The great majority of studies exploring RNFL in MS patients have been performed using a 'time-domain' OCT (considered the 'old' OCT model), which produces less accurate images than the 'spectral domain' OCT (SD-OCT), especially in longitudinal studies [16–19].

BICAMS and OCT share three important qualities for MS assessment in a clinical setting: brevity, ease of use, and low cost.

The present study entails a cross-sectional and longitudinal assessment of the use of SD-OCT and BICAMS in the evaluation of the neurodegenerative aspects of MS. These procedures are compared with MRI brain atrophy measurements, which are currently considered the gold standard among neurodegenerative markers in MS patients.

Methods

MS-relapsing patients consecutively referred to the MS Centre of the University of Cagliari/Binaghi Hospital from March to July 2015 were prospectively included in the study. A group of healthy controls working in the Binaghi hospital was also recruited over the same time period. All the subjects signed an informed consent. The inclusion criteria for MS patients were: 18-65 years of age; relapsing remitting course; no relapses and/or steroids intake in the 30 days before enrolment and follow-up evaluation. All patients started a disease-modifying drug (DMD) prior to enrolment. Psychoactive drugs or substances that might interfere with neuropsychological performance were forbidden for both patients and healthy controls.

The ethics committee of the University of Cagliari approved the study.

At baseline, after written informed consent was given, all the subjects underwent neuropsychological assessment, brain MRI, and OCT. These three evaluations were carried out within a maximum period of three

months. The evaluations were repeated for a group of MS patients after 12 months ±3. The changes from baseline and follow-up (difference between follow-up and baseline) were calculated for all of the collected MRI, OCT and BICAMS parameters collected.

Gender and age were collected for the whole cohort. In the MS group, the following clinical data were also recorded from medical records by a neurologist with expertise in MS: age at onset; clinical course; expanded disability status scale score (EDSS) at baseline; all DMD from six months before baseline until the end of the study; presence of relapses and steroid therapy in the 30 days before baseline and before the follow-up evaluation; and optic neuritis in the clinical history with indication of the affected eye. Eyes affected by previous optic neuritis were excluded from the statistical analysis.

Neuropsychological evaluation

An expert neuropsychologist (G.F.) performed the neuropsychological evaluation in a quiet room using the BICAMS. This assessment was recently developed by an expert consensus group and included: the Symbol Digit Modality Test (SDMT) to evaluate processing speed (or working memory); the California Verbal Learning Test II (CVLT-II) to evaluate verbal learning and memory; and the Brief Visual Memory Test Revised (BVMT-R) to evaluate visual learning and memory [8, 20]. All tests were considered normal or altered according to the authors' definition (T score equal or inferior to 35). T score estimations were made using available normative values, with corrections for age, gender and education among the Italian population [20]. Patients were categorized as either cognitive impaired (at least one test altered) or cognitive preserved (no tests altered).

The neuropsychologist was blinded to clinical and radiological findings.

Brain MR acquisition

Brain MRI acquisition and analysis was performed at the Radiology Unit of Binaghi Hospital, Cagliari, Italy. The operator was blinded to the clinical and neuropsychological status of the subjects. The acquisition of brain MRIs was obtained in a single session, using a Siemens Magneton Avanto Scan at 1.5 T. A sagittal survey image was used to identify the anterior and posterior commissures. A dual-echo, turbo spin-echo sequence (repetition time/echo time 1/echo time 2 5 2075/30/90 milliseconds, 256 X 256 matrix, 1 signal average, 250 mm field of view, 50 contiguous 3 mm slices) yielding proton density–weighted and T2-weighted images were acquired in the transverse plane parallel to the line connecting the anterior and posterior commissures. Transverse T1-weighted (T1W) images (repetition time 35 milliseconds; echo time 10 milliseconds; 256 X 256 matrix; 1

signal average; 2,503,250 mm field of view) were acquired, yielding images of 176 contiguous 1 mm-thick slices, oriented to match the proton density of the T2-weighted image.

Brain parenchyma volumes were measured on T1W gradient echo images by using the cross-sectional version of the SIENA (*structural image evaluation using normalization of atrophy*) software, named SIENAX (part of FSL 4.0: http://www.fmrib.ox.ac.uk/fsl/), a previously described method to estimate global brain volume normalized for head size [21]. MRI analysis allowed for Normalized Brain Volume (NBV), Normalized Grey Matter Volume (NGV), peripheral NGV (p-NGV), and Normalized White Matter Volume (NWV) to be obtained. Lesion refilling was performed as described previously [22].

Longitudinal evaluation of the percentage of brain volume change (PBVC) was performed using SIENA software only in patients not showing new T2 and/or gadolinium enhancing lesions during follow-up. To evaluate annualized PBVC (a-PBVC), the following formula was used: PBVC/months from baseline to follow-up * 12.

Optical coherence tomography

OCT evaluations were performed using a Spectralis SD-OCT (Heidelberg Engineering; Heidelberg, Germania). The machine is able to record ocular movements via a confocal scanning laser ophthalmoscope (TrueTrac ®; Heidelberg Engineering, Heidelberg, Germany). True-Trac have adapted the software to ocular movements, allowing a correct examination. Eyes that were blind due to reasons other than MS were excluded. The RNFL examination was performed by a ring scan centred on the optic nerve head. The follow-up study was made using the automatic rescan mode. The thickness of global RNFL, the temporal sector (TEMP) and the papillomacular bundle sector (PMB) were calculated using the machine's software, and an evaluation of subclinical previous optic neurotis was performed [23]. After excluding previous clinical and subclinical ON, the minimum value between right and left eye for the same subject was entered for analysis. Two neurologists trained in the use of the Spectralis SD-OCT performed all examinations.

Sample size and statistical analysis

At an alpha level of 5%, and for a statistical power of 90%, a minimum of 61 patients was needed to observe a significant correlation of at least 0.4 (threshold between a weak and moderate correlation).

Comparisons between MS patients and healthy controls at baseline were made using independent samples Student's t-test for age, chi-square test for gender, Mann-Whitney for education, and linear regression models for MRI parameters and SDMT. Regression models were adjusted for age (MRI parameters) and education (SDMT).

Partial correlation coefficients were estimated to assess the cross-sectional correlations at baseline between cognitive functions, RNFL and MRI characteristics. These correlations were adjusted for age, gender, EDSS (MRI and RNFL), and education.

A multivariable model for each MRI volume (considered as dependent variable) was performed to assess the impact, quantified by R^2 value, of each RNFL and cognitive functions characteristics on MRI parameters. Only variables for which univariable analysis showed a p value < 0.10 were considered for the multivariable model, and a stepwise approach was adopted to select those included in the model.

One-year changes in MRI, cognitive functions and RNFL were assessed using paired samples Student's t-test.

To assess the correlations between the longitudinal changes in cognitive functions, RNFL and MRI characteristics, partial correlation coefficients were estimated using delta changes between baseline and one year. Correlations between baseline and longitudinal changes were also assessed. These were adjusted for age, gender, EDSS (MRI and RNFL) and education.

Stata (v.14; StataCorp.) was used for the computation of results.

Results

We included 66 MS subjects (female: 48; 72.7%) and 16 healthy controls (female: 9; 56.25%). Mean age at baseline was 43.4 years (SD: 12) in patients, and 46.8 years (SD: 9) in healthy controls. Mean education was 11.6 years (SD: 4.16) in patients, and 14.3 years (SD: 4.19) in healthy subjects. In the MS group, the mean duration of the disease was 10.8 years and the median EDSS was 2 (range: 0 - 7.5). Ten patients were not included in the OCT study due to poor compliance. In 4 other patients, the OCT evaluation was made only in 1 eye, as the other eye was blind for reasons other than MS.

Baseline values of NBV, NWV, NGV, p-NGV, SDMT, CVLT-II, BVMT-R, average-RNFL, TEMP-RNFL, and PMB-RNFL are reported in Table 1.

The comparison between healthy controls and patients at baseline showed higher NBV ($p = 0.006$), higher NWV ($p = 0.003$), and higher RNFL thickness ($p = 0.014$) in the first group. The healthy subjects group also demonstrated better performance at SDMT ($p = 0.037$). No significant differences were found in NGV and p-NGV.

Cross sectional analysis in MS patients at baseline

In Table 2 were reported all baseline correlations. A significant correlation between: p-NGV and SDMT ($p = 0.022$); NGV and SDMT ($p = 0.013$); NGV and BVMT ($p = 0.048$); TEMP-RNFL and NBV ($p = 0.007$); TEMP-RNFL and

Table 1 Clinical and demographic features

	MS ($n = 66$)	HC ($n = 16$)	p-value
Age, mean (SD)	43.4 (12)	46.8 (9)	0.32
Gender, n(%)			0.21
Females	48 (72.7)	9 (56.3)	
Males	18 (27.3)	7 (43.7)	
Education (years), median (range)	13 (5-21)	13 (8-19)	0.096
Disease duration, mean; median (range)	10.8; 8.5 (0-34)		
EDSS, median (range)	2 (0-7.5)		
NBV, mean (SD)	1473.5 (81.9)	1519.6 (38.4)	0.006^
NWV, mean (SD)	694 (39.9)	728.1 (19.1)	0.003^
NGV, mean (SD)	777.7 (72)	791.5 (33.1)	0.14^
p-NGV, mean (SD)	609.6 (52.1)	616.2 (28.7)	0.11^
SDMT, mean (SD)	45.1 (12.3)	53.3 (8.4)	0.037*
CVLT-II, mean (SD)	41.6 (10.3)	–	
BVMT-R, mean (SD)	47.6 (10.8)	–	
RNFL, mean (SD)	93.8 (10.7)	101.8 (9.9)	0.014
TEMP-RNFL, mean (SD)	63.3 (11)	–	
PMB-RNFL, mean (SD)	49.6 (9.4)	–	

^ - linear regression model adjusted for Age; *linear regression model adjusted for education
MRI measures (NBV, NWV, NGV, p-NGV) are expressed in ml
Cognitive measures (SDMT, CVLT-II, BVMT-R) are expressed in T score

Table 2 Partial correlations among OCT, cognitive and MRI parameters

Neurodegenerative assessment	Variables	r	p-value
SD-OCT			
Average-RNFL	SDMT	0.01	0.96
	CVLT-II	0.20	0.18
	BVMT-R	0.08	0.60
	NBV	0.25	0.095
	NWV	0.16	0.28
	NGV	0.22	0.14
	p-NGV	0.29	0.06
TEMP-RNFL	SDMT	0.01	0.95
	CVLT-II	0.09	0.57
	BVMT-R	0.08	0.58
	NBV	0.40	0.007
	NWV	0.37	0.012
	NGV	0.30	0.048
	p-NGV	0.36	0.021
PMB-RNFL	SDMT	0.044	0.78
	CVLT-II	0.09	0.55
	BVMT-R	0.13	0.38
	NBV	0.37	0.013
	NWV	0.35	0.02
	NGV	0.30	0.049
	p-NGV	0.33	0.032
SDMT	NBV	0.20	0.10
	NWV	−0.07	0.56
	NGV	0.21	0.11
	p-NGV	0.31	0.022
CVLT-II	NBV	0.09	0.48
	NWV	0.06	0.66
	NGV	0.04	0.78
	p-NGV	0.01	0.97
BVMT-R	NBV	0.11	0.38
	NWV	0.05	0.68
	NGV	0.18	0.17
	p-NGV	0.22	0.11

NWV ($p = 0.012$); TEMP-RNFL and NGV ($p = 0.048$); TEMP-RNFL and p-NGV ($p = 0.021$); PMB-RNFL and NBV (p = 0.013); PMB-RNFL and NWV ($p = 0.02$); PMB-RNFL and NGV ($p = 0.049$); PMB-RNFL and p-NGV ($p = 0.032$). The correlations between SDMT and p-NGV are shown in Fig. 1, while the correlations between TEMP-RNFL and MRI parameters in Fig. 2.

Average-RNFL thickness displayed a correlation with both NBV ($p = 0.10$), and p-NGV ($p = 0.06$) even thought it did not reach the statistical significance. The OCT measures did not correlate with the results of BICAMS tests.

Since p-NGV correlated with both OCT and cognitive performances, a multivariable model was implemented. After selection, SDMT and TEMP-RNFL, together with age and disease duration, were significantly associated with p-NGV (Table 3). The multivariable model increased R^2 from 38.3% (with age) to 48.5% with the inclusion of SDMT (ΔR^2 of 10.2%), and to 65.2% with the inclusion of TEMP-RNFL (ΔR^2 of 16.7%).

Longitudinal analysis
At follow-up, 26 patients did not repeat the OCT, 30 did not repeat the brain MRI, and 25 did not repeat the neuropsychological evaluation. The longitudinal evaluations of all the three measures were therefore available for 36 patients, while in a further 4 subjects only OCT and BICAMS, but not MRI, were performed at follow-up.

The mean percentage of brain volume change from baseline to follow-up was 0.57 (SD: 0.54, p: < 0.001). All the OCT parameters changed significantly from baseline to follow-up. A mean decrease of 1.3 (SD: 1.7) for average-RNFL ($p < 0.001$); 1.2 (SD: 1.9) for TEMP ($p = 0.001$); and 1.4 (SD: 2.2) for PMB (p = 0.001) was observed. No significant changes were detected in all the BICAMS tests results.

No significant correlation was found between OCT, MRI and cognitive changes.

A cross-sectional and longitudinal study evaluating brain volumes, RNFL, and cognitive functions...

5

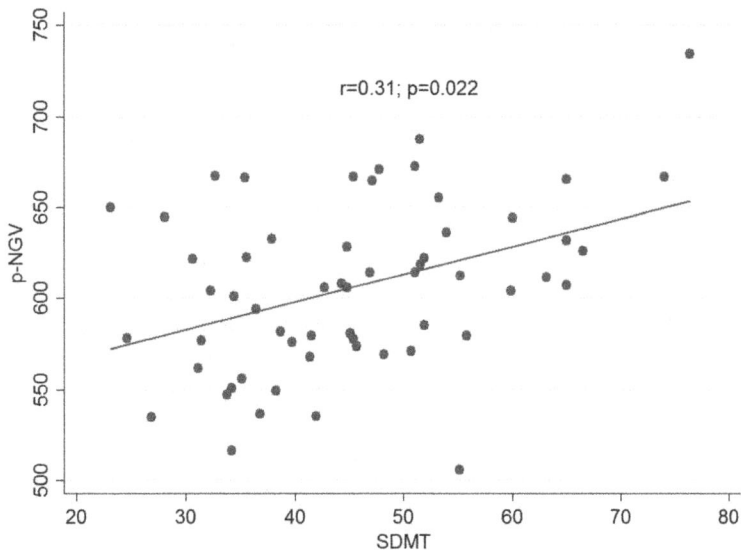

Fig. 1 Correlation between SDMT and p-NGV

Discussion

We found that the evaluation of RNFL thickness by SD-OCT and cognitive functions by BICAMS are able to differentiate the group of MS patients from that of healthy controls, as previously shown by numerous studies [8–11], as well as being independent markers of neurodegeneration. These were compared with brain volume evaluation performed with MRI - the most commonly used instrument for MS follow-up and what is generally considered the gold standard

marker for monitoring the degenerative component of the pathology.

Our data confirmed the association between both assessments and brain volume measures [5, 10–14]. In particular, we found that the BICAMS tests correlate with NGV, especially with cortical atrophy, which is notoriously associated with cognitive decline [5]. Moreover, we found a significant correlation between specific OCT parameters (temporal quadrant and PMB thickness) and brain volume measurements. This correlation appears to

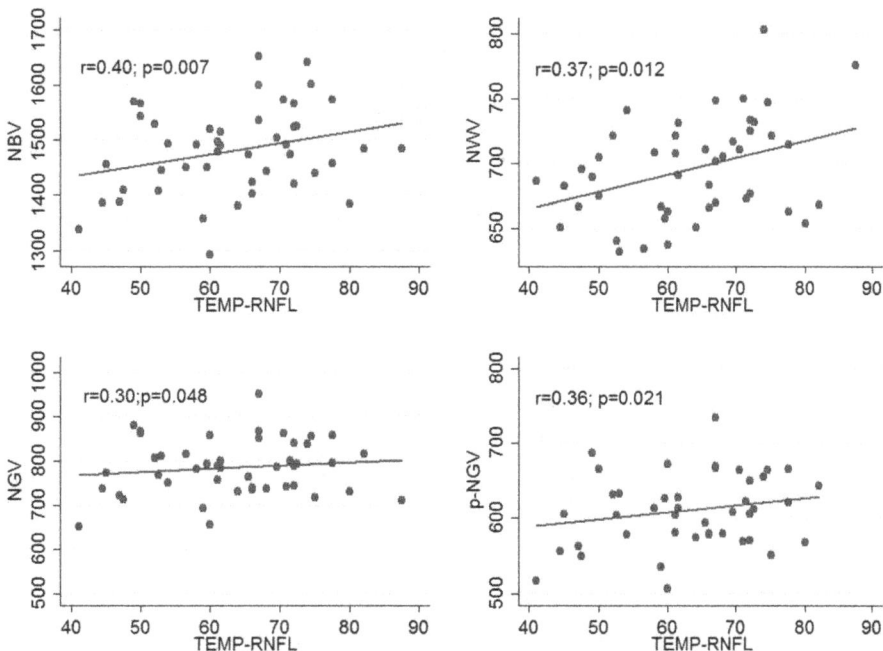

Fig. 2 Correlation between TEMP-RNFL and the following brain volume measures: NGV, NBV, NWV, and p-NGV

Table 3 Effect of cognitive and OCT characteristics on p-NGV at baseline. The increase of R^2 associated with the inclusion of significant characteristics in the model was reported

	B (95% CI); p-value	ΔR^2
Model 1		
SDMT (T-score)	1.20 (0.46-1.95); p = 0.002	+ 0.102
Model 2		
SDMT (T-score)	1.20 (0.44-1.95); p = 0.003	
TEMP-RNFL	1.26 (0.35-2.16); p = 0.008	+ 0.167

Both models include age and disease duration at baseline

be stronger with global and white brain volume than grey matter volume. This result is in line with previous studies in which OCT measures were found to be associated with total brain volume and normalized white matter volume [12, 24], or both normalized white and grey matter volumes [11].

An innovative aspect of our work was the combined analysis of brain atrophy, RNFL thickness, and cognitive functions. Indeed, while the association between brain volume and the other two parameters has been clearly assessed previously, and confirmed by our data, there is less evidence of a possible correlation between RNFL thickness and cognitive impairment. Toledo et al. performed a unique study exploring this issue [25]. They found a significant correlation between SDMT and RNFL thickness, both for the average and the temporal quadrant. However, this result was not confirmed by our work, and we did not observe any correlation between RNFL (average, temporal and PMB) and BICAMS tests. It is worth noting that Toledo et al. performed their OCT analysis with a smaller sample and using a less accurate time-domain machine.

The lack of association between RNFL thickness and cognitive impairment, as for their correlation with different brain volume regions (only grey matter for BICAMS tests, both grey and white matter for TEMP-RNFL and PMB-RNFL), leads us to hypothesize that RNFL and cognitive impairment may represent different aspects of neurodegeneration in MS. Indeed, cognitive decline is secondary to axonal loss, dendritic transection and apoptosis [26]. Moreover, as well as the grey matter pathology, cognitive impairment is mainly associated with primitive degeneration present from the initial stages of the disease, as entirely independent degenerative process, and only partially it is secondary to inflammation. [6, 27]. Otherwise, RNFL thickness may equally be associated with both primitive degeneration and degeneration due to an inflammatory component. In particular, the thinning observed by OCT may be due to clinical and subclinical episodes of ON, primary neurodegeneration of the retinal ganglion cells and their axons, or retrograde transsynaptic degeneration of the

ganglion cells and their axons due to MS lesions in the posterior visual pathways [28].

Longitudinally, no significant changes in BICAMS tests scores emerged. This was probably due to a well-known practice effect [20].

A reduction was observed in the mean percentage of brain volume, and in all the OCT parameters considered. However, the longitudinal trend of the two measures did not correlate, perhaps due to the fact that they do not reflect the same specific inflammatory and degenerative brain damage in MS pathology. When considering the brain atrophy measure, we also need to take into account the well-known phenomenon of so-called 'pseudo-atrophy' [4], which hinders the correct evaluation of the degenerative and inflammatory components. Thus, some patients could have a 'false' light reduction of brain volume over the course of one year due to the presence of inflammatory oedema. To note that all the patients were clinically stable between baseline and follow-up, and no active lesions in brain MRI were observed.

The study was also subject to some limitations.

First, follow-up may have been too short to observe significant changes in the degenerative component, which is present since the initial stages of the disease and is characterized by slow progression.

Second, while our cohort of participants is of a comparable size to that of previous cross-sectional studies, it may be too small to provide clear longitudinal results. Moreover, patients were heterogeneous for the duration of disease, DMD, and grade of inflammation at MRI. However, the great majority of them were clinically stable during the observational period, and no optic neuritis was recorded between baseline and follow-up.

Conclusions

Our study shows that the evaluation of brain volume, cognitive functions, and RNFL thickness are different continuous measures of neurodegeneration. Unconventional MRI, with its significant costs and requirement for qualified personnel, is more difficult to use in all MS settings. BICAMS and OCT, however, which can be performed at low cost after minimal training, may be suitable for use in clinical practice to assess different aspects of neurodegeneration.

Abbreviations
a-PBVC: Annualize of percentage of brain volume change; BICAMS: Brief international cognitive assessment for multiple sclerosis; BVMT-R: Brief visual memory test revised; CVLT-II: California verbal learning test II; DMD: Disease-modifying drug; EDSS: Expanded disability status scale; MRI: Magnetic resonance imaging; MS: Multiple sclerosis; NBV: Normalized volume of brain; NGV: Normalized volume of grey; NWV: Normalized volume of white; OCT: Optical coherence tomography; PBVC: Percentage of brain volume change; PMB: Papillo-macular bundle; pNGV: Normalized volume of peripheral grey; RNFL: Retinal nerve fibre layer; SD: Spectral domain; SD: Standard deviation; SDMT: Symbol digit modalities test; TEMP: Temporal

Acknowledgements
The authors wish to thank the patients and their caregivers for their time and commitment to this research.

Funding
The author(s) received no financial support for the research, authorship, and/or publication of this article.

Authors' contributions
JF, GF, GC participated in the design of the study and drafted the manuscript. AS performed the statistical analysis. JF, GC carried out the OCT acquisition, performed MRI data analysis and interpretation. VS, MAB, FC carried out the MRI acquisition. GF, LL performed MRI data analysis and interpretation. GF, MB carried out the neuropsychological evaluation. EC, MGM helped draft the manuscript and revise it critically for important intellectual content. All authors read and approved the final manuscript.

Competing interests
The author(s) declared no potential conflicts of interest with respect to the research, authorship, and/or publication of this article.

Author details
[1]Multiple Sclerosis Center Binaghi Hospital, Department of Medical Sciences and Public Health, University of Cagliari, via Is Guadazzonis 2, 09126 Cagliari, Italy. [2]Department of Health Sciences, Section of Biostatistics, University of Genova, Via Pastore, 1, 16132 Genoa, Italy. [3]Unit of Radiology, Binaghi Hospital, ATS Sardegna, via Is Guadazzonis 2, 09126 Cagliari, Italy.

References
1. Kamm CP, Uitdehaag BM, Polman CH. Multiple sclerosis: current knowledge and future outlook. Eur Neurol. 2014;72(3-4):132–41.
2. Río J, Rovira À, Tintoré M, Otero-Romero S, et al. Disability progression markers over 6-12 years in interferon-β-treated multiple sclerosis patients. Mult Scler. 2017;1:1352458517698052.
3. Sastre-Garriga J, Pareto D, Rovira À. Brain atrophy in multiple sclerosis: clinical relevance and technical aspects. Neuroimaging Clin N Am. 2017; 27(2):289–300.
4. De Stefano N, Airas L, Grigoriadis N, et al. Clinical relevance of brain volume measures in multiple sclerosis. CNS Drugs. 2014;28(2):147–56.
5. Rocca MA, Amato MP, De Stefano N, et al. Clinical and imaging assessment of cognitive dysfunction in multiple sclerosis. Lancet Neurol. 2015;14(3):302–17.
6. Chiaravalloti ND, DeLuca J. Cognitive impairment in multiple sclerosis. Lancet Neurol. 2008;7(12):1139–51.
7. Ruano L, Portaccio E, Goretti B, et al. Age and disability drive cognitive impairment in multiple sclerosis across disease subtypes. Mult Scler. 2017; 23(9):1258–67.
8. Langdon D. Cognitive assessment in MS. Neurodegener Dis Manag. 2015; 5(6 Suppl):43–5.
9. Parisi V, Manni G, Spadaro M, et al. Correlation between morphological and functional retinal impairment in multiple sclerosis patients. Invest Ophthalmol Vis Sci. 1999;40(11):2520–7.
10. Gordon-Lipkin E, Chodkowski B, Reich DS, et al. Retinal nerve fiber layer is associated with brain atrophy in multiple sclerosis. Neurology. 2007; 69(16):1603–9.
11. Sepulcre J, Murie-Fernandez M, Salinas-Alaman A, et al. Diagnostic accuracy of retinal abnormalities in predicting disease activity in MS. Neurology. 2007; 68(18):1488–94.
12. Grazioli E, Zivadinov R, Weinstock-Guttman B, et al. Retinal nerve fiber layer thickness is associated with brain MRI outcomes in multiple sclerosis. J Neurol Sci. 2008;268(1-2):12–7.
13. Siger M, Dziegielewski K, Jasek L, et al. Optical coherence tomography in multiple sclerosis: thickness of the retinal nerve fiber layer as a potential measure of axonal loss and brain atrophy. J Neurol. 2008;255(10):1555–60.
14. Dörr J, Wernecke KD, Bock M, et al. Association of retinal and macular damage with brain atrophy in multiple sclerosis. PLoS One. 2011;6(4): e18132.
15. Lamirel C, Newman NJ, Biousse V. Optical coherence tomography (OCT) in optic neuritis and multiple sclerosis. Rev Neurol (Paris). 2010;166(12):978–86.
16. Lange AP, Sadjadi R, Saeedi J, et al. Time-domain and spectral-domain optical coherence tomography of retinal nerve Fiber layer in MS patients and healthy controls. J Ophthalmol. 2012;2012:564627.
17. Knight OJ, Chang RT, Feuer WJ, et al. Comparison of retinal nerve fiber layer measurements using time domain and spectral domain optical coherent tomography. Ophthalmology. 2009;116(7):1271–7.
18. Watson GM, Keltner JL, Chin EK, et al. Comparison of retinal nerve fiber layer and central macular thickness measurements among five different optical coherence tomography instruments in patients with multiple sclerosis and optic neuritis. J Neuro-Oncol. 2011;31(2):110–6.
19. Arthur SN, Smith SD, Wright MM, et al. Reproducibility and agreement in evaluating retinal nerve fibre layer thickness between stratus and Spectralis OCT. Eye (Lond). 2011;25(2):192–200.
20. Goretti B, Niccolai C, Hakiki B, et al. The brief international cognitive assessment for multiple sclerosis (BICAMS): normative values with gender, age and education corrections in the Italian population. BMC Neurol. 2014;14:171.
21. Smith SM, Zhang Y, Jenkinson M, et al. Accurate, robust, and automated longitudinal and cross-sectional brain change analysis. NeuroImage. 2002; 17(1):479–89.
22. Battaglini M, Jenkinson M, De Stefano N. Evaluating and reducing the impact of white matter lesions on brain volume measurements. Hum Brain Mapp. 2012;33(9):2062–71.
23. Martinez-Lapiscina EH, Arnow S, Wilson JA, et al. Retinal thickness measured with optical coherence tomography and risk of disability worsening in multiple sclerosis: a cohort study. Lancet Neurol. 2016;15(6):574–84.
24. Young KL, Brandt AU, Petzold A, et al. Loss of retinal nerve fibre layer axons indicates white but not grey matter damage in early multiple sclerosis. Eur J Nurol. 2013;20(5):803–11.
25. Toledo J, Sepulcre J, Salinas-Alaman A, et al. Retinal nerve fiber layer atrophy is associated with physical and cognitive disability in multiple sclerosis. Mult Scler. 2008;14(7):906–12.
26. Peterson JW, Bö L, Mörk S, Chang A, et al. Transected neurites, apoptotic neurons, and reduced inflammation in cortical multiple sclerosis lesions. Ann Neurol. 2001;50(3):389–400.
27. Benedict RH, Shucard JL, Zivadinov R, et al. Neuropsychological impairment in systemic lupus erythematosus: a comparison with multiple sclerosis. Neuropsychol Rev. 2008;18(2):149–66.
28. Britze J, Pihl-Jensen G, Frederiksen JL. Retinal ganglion cell analysis in multiple sclerosis and optic neuritis: a systematic review and meta-analysis. J Neurol. 2017; https://doi.org/10.1007/s00415-017-8531-y.

The Turkish validation of the Brief International Cognitive Assessment for Multiple Sclerosis (BICAMS) battery

Serkan Ozakbas[1], Pinar Yigit[1], Bilge Piri Cinar[2*], Hatice Limoncu[1], Turhan Kahraman[3] and Görkem Kösehasanoğulları[4]

Abstract

Background: Cognitive impairment may be seen in as many as 43–70% of patients with multiple sclerosis (MS) and may be observed in all MS subtypes. The Brief International Cognitive Assessment in Multiple Sclerosis (BICAMS) battery may be used to evaluate cognition status. The purpose of the current study is to validate the BICAMS battery in Turkish.

Methods: Patients with MS attending our clinic between September 2014 and April 2015 were invited to participate. Healthy control participants were matched in terms of age, gender and years of education.

Results: One hundred seventy-three MS patients and 153 healthy control participants were enrolled in the study. MS patients performed significantly worse in all trials than the members of the healthy control group. In addition, cognitive dysfunction was identified in 78 of the 173 (45.1%) patients. In the MS with cognitive impairment group, 64 out of 151 (42.4%) subjects were RRMS patients, 12 out of 18 (66.7%) were secondary progressive MS patients, and 2 out of 4 (50%) were primer progressive MS patients.

Conclusions: The BICAMS has been proposed for assessing cognitive impairment in MS patients. This study shows that the battery is suitable for use in Turkey.

Keywords: Multiple sclerosis, BICAMS battery, Cognitive impairment

Background

Cognitive impairment is common in multiple sclerosis (MS), and approximately half of patients with MS present with cognitive impairment that adversely impacts on aspects of both patients' and caregivers' everyday lives [1, 2]. It is demonstrable in all disease stages and subtypes, in up to 40% of newly diagnosed individuals with clinically isolated syndrome and relapsing remitting MS (RRMS) [3] and in up to 60% of those with secondary progressive MS (SPMS) [4]. It can have a significant impact on quality of life and can influence employment status, physical independence, communications, treatment adherence and even rehabilitation benefit [2]. The assessment of MS-related cognitive decline has received increasing attention in recent decades. Many different neuropsychological batteries have been proposed. However, the Brief Repeatable Battery of Neuropsychological tests (BRB-N) [5] and the Minimal Assessment of Cognitive Function in MS (MACFIMS) [4, 6] are the most popular tools. While both batteries are known to be highly specific for the evaluation of cognitive impairment in MS patients, their implementation in everyday clinical practice remains limited due to their high time demands (at least 45 min are required for BRB-N and 90 min for MACFIMS) and the need for surveillance and interpretation by specialist neuropsychologists [4–7]. Various neuropsychological batteries have been proposed for the assessment of cognitive impairment in MS as the interest in this area has increased over recent years. The Brief International Cognitive Assessment in Multiple Sclerosis (BICAMS) was proposed by an expert panel as a tool for brief cognitive monitoring of MS patients in clinical settings in 2012 [8]. It can be administered by healthcare

* Correspondence: bilge.cinarpiri@gmail.com
[2]Department of Neurology, Samsun Training and Researce Hospital, Samsun, Turkey
Full list of author information is available at the end of the article

professionals without any formal neuropsychological training to identify early or subtle cognitive impairment. The BICAMS battery is a fast, reliable, sensitive and specific tool that has been validated and applied in many countries [9–14]. The primary objective of our study was the cross-cultural validation of the BICAMS battery to Turkish. The secondary objective was to measure the impact of cognitive impairment on patients' quality of life and the effect of fatigue on patients' cognitive state by assessing correlations between BICAMS performance and the Modified Fatigue Impact Scale (MFIS) and the Multiple Sclerosis International Quality of Life (MUSIQoL) questionnaire.

Methods

Patients

Patients with a diagnosis of MS according to the 2010 revised McDonald criteria [15] attending our clinic between September, 2014, and April, 2015, were invited to participate. Patients were recruited cross-sectionally, and no pre-selection was applied for cognitive impairment. The inclusion criteria were age over 18 years, the ability to give informed consent, neurological stability with no evidence of relapse, being steroid and/or plasmapheresis-free for at least 4 weeks preceding enrollment, and proficiency in the Turkish language. Patients were excluded if they had a current or previous neurological disorder other than MS, a current psychiatric disorder unrelated to that diagnosis, a coexistent medical condition that might influence cognition, a previous history of developmental disorder unrelated to MS, a history of learning disability, any vision or hearing problems that might influence performance on the tests, or a current or past history of alcohol or drug abuse. Control participants were recruited from unaffected relatives or friends of MS patients or from other individuals attending the neurology outpatient clinic for other reasons, such as migraine or vertigo. All relatives were matched in terms of age, gender and years of education. All patients and all healthy control subjects provided verbal informed consent to participation in the study. Approval for the research project was granted by the Ethics Committee of Dokuz Eylul University of Izmir.

Study instruments and procedures

The methodology employed followed the recommendations for BICAMS national validation (step 1; standardization and translation of test stimuli, step 2; standardization and translation of test instructions, step 3; normalization, step 4; test-retest reliability, step 5; criterion-related validity) [16]. Age, sex, handedness, years of education, occupation and employment status were recorded for all participants. In the MS group, disease subtype, expanded disability status scale (EDSS) [17] and disease duration from onset of symptoms were also noted. Depression was assessed using the Beck Depression Inventory (BID) [18], and the (MFIS) [19] was used to measure fatigue.

All participants were administered the BICAMS, and test re-test reliability was confirmed for all patients and controls. The BICAMS is composed of the Symbol Digit Modalities Test (SDMT), California Verbal Learning Test (CVLT-II) and Brief Visuospatial Memory Test Revised (BVMTR) [8]. The SDMT measures the working memory and information processing speed. It consists of nine symbols, each representing a number from 1 to 9. These pairs are visible in a key at the top of an A4-size page. Below are a number of rows of the same symbols arranged in random order. After a short practice session, subjects are asked to match as many of the symbols with the digits as they can in 90 s. The answers can be written or orally. We used the oral version, and number of correct answers recorded within 90 s [20].

The CVLT-II is composed of a list of 16 words in 4 semantic categories. The examiner reads out the list of words at a steady pace of in approximately 20 s. The patient listens to the complete list and is then asked to repeat as many of the words as possible, in any order, which the examiner records on a piece of paper. Five trials in total are performed, and the final score is composed of the total number of words recorded across these trials. On each occasion the patient is asked to remember the answers given in the preceding trial. The BVMT-R consists of 6 abstract symbols on an A4-size page. Patients are given 10 s to look at the page, which is then removed from view. They are then asked to draw as many symbols as they can remember in the order given on a blank page. These symbols are then scored from 0 to 2, depending on accuracy and location. This is performed 3 times, and the total score consists of the sum of scores from all 3 trials.

Quality of life (QoL) was assessed using the MUSIQoL questionnaire [21]. This consists of 31 questions in 9 dimensions (subscales): activities of daily living (8 items), psychological well-being (4), symptoms (4), relationships with friends (3), relationships with family (3), sentimental and sexual life (2), coping (2), rejection (2), and relationships with the healthcare system (3). The index score is computed as the mean of these subscale scores. We used only the index score, which was linearly transformed and standardized on a 0 to 100 scale, where 0 indicates the worst possible level of QoL and 100 indicates the best possible level. The MFIS battery consists of 40 questions (3 subscales; social functions, physical functions and cognitive functions). Each question is scored from 0 (minimal problems) to 4 (severe) [19].

Statistical analysis

Comparisons between groups were performed using paired-sample t-tests and the Mann–Whitney U test for continuous variables where appropriate. The chi square test was used for categorical variables. Normal distribution of data was verified using the Shapiro-Wilk test.

Multinomial logistic regression was performed to evaluate associations among the individual neuropsychological tests, and depression, education status, disability level, duration of the disease, and the relapse rate. Correlation of BICAMS test-retest scores was evaluated using Pearson correlation coefficient r. Statistical analysis was performed on SPSS 15.0 software. Statistical significance was set at $p < 0.05$.

Results

One hundred seventy-three MS patients and 153 healthy controls were recruited to the study. Baseline characteristics are outlined in Table 1. Of the MS patient group, 151 (87.3%) were classified as having RRMS, 18 (10.4%) with SPMS and 4 (2.3%) with primary progressive MS (PPMS). Mean EDSS scores were 2.1 (SD: 1.1), 4.6 (SD: 1.5) and 5.3 (SD: 1.6), respectively, with disease durations of 7.1 (SD: 5.6), 14.9 (SD: 9.1) and 11.5 (SD: 8.4) years. Table 2 shows the group data and the differences between the patient and healthy groups' raw scores in all 3 trials and during the retests. The MS patients performed significantly worse in all trials than the members of the healthy group. As no validated threshold of cognitive impairment for BICAMS was available, we identified the 5th percentile on each performance of the healthy group in order to evaluate how many MS patients were impaired on each of the three components of BICAMS. Based on the proposed criterion of one or more test performances being below the 5th percentile of the healthy controls' performance, we identified cognitive dysfunction in 78 of the 173 (45.1%) patients. Of the MS with cognitive impairment group, 64 out of 151 (42.4%) subjects were RRMS patients, 12 out of 18 (66.7%) were SPMS patients, and 2 out of 4 (50%) were PPMS patients. When the MS group was further subdivided into RRMS and progressive MS (SPMS and PPMS) groups,

statistically significant differences were observed between the groups in each of the individual tests (p 0.05). Using the cut-off of one or more impaired tests, 41.7% of the RRMS and 77.3% of the progressive MS patients met the criterion for cognitive impairment. Table 3 summarizes the results and the estimation of impaired MS patients on one, two, and three tests.

When the patient group was subdivided in terms of disease duration, 36.6% of those diagnosed < 10 years previously (45 out 14 of 123) and 64% diagnosed ≥10 years (32 out of 50) previously also met the criterion for cognitive impairment (data not shown). Significant negative correlations were determined between SDMT scores and EDSS ($r = -0.46$, $p = 0.003$), and between CVLT II 17 scores and EDSS (r = -0.4, $p = 0.024$). No significant correlation was determined with BVMT-R ($r = -0.24$, $p > 0.05$). As expected, higher rates of unemployment were seen amongst the patient population compared to the control participants. We also determined higher rates of unemployment or inability to work due to MS in patients with cognitive impairment (34 vs 11 patients, respectively, p0.05). The test-retest interval was calculated as a median value of 15 days, with a mean value of 14.2 ± 4 days (10–21 days). We evaluated the difference between the patient and the healthy group test-retest scores (Table 4). Table 4 shows that the r values in the patient group were higher than those of the healthy controls ($r = 0,814$ vs r = 0,714).

In order assess the impact of fatigue on patients' cognitive status, we examined the correlations between their scores during the BICAMS battery and the MFIS battery scores. We determined significant negative correlations between the patients' overall subjective fatigue scores and their cognitive performance in all parts of the BICAMS (Table 5). The decline in cognitive functions measured by the BICAMS correlated best with the

Table 1 Baseline characteristics of patient and control participants

	MS Patients	Control Group	P
Gender n (%)			
Female	124 (71.7)	109 (71.2)	NS
Male	49 (28.3)	44 (28.8)	NS
Age (years) mean ± SD	37.5 ± 10.7	36.9 ± 8.9	NS
Education (years) mean ± SD	13.9 ± 7.3	15.4 ± 8.8	NS
Employment n (%)			
Employed	41 (23.7)	59 (39.1)	0.008
Unemployment or not working due to MS	45 (26)	20 (13.2)	0.024
Not working by choice/housewife/retired	71 (39.7)	58 (38.4)	NS
Student	16 (9.2)	14 (9.3)	NS
Disease duration (years), mean ± SD	9.2 ± 6.1	–	–
EDSS score, mean ± SD	2.4 ± 1.7	–	–

NS not significant, *SD* standard deviation, *EDSS* expanded disability status scale

Table 2 Differences between the patient and healthy groups'raw scores in all 3 trials and during the retests

| | Raw Score (SD) | | |
	MS Patients	Healthy Controls	p
SDMT	43.2 (12.5)	53.5 (9.5)	<0.001
SDMT retest	46.6 (16.4)	56.1 (10.2)	<0.001
CVLT-II	45.7 (11.3)	53.9 (7.7)	0.002
CVLT-II retest	47.9 (16.2)	60.2 (9.2)	0.003
BVMT-R	16.9 (8.5)	22.5 (9.2)	0.002

cognitive dimension subscale of the MFIS, followed by the physical subscale. We only determined meaningful correlation between the SDMT and the social subscale of the MFIS. As shown in Table 6, cognitive impairment correlated significantly with all MUSIQoL subscales. The most prominent correlations were with "activities of daily living", "psychological well-being" and "sentimental and sexual life".

Discussion

The assessment of cognitive status and characterization of damaged domains are useful for all MS patients in terms of appropriate rehabilitation, vocational counseling, and quantification of disability, beginning from the initial stages of the disease. It is now recognized that assessments and follow-ups should be as much as a priority as the evaluation of physical disability. Many diagnostic batteries have been used for these purposes. The most commonly used batteries of neuropsychological tests in MS are the BRB-N and MACFIMS, which are accurate, but may be time-consuming to administer. These batteries are not, therefore, suitable for everyday clinical practice, especially in centers without a resident neuropsychologist.

There is a need for a brief cognitive assessment tool with adequate reliability, validity, specificity and sensitivity, capable of provide comprehensive and accurate cognitive evaluations. The BICAMS has been proposed for

Table 3 Prevalence of cognitive impairment in MS patients according to the 5th percentile value of HC on BICAMS tests

	RRMS n (%)	SPMS n (%)	PPMS n (%)	Total)
SDMT	56 (37.1)	13 (72)	2 (50)	71 (41)
SDMT retest	55 (36.4)	13 (72)	2 (50)	70 (40.5)
CVLT-II	54 (35.7)	11 (60.6)	1 (25)	66 (38.2)
CVLT-II retest	56 (37.1)	10 (55.6)	1 (25)	67 (38.7)
BVMT-R	48 (31.8)	9 (50)	1 (25)	58 (33.5)
BVMT-R retest	46 (30.5)	10 (55.6)	1 (25)	57 (32.9)
On 1 test	63 (41.7)	14 (77.8)	3 (75)	80 (46.2)
On 2 tests	35 (23.2)	8 (44.4)	1 (25)	44 (25.4)
On 3 tests	21 (13.9)	5 (27.8)	1 (25)	27 (15.6)

SDMT symbol digit modalities test, CVLT-II California verbal learning test II, BVMT-R the brief visuospatial memory test revised

Table 4 Correlation coefficients between the tests and the retests

| | Overall | | Patient | | Healthy controls | |
	R	P	R	P	R	P
SDMT	0.814	<0.001	0.862	<0.001	0.714	<0.001
CVLT-II	0.892	<0.001	0.904	<0.001	0.792	<0.001
BVMT-R	0.828	<0.001	0.869	<0.001	0.706	<0.001

SDMT symbol digit modalities test, CVLT-II California verbal learning test II, BVMT-R the brief visuospatial memory test revised

assessing cognitive impairment in MS patients [8, 16]. The BICAMS battery can be used in small MS centers without a resident neuropsychologist [22]. Translation and validation studies of the BICAMS battery are currently being performed in several countries.

In our study, we assessed the cognitive status of MS patients using the Turkish translation of the BICAMS and measured the impact of cognitive impairment on the demographic and clinical characteristics. In our validation process, we observed significant differences in all tests between the MS group and the healthy group. The most significant difference was determined in the SDMT. We also determined strong correlations ($p < 0.001$) when assessing the test-retest reliability in both the patient and HC groups. Correlations were stronger in the patient group ($r > 0.8$) than in the HC group (r between 0.7 and 0.8).

In agreement with many other studies [3, 23], level of disability and duration of disease were associated with severity of cognitive impairment in the present research. However, some studies have also reported that duration of disease was not correlated with cognitive impairment [10]. Unemployment or inability to work due to MS was also correlated with cognitive impairment. Although patients often report that fatigue impairs their cognitive abilities [24], the majority of studies have failed to identify any correlation between fatigue and cognitive involvement [25–29]. But, fatigue has been reported to be capable of an adverse impact on patients' cognition [12, 30]. We observed significant negative correlations between patients' overall subjective fatigue scores and their cognitive performance in all parts of the BICAMS. Sandi et al. reported that all FIS scores exhibited meaningful negative correlations with patients' BICAMS performances. The strongest correlation was determined in SDMT [12]. In terms of the FIS subscales, they

Table 5 Correlations between the FIS battery and its subscales with the parts of the BICAMS battery

| | Total | | Cognitive | | Physical | | Social | |
	R	P	r	P	r	p	R	p
SDMT	−0.428	<0.001	−0.463	<0.001	−0.386	0.002	−0.302	0.046
CVLT-II	−0.382	0.003	−0.414	0.004	−0.362	0.021	−0.268	0.076
BVMT-R	−0.316	0.026	−0.396	0.034	−0.298	0.045	−0.245	0.081

SDMT symbol digit modalities test, CVLT-II California verbal learning test II, BVMT-R the brief visuospatial memory test revised

Table 6 Correlations between performance in BICAMS battery and score in MUSIQoL battery

	SDMT		CVLT-II		BVMT-R	
	r	p	r	p	r	p
Activities of daily living	0.445	<0.001	0.412	<0.001	0.403	<0.001
Psychological well-being	0.489	<0.001	0.398	<0.001	0.387	<0.001
Symptoms	0.402	0.004	0.378	0.008	0.335	0.012
Relationships with friends	0.389	0.014	0.316	0.024	0.372	0.014
Relationships with family	0.394	0.002	0.332	0.009	0.368	0.008
Sentimental and sexual life	0.512	<0.001	0.438	<0.001	0.475	<0.001
Coping	0.342	0.023	0.316	0.044	0.325	0.018
Rejection	0.358	0.028	0.318	0.041	0.340	0.007
Relationships with the healthcare system	0.306	0.042	0.322	0.048	0.314	0.04

SDMT symbol digit modalities test, *CVLT-II* California verbal learning test II, *BVMT-R* the brief visuospatial memory test revised

observed that the physical subscale exhibited the strongest correlation with cognitive status, while the cognitive subscale exhibited meaningful correlation both the SDMT and the CVLT-II tests. In our study, however, the decline in cognitive functions measured using BICAMS correlated best with the cognitive dimension subscale of the FIS, followed by the physical subscale. The SDMT was only significantly correlated with the FIS social subscale.

Several studies have reported that a decline in cognitive status is associated with poorer QoL [12, 31, 32]. Our study yielded similar results. All MUSIQoL subscales exhibited significant correlation with scores on the BICAMS battery. The most prominent correlations were with "activities of daily living", "psychological well-being" and "sentimental and sexual life". Sexual life is the subscale-most commonly correlated with cognitive status in ours and previous studies [12, 31–34].

The BICAMS is useful as a monitoring test for identifying MS patients with cognitive impairment. The Turkish version of the BICAMS is a short, easily administered, and specific tool for the clinical evaluation of cognitive impairment in MS patients, and is as reliable as the original English version. However, there are a number of limitations to our study. Some of the healthy control group being relatives of MS patients may be one such limitation, because there is a known greater incidence of MS in the relatives of MS patients. However, no significant difference was determined between this control subgroup and the other healthy control group in any tests. Moreover, alternative forms were used for the BVMT-R and SDMT testretest applications in order to avoid the practice effect. However, since there is only one CVLTII form, that single form was used. This may have led to a practice effect for CVLTII, and may constitute a limitation.

Conclusions

The present study contained the highest number of patients and healthy subjects to date. We want to emphasize that fatigue can have a negative effect on patients' cognitive status, while cognitive impairment can impact on employment status among patients with MS.

Abbreviations
BICAMS: Brief International Cognitive Assessment In Multiple Sclerosis; BID: Beck depression inventory; BRB-N: Brief repeatable battery of neuropsychological test; BVMTR: Brief visuospatial memory test revised; CVLT-II: California verbal learning test; EDSS: Expanded disability status scale; MACFIMS: Minimal assessment of cognitive function in multiple sclserosis; MFIS: Modified fatigue impact scale; MS: Multiple sclerosis; MUSIQoL: Multiple sclerosis international quality of life; PPMS: Primary progressive multiple sclerosis; RRMS: Relapsing remitting multiple sclerosis; SDMT: Symbol digit modalities test; SPMS: Secondary progressive multiple sclerosis

Acknowledgments
This study was sponsored by the Multiple Sclerosis Research Society, to whom we are most grateful. We would also like to thank all the patients and members of the healthy control group for their co-operation in the validation process.

Funding
The authors declared that no grants were involved in supporting this work.

Authors' contributions
SO and made substantial contributions to conception, design and acquisition of data. PY, GK, HL and TK agreed to be accountable for all aspects of the work in ensuring that questions related to the accuracy. BPC, SO been involved in drafting the manuscript or revising it critically for important intellectual content and wrote the paper. Each author have participated sufficiently in the work to take public responsibility for appropriate portions of the content and all authors read and approved the final manuscript.

Competing interests
The authors declare that they have no competing interests.

Author details
[1]Department of Neurology, Dokuz Eylul University, Izmir, Turkey. [2]Department of Neurology, Samsun Training and Researce Hospital, Samsun, Turkey. [3]School of Physical Therapy and Rehabilitation Department, İzmir Katip Celebi University, Izmir, Turkey. [4]Department of Neurology, Usak State Hospital, Usak, Turkey.

References

1. Chiaravalloti ND, DeLuca J. Cognitive impairment in multiple sclerosis. Lancet Neurol. 2008;7:11391151.
2. Langdon DW. Cognition in multiple sclerosis. Curr Opin Neurol. 2011 Jun;24(3):244–9.
3. Amato MP, Portaccio E, Goretti B, Zipoli V, Iudice A, Della Pina D, Malentacchi G, Sabatini S, Annunziata P, Falcini M, Mazzoni M, Mortilla M, Fonda C, De Stefano N, TuSCIMS Study Group. Relevance of cognitive deterioration in early relapsing-remitting MS: a3-year follow-up study. MultScler. 2010;16:1474–82.
4. Benedict RH, Cookfair D, Gavett R, Gunther M, Munschauer F, Garg N, Weinstock-Guttman B. Validity of the minimal assessment of cognitive function in multiple sclerosis (MACFIMS). J Int Neuropsychol Soc. 2006;12(4):549–58.
5. Rao SM. A manual for the brief repeatable battery of neuropsychological tests in multiple sclerosis. Milwaukee: Medical College of Wisconsin; 1990.
6. Benedict RH, Fischer JS, Archibald CJ, Arnett PA, Beatty WW, Bobholz J, Chelune GJ, Fisk JD, Langdon DW, Caruso L, Foley F, LaRocca NG, Vowels L, Weinstein A, DeLuca J, Rao SM, Munschauer F. Minimal neuropsychological assessment of MS patients: a consensus approach. Clin Neuropsychol. 2002;16(3):381–97.
7. Takeda A. Neuropsychological tests in multiple sclerosis. Nihon Rinsho. 2014;72(11):1989–94.
8. Langdon DW, Amato MP, Boringa J, Brochet B, Foley F, Fredrikson S, Hämäläinen P, Hartung HP, Krupp L, Penner IK, Reder AT, Benedict RH. Recommendations for a brief international cognitive assessment for multiple sclerosis (BICAMS). Mult Scler. 2012;18:891–8.
9. Walker LA, Osman L, Berard JA, Rees LM, Freedman MS, MacLean H, Cousineau D. Brief international cognitive assessment for multiple sclerosis (BICAMS): Canadian contribution to the international validation project. J Neurol Sci. 2016;362:147–52.
10. Giedraitienė N, Kizlaitienė R, Kaubrys G. The BICAMS battery for assessment of LithuanianSpeaking multiple sclerosis patients: relationship with age, education, disease disability, and duration. Med Sci Monit. 2015;21:3853–9.
11. O'Connell K, Langdon D, Tubridy N, Hutchinson M, McGuigan C. A preliminary validation of the brief international cognitive assessment for multiple sclerosis (BICAMS) tool in an Irish population 40 with multiple sclerosis (MS). Mult Scler Relat Disord. 2015;4(6):521–5.
12. Sandi D, Rudisch T, Füvesi J, Fricska-Nagy Z, Huszka H, Biernacki T, Langdon DW, Langane É, Vécsei L, Bencsik K. The Hungarian validation of the brief international cognitive assessment for multiple sclerosis (BICAMS) battery and the correlation of cognitive impairment with fatigue and quality of life. Mult Scler Relat Disord. 2015;4(6):499–504.
13. Spedo CT, Frndak SE, Marques VD, Foss MP, Pereira DA, Carvalho Lde F, Guerreiro CT, Conde RM, Fusco T, Pereira AJ, Gaino SB, Garcia RB, Benedict RH, Barreira AA. Cross-cultural adaptation, reliability, and validity of the BICAMS in Brazil. Clin Neuropsychol. 2015;29(6):836–46.
14. Dusankova JB, Kalincik T, Havrdova E, Benedict RH. Cross cultural validation of the minimal of cognitive function in multiple sclerosis (MACFIMS) and the brief international cognitive assessment for multiple sclerosis (BICAMS). Clin Neuropsychol. 2012;26(7):1186–200.
15. Polman CH, Reingold SC, Banwell B, Clanet M, Cohen JA, Filippi M, Fujihara K, Havrdova E, Hutchinson M, Kappos L, Lublin FD, Montalban X, O'Connor P, Sandberg-Wollheim M, Thompson AJ, Waubant E, Weinshenker B, Wolinsky JS. Diagnostic criteria for multiple sclerosis: 2010 revisions to the McDonald criteria. Ann Neurol. 2011;69(2):292–302.
16. Benedict RH, Amato MP, Boringa J, Brochet B, Foley F, Fredrikson S, Hamalainen P, Hartung H, Krupp L, Penner I, Reder AT, Langdon D. Brief international cognitive assessment for MS (BICAMS): international standards for validation. BMC Neurol. 2012;12:55.
17. Kurtzke JF. Disability rating scales in multiple sclerosis. Ann N Y Acad Sci. 1984;436:347–60.
18. Beck AT, Steer RA, Brown GK. Beck depression inventory-second edition manual. San Antonio: The Psychological Corporation S; 1996.
19. Schwid SR, Covington MMSB, Segal BM, Goodman AD. Fatigue in multiple sclerosis: current understanding and future directions. J Rehabil Res Dev. 2002;39(2):211–24.
20. Smith A. Symbol digit modalities test manual. Los Angeles: Western Psychological Services; 1982.
21. Simeoni M, Auquier P, Fernandez O, Flachenecker P, Stecchi S, Constantinescu C, Idiman E, Boyko A, Beiske A, Vollmer T, Triantafyllou N, O'Connor P, Barak Y, Biermann L, Cristiano E, Atweh S, Patrick D, Robitail S, Ammoury N, Beresniak A, Pelletier J, MusiQol study group. Validation of the multiple sclerosis international quality of life questionnaire. Mult Scler. 2008;14:219–30.
22. Goverover Y, Chiaravalloti N, DeLuca J. Brief international cognitive assessment for multiple sclerosis (BICAMS) and performance of everyday life tasks: actual reality, multiple 17. Sclerosis Journal. 2015;
23. Smestad C, Sandvik L, Landrø NI, Celius EG. Cognitive impairment after three decades of multiple sclerosis. Eur J Neurol. 2010;17(3):499–505.
24. Krupp LB, Alvarez LA, LaRocca NG, Scheinberg LC. Fatigue in multiple sclerosis. Arch Neurol. 1988;45(4):435–7.
25. Johnson SK, Lange G, DeLuca J, Korn LR, Natelson B. The effects of fatigue on neuropsychological performance in patients with chronic fatigue syndrome, multiple sclerosis, and depression. ApplNeuropsychol. 1997;4(3):145–53.
26. Paul RH, Beatty WW, Schneider R, Blanco CR, Hames KA. Cognitive and physical fatigue in multiple sclerosis: relations between self-report and objective performance. Appl Neuropsychol. 1998;5(3):143–8.
27. Bailey A, Channon S, Beaumont JG. The relationship between subjective fatigue and cognitive fatigue in advanced multiple sclerosis. Mult Scler. 2007;13(1):73–80.
28. Bol Y, Duits AA, Hupperts RM, Verlinden I, Verhey FR. The impact of fatigue on cognitive functioning in patients with multiple sclerosis. Clin Rehabil. 2010;24(9):854–62.
29. Morrow SA, Drake A, Zivadinov R, Munschauer F, Weinstock-Guttman B, Benedict RH. Predicting loss of employment over three years in multiple sclerosis: clinically meaningful cognitive decline. Clin Neuropsychol. 2010;24(7):1131–45.
30. Andreasen AK, Spliid PE, Andersen H, Jakobsen J. Fatigue and processing speed are related in multiple sclerosis. Eur J Neurol. 2010;17(2):212–8.
31. Mitchell AJ, Benito-León J, González JM, Rivera-Navarro J. Quality of life and its assessment in multiple sclerosis: integrating physical and psychological components of well-being. Lancet Neurol. 2005;4(9):556–66.
32. Glanz BI, Holland CM, Gauthier SA, Amunwa EL, Liptak Z, Houtchens MK, Sperling RA, Khoury SJ, Guttmann CR, Weiner HL. Cognitive dysfunction in patients with clinically isolated syndromes or newly diagnosed multiple sclerosis. Mult Scler. 2007;13(8):1004–10.
33. Benito-León J, Morales JM, Rivera-Navarro J. Health-related quality of life and its relationship to cognitive and emotional functioning in multiple sclerosis patients. Eur J Neurol. 2002;9(5):497–502.
34. Turpin KV, Carroll LJ, Cassidy JD, Hader WJ. Deterioration in the health-related quality of life of persons with multiple sclerosis: the possible warning signs. Mult Scler. 2007;13(8):1038–45.

Effectiveness, safety and health-related quality of life of multiple sclerosis patients treated with fingolimod: results from a 12-month, real-world, observational PERFORMS study in the Middle East

Anat Achiron[1*], Hany Aref[2], Jihad Inshasi[3], Mohamad Harb[4], Raed Alroughani[5], Mahendra Bijarnia[6], Kathryn Cooke[7] and Ozgur Yuksel[7]

Abstract

Background: Evidence on the use of fingolimod in real-world clinical practice and data on patient-reported health-related quality of life (HRQoL) in countries such as the Middle East are sparse. The Prospective Evaluation of Treatment with Fingolimod for Multiple Sclerosis (PERFORMS) study assessed HRQoL and effectiveness and safety of fingolimod in patients with relapsing-remitting multiples sclerosis (RRMS), primarily in Middle Eastern countries.

Methods: This 12-month, observational, multicentre, prospective, real-world study was conducted in patients with RRMS who initiated fingolimod or another approved disease-modifying treatment (DMT) within 4 weeks before study entry. Patients were enrolled in a 2:1 ratio to obtain more data in fingolimod and parallel in other DMTs cohort by physicians during routine medical care. Key study outcomes included HRQoL assessed using MS International QoL (MusiQoL), MS relapses and disability. Safety was assessed throughout the study period. Due to the observational nature of the study, no neuroimaging assessments were mandated and central reading was not performed.

Results: Of 249 enrolled patients, 247 were included in the analysis (fingolimod cohort 172; other DMTs cohort 75). Overall, the mean age of patients was 36.5 years, 64.4% were women and ~90% were Caucasians. At baseline, mean MS duration since diagnosis was 7.2 years in the fingolimod and 4.8 years in the other DMTs cohorts. Overall, mean changes in MusiQoL index scores were −2.1 in the fingolimod cohort and −0.7 in the other DMTs cohort at Month 12, but improvement was not significant vs. baseline in both cohorts. Proportion of relapse-free patients increased significantly during the study vs. 0–12 months before the study in the fingolimod cohort (80.2% vs. 24.4%; $p < 0.0001$). Proportion of patients free from disability progression was 86.5% in the fingolimod cohort. The incidences of AEs were 59.9% and 50.6% in the fingolimod and other DMTs cohorts, respectively. First-dose monitoring of fingolimod observed no cases of symptomatic bradyarrhythmia. Three cases of bradycardia were reported in the fingolimod cohort: one after the first dose and two during the study. No cases of macular oedema were observed during the study.

Conclusions: Fingolimod treatment maintained QoL over 12 months and was effective in reducing relapse rate and disability progression. No new safety findings were observed in this real-world observational study in Middle Eastern countries.

Keywords: Real-world, Observational, Fingolimod, Other DMTs, Health-related quality of life, Effectiveness, Safety, PERFORMS

* Correspondence: Anat.Achiron@sheba.health.gov.il
[1]Multiple Sclerosis Center, Sheba Medical Center, 52621 Tel-Hashomer, Israel
Full list of author information is available at the end of the article

Effectiveness, safety and health-related quality of life of multiple sclerosis patients treated...

15

Background

Multiple sclerosis (MS), a chronic, auto-immune disease of the central nervous system (CNS), is characterised by inflammation, demyelination and axonal/neuronal destruction, which may lead to residual disability [1, 2]. Approximately 2.5 million people worldwide are affected with MS [3]. The prevalence of MS is increasing in the Middle Eastern countries, probably due to the influence of lifestyle changes from Western countries and environmental and genetic factors [4, 5]. The overall prevalence of MS in this region is 51.52/100000, with the female/male ratio ranging from 0.8 to 4.3 and an overall mean age at disease onset of 28.54 years [4].

Several disease-modifying treatments (DMTs) exist for MS, i.e. drugs that have the potential to modify or change the course of MS by acting on its underlying pathophysiology [6]. Fingolimod (FTY720, Gilenya®) is a first-in-class, oral sphingosine-1-phosphate (S1P) receptor immunomodulator that acts as a functional antagonist by internalising activated receptors [7].

Fingolimod has been approved in several countries for treatment of patients with relapsing forms of MS. The three large Phase 3 clinical trials of fingolimod—FREEDOMS [8], FREEDOMS II [9] and TRANSFORMS [10]—showed a significant reduction in relapse rate, magnetic resonance imaging-related lesion counts and brain volume loss vs. placebo and interferon β-1a in patients with relapsing-remitting MS (RRMS). These effects were sustained in the respective extension studies [11, 12], as reflected by low levels of MS disease activity and disability progression. Moreover, several observational studies reported that treatment with fingolimod showed improvement in patients' quality of life (QoL) and satisfaction [13–20].

The safety and efficacy of fingolimod in MS patients have been established in clinical development programmes [8–12] as well as in a few non-interventional observational studies [21–26].

It is essential to assess the health-related QoL (HRQoL) outcome in patients with MS and evaluate the impact of treatments and care management in these patients. In 2008, Simeoni and colleagues developed the MS International QoL (MusiQoL) specifically to account for patients' viewpoint on the impact of disease on their daily life and assess patient-reported HRQoL [27], which has been globally accepted by physicians. The importance of HRQoL outcome in the management of patients with MS using MusiQoL was also emphasised and recommended by the Middle East MS Advisory Group as part of routine care [28]. However, evidence on the use of fingolimod in real-world clinical practice in countries such as the Middle East is limited, and data are sparse on patient-reported HRQoL, particularly using the MS-specific MusiQoL questionnaire.

The present Prospective Evaluation of Treatment with Fingolimod for Multiple Sclerosis (PERFORMS) non-interventional study was conducted to assess the HRQoL of RRMS patients and expand the knowledge of fingolimod effectiveness and safety in real-world clinical practice, primarily in the Middle Eastern countries. The objectives of the present study were to explore the effect of fingolimod on patients' HRQoL in relation to other DMTs, assess the effectiveness of fingolimod in relation to other DMTs, assess the incidence of selected safety outcomes, describe the overall safety profile of fingolimod and describe physicians' impression of treatment with fingolimod in routine clinical practice.

Methods

Patient population

Men and women aged ≥18 years who were diagnosed with RRMS and were started on MS therapy with fingolimod or other approved DMTs within 4 weeks prior to study entry and who provided written informed consent were included in the study. The MS therapy was part of the patients' routine medical care and was prescribed in compliance with the local prescribing information. In countries where fingolimod was approved as a second-line therapy, only patients who had switched from MS treatment to either fingolimod or other DMTs within 4 weeks prior to study entry were included.

Patients with contraindications mentioned in the local prescribing information for the treatment were not included in the study.

Study design

This was a 12-month, observational, multicentre, prospective-cohort, real-world study. The study was conducted in 27 outpatient centres across Egypt, Israel, Kuwait, Lebanon, United Arab Emirates, Saudi Arabia and Thailand from March 2012 to January 2015. Patients with RRMS were enrolled at a ratio of 2:1 (fingolimod:other DMTs) to obtain more data on fingolimod (hereafter, fingolimod cohort refers to patients taking fingolimod at study entry), while additionally obtaining data in a parallel cohort (hereafter, other DMTs cohort refers to patients taking another MS DMT at study entry). This ratio was controlled primarily at the investigator site level and secondarily at the country level. The choice of MS treatment was made within the context of the patient's routine medical care and independent of the decision to include the patient in the study.

Data collected for the study originated from the routine care of patients and were recorded by physicians at study entry (baseline) and at Months 3, 6 and 12. Completion of the MusiQoL questionnaire by patients and the Clinical Global Impression-Improvement scale (CGI-I) by physicians were the only study-specific requirements. No additional visits or diagnostic or monitoring procedures were mandated by the protocol. Due to the observational nature of the study, no neuroimaging assessments were mandated and central reading was not performed.

Study outcomes and endpoints

Effectiveness

Health-related quality of life Patient-reported HRQoL was assessed at baseline and at Months 6 and 12 using MusiQoL. This multidimensional (nine dimensions) self-administered questionnaire consists of 31 items, with responses describing frequency/extent of an event on a 5-point scale ranging from 1 (never/not at all) to 5 (always/very much) [27]. If a patient changed or discontinued the medication of interest (MOI), then the questionnaire was requested to be completed at the time of the MS therapy change. The change in MusiQoL scores from baseline to Months 6 and 12 was reported in the study.

Physician impression of treatment At the study completion, physicians were asked to provide a subjective evaluation of the improvement of patients over the study period using the CGI-I. The CGI-I is a 7-point Likert-type scale, allowing physicians to rate the change in the patient's condition over time (from 'very much improved' to 'very much worse') and has been a robust tool for physicians, accounting for both therapeutic efficacy and treatment-emergent adverse events (AEs) response/rates [29].

Multiple sclerosis relapses MS relapses were reported according to the physician's judgement, with the recommendation to apply the international definition of a relapse [30]. The proportion of patients with MS relapses at 12–24 months and 0–12 months prior to study and during the 12 months of study duration was reported. Kaplan-Meier plot was provided to report time to the first relapse during the study.

Disability Neurologic disability was measured by the Expanded Disability Status Scale (EDSS) score [31]. Disability progression was determined according to the baseline severity of symptoms and based on previously used criteria [32, 33], and was defined as a sustained increase in the EDSS score by 1 point if baseline EDSS was ≤5.0 or by 0.5 points if baseline EDSS was ≥5.5. The change in EDSS scores from baseline to Months 6 and 12/end of study (EOS) and proportions of patients free from disability progression at Months 6 and 12/EOS were reported.

Disability was also assessed by reporting patients' walking ability. Physicians used the four-level Likert-type measure to determine whether the patient was able to walk unrestricted/unable to walk unrestricted but no assistive device used/unable to walk unrestricted and assistive device used/unable to walk at all. Patients' walking ability at baseline and Months 6 and 12 was reported.

Safety

Safety assessments consisted of collecting all AEs and serious AEs (SAEs) and assessing their severity and relationship to the study drug. Clinically significant abnormalities in haematology and clinical chemistry were reported. The proportion of patients with AEs, SAEs, AEs leading to treatment discontinuation and selected AEs (such as symptomatic bradyarrhythmia, macular oedema, increase in liver enzymes and infections) by Month 12/EOS were reported. Ophthalmic examinations were performed at each time point, including the presence of macular oedema and the assessment of visual acuity for both eyes.

First-dose monitoring of fingolimod included haemodynamic assessments at several pre- and post-dose time points: sitting pulse (beats per minute, continuous variable) and blood pressure (mm Hg, continuous variable) per usual clinical practice. Additionally, any new incidence of bradycardia, new or worsening electrocardiography findings and the need for concomitant treatment were monitored at first fingolimod dose for the fingolimod cohort.

Statistical analysis

The target sample size of 246 patients, with a 2:1 ratio (fingolimod:other DMTs), was determined empirically. All effectiveness outcomes were determined on the full analysis set (FAS), defined as patients who were assigned to either the fingolimod or the other DMTs cohort at baseline and remained in the same cohort (MOI) throughout the study as well as patients who switched cohort or discontinued the MOI but remained in the study up to Month 12. All the safety analyses were performed on the safety set, defined as the set of patients included in the analyses and who used fingolimod or other DMTs for at least 1 day and at any time during the study. The safety set considered patients who switched from their original cohort (from 'fingolimod' to 'other DMTs' or vice versa) during the study. The MOI was defined as the MS DMT initiated prior to study entry (baseline) or within a month prior to baseline.

The statistics were summarised descriptively in the study, except for the few comparisons performed in the two cohorts separately (no comparisons between cohorts). The mean MusiQoL (for each dimension and for the index score) and EDSS scores at Months 6 and 12/EOS vs. baseline were analysed using paired t-tests, providing 95% confidence intervals (CIs) of the mean difference and the p value for the test. The mean change in MusiQoL was calculated from baseline to Months 6 and 12/EOS. The proportion of patients with at least one MS relapse during the study vs. 0–12 months before study was analysed using a McNemar test for repeated measures. The time to first relapse was computed to provide Kaplan-Meier estimates. Missing data on drug discontinuation date and drug initiation date were imputed using the next drug initiation date and preceding drug date, respectively. Missing data in the self-reported MusiQoL were imputed as suggested by Simeoni and colleagues in 2008 [27]. To minimise the risk of self-selection bias, participating physicians were encouraged to enrol patients in both cohorts in a consecutive manner during a regular visit.

Ethical and good clinical practice
The study protocol and amendment were approved by the Independent Ethics Committees and Institutional Review Boards for each centre per local regulations. All patients provided written informed consent before study entry. The study was conducted in compliance with the ethical principles of the Declaration of Helsinki and the International Conference on Harmonization Good Clinical Practice Guidelines [34].

Results
Patient disposition and baseline characteristics
Of the 249 enrolled patients (fingolimod cohort, 174; other DMTs cohort, 75), 247 were included in the FAS (fingolimod cohort, 172; other DMTs cohort, 75). Two patients in the fingolimod cohort were excluded from the FAS, as fingolimod was not newly initiated (within 4 weeks) prior to study entry. The safety set consisted of 177 patients in the fingolimod cohort and 87 in the other DMTs cohort. The majority of the patients (88.7%) completed the 12-month follow-up (Additional file 1: Table S1).

Patients' demographics and baseline characteristics are described in Table 1. The overall mean age of patients was 36.5 years, 64.4% were women and Caucasians were predominant (~90%). At baseline, the mean duration since diagnosis of MS was 7.2 years in the fingolimod cohort and 4.8 years in the other DMTs cohort. Overall, 113 (65.7%) patients in the fingolimod cohort and 62 (82.7%) in the other DMTs cohort had at least one MS relapse in the previous year before study entry. The mean ± standard deviation (SD) number of relapses in the 12 months before study start was 1.1 ± 0.9 and

1.2 ± 0.8 in the fingolimod and other DMTs cohorts, respectively. Before study entry, the proportion of treatment-naïve patients was 14.0% in the fingolimod cohort and 61.3% in the other DMTs cohort. Among the patients who were on MS DMTs before the study, the majority in both cohorts were on interferon β therapies (Table 1). At the study start, most of the patients in the other DMTs cohort (~73%) were prescribed interferon β therapies, followed by natalizumab (20.0%) and glatiramer acetate (6.7%).

Drug exposure
The mean duration of drug exposure during the study was 321.8 ± 147.7 days (151.6 patient-years) in the fingolimod cohort and 337.6 ± 117.0 days (69.3 patient-years) in the other DMTs cohort.

Effectiveness
Health-related quality of life
Overall, >97% patients completed the MusiQoL questionnaire at baseline. At Month 12/EOS, 94.6% patients completed this questionnaire in the fingolimod cohort and 87.7% in the other DMTs cohort.

During the study, overall mean change (CI; p value) in the MusiQoL index score was -0.2 [-2.5 to 2.1; $p = 0.868$] at Month 6 and -2.1 [-4.7 to 0.5; $p = 0.112$] at Month 12 for the fingolimod cohort and -0.8 [-3.7 to 2.2; $p = 0.598$] at Month 6 and -0.7 [-4.6 to 3.2; $p = 0.719$] at Month 12 for the other DMT cohort, but the improvement was not statistically significant vs. baseline in both cohorts (Fig. 1). The fingolimod cohort showed significant improvements in MusiQoL sub-scores of -6.4 (-10.5 to -2.3; $p = 0.002$) for the 'psychological well-being' dimension at Month 6 and -5.2 (-9.0 to -1.4; $p = 0.008$) for the 'activity of daily living' and -5.8 (-10.1 to -1.5; $p = 0.009$) for 'psychological well-being' dimensions at Month 12 (both $p < 0.01$ vs. baseline). There was a significant improvement in the sub-score for the 'relationship with healthcare system' dimension at Month 12 (-5.6 [-11.0 to -0.2]; $p = 0.043$ vs. baseline) in the other DMTs cohort.

The questions to patients under the 'psychological well-being' dimension included if they felt anxious; felt depressed or gloomy; felt like crying; or felt nervous or irritated by a few things or situations. The questions to patients under the 'activity of daily living' dimension included if they had difficulty walking or moving outside; difficulty with outdoor activities, i.e. shopping, going out to a movie, etc.; difficulty walking or moving around at home; been troubled by their balance or walking problems; difficulty with leisure activities at home, i.e. do-it-yourself, gardening, etc.; difficulty with their occupational activities, i.e. integration, interruption, limitation,

Table 1 Patient demographics and baseline characteristics

	Fingolimod cohort N = 172	Other DMTs cohort N = 75	Total N = 247
Age (years)			
Mean	36.7 ± 11.2	36.2 ± 12.2	36.5 ± 11.5
Median (min–max)	35.0 (18.0–64.0)	34.0 (18.0–68.0)	34.0 (18.0–68.0)
Women, n (%)	112 (65.1)	47 (62.7)	159 (64.4)
BMI (kg/m²), n (%)			
Overweight (25 ≤ BMI < 30)	47 (27.3)	14 (18.7)	61 (24.7)
Obese (BMI ≥30)	18 (10.5)	12 (16.0)	30 (12.1)
Race, n (%)			
Caucasian	153 (89.0)	68 (90.7)	221 (89.5)
Asian	4 (2.3)	1 (1.3)	5 (2.0)
Other	15 (8.7)	6 (8.0)	21 (8.5)
MS disease history			
Duration since MS diagnosis (years)			
Mean	7.2 ± 6.1	4.8 ± 6.8	6.5 ± 6.4
Median (min–max)	5.3 (0.0–32.0)	1.2 (0.0–23.9)	4.2 (0.0–32.0)
Duration since the first MS symptoms (years)			
Mean	9.4 ± 7.6	7.5 ± 9.1	8.9 ± 8.1
Median (min–max)	7.3 (0.1–34.7)	3.2 (0.0–44.1)	6.6 (0.0–44.1)
Duration since the most recent MS relapse (months)			
Mean	10.4 ± 14.8	6.1 ± 8.6	9.0 ± 13.2
Median (min–max)	5.0 (0.0–87.0)	3.0 (0.0–50.0)	4.0 (0.0–87.0)
Number of MS relapses in the 12 months before baseline			
Mean	1.1 ± 0.9	1.2 ± 0.8	1.1 ± 0.9
Median (min–max)	1.0 (0.0–5.0)	1.0 (0.0–3.0)	1.0 (0.0–5.0)
Number of MS relapses 12–24 months before baseline			
Mean	0.9 ± 1.1	0.5 ± 0.8	0.8 ± 1.0
Median (min–max)	1.0 (0.0–5.0)	0.0 (0.0–3.0)	0.0 (0.0–5.0)
History of MS patients before study, n (%)			
Treatment-naïve patients [a]	24 (14.0)	46 (61.3)	-
Patients on any approved MS DMT	148 (86.0)	29 (38.7)	-
Type of DMTs prescribed before study entry, n (%)			
Fingolimod	8 (5.4)	4 (13.8)	-
Any interferon β	103 (69.6)	15 (51.7)	-
Glatiramer acetate	17 (11.5)	8 (27.6)	-
Natalizumab	16 (10.8)	2 (6.9)	-
Other	4 (2.7)	0 (0.0)	-

Data are presented as mean ± SD, unless stated otherwise; percentages were calculated based on the total number of patients in each treatment cohort (n)
BMI body mass index, DMT disease-modifying treatment, MS multiple sclerosis, min minimum, max maximum, SD standard deviation
[a]Treatment-naïve patients are patients who had never received any MS DMT before study entry (±4 weeks)

been quickly tired, etc.; or been short of energy. The questions to patients under the 'relationship with healthcare system' dimension included if they were satisfied with the information on their disease or the treatment given by the doctors, nurses, psychologists taking care of their MS; felt understood by the doctors, nurses, psychologists taking care of their MS; or were satisfied with their treatments [28].

Physician impression of treatment

The CGI-I score was completed in >90% of patients at EOS. Physicians indicated that 88.5% of patients in the

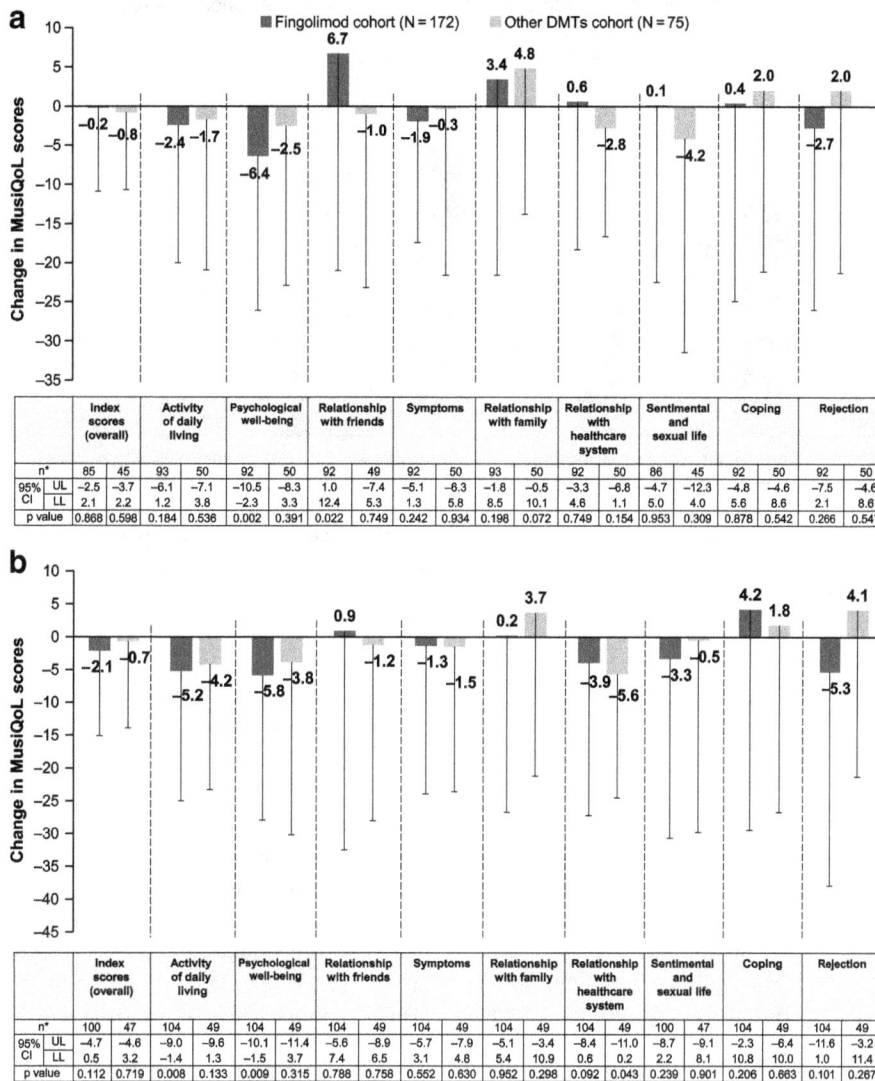

Fig. 1 Mean (±SD) change in MusiQoL scores from baseline to Months (**a**) 6 and (**b**) 12 (FAS). *No. of pairs. Displayed is the difference in mean between the baseline score and the score of the evaluation time (a negative difference indicates a QoL improvement and a positive difference indicates a QoL deterioration). DMT, disease-modifying treatment; CI, confidence interval; FAS, full analysis set; LL, lower limit; MusiQoL, Multiple Sclerosis International Quality of Life; QoL, quality of life; SD, standard deviation; UL, upper limit

a

	Index scores (overall)		Activity of daily living		Psychological well-being		Relationship with friends		Symptoms		Relationship with family		Relationship with healthcare system		Sentimental and sexual life		Coping		Rejection	
n*	85	45	93	50	92	50	92	49	92	50	93	50	92	50	86	45	92	50	92	50
95% CI UL	-2.5	-3.7	-6.1	-7.1	-10.5	-8.3	1.0	-7.4	-5.1	-6.3	-1.8	-0.5	-3.3	-6.8	-4.7	-12.3	-4.8	-4.6	-7.5	-4.6
LL	2.1	2.2	1.2	3.8	-2.3	3.3	12.4	5.3	1.3	5.8	8.5	10.1	4.6	1.1	5.0	4.0	5.6	8.6	2.1	8.6
p value	0.868	0.598	0.184	0.536	0.002	0.391	0.022	0.749	0.242	0.934	0.196	0.072	0.749	0.154	0.953	0.309	0.878	0.542	0.266	0.547

b

	Index scores (overall)		Activity of daily living		Psychological well-being		Relationship with friends		Symptoms		Relationship with family		Relationship with healthcare system		Sentimental and sexual life		Coping		Rejection	
n*	100	47	104	49	104	49	104	49	104	49	104	49	104	49	100	47	104	49	104	49
95% CI UL	-4.7	-4.6	-9.0	-9.6	-10.1	-11.4	-5.6	-8.9	-5.7	-7.9	-5.1	-3.4	-8.4	-11.0	-8.7	-9.1	-2.3	-6.4	-11.6	-3.2
LL	0.5	3.2	-1.4	1.3	-1.5	3.7	7.4	6.5	3.1	4.8	5.4	10.9	0.6	0.2	2.2	8.1	10.8	10.0	1.0	11.4
p value	0.112	0.719	0.008	0.133	0.009	0.315	0.788	0.758	0.552	0.630	0.952	0.298	0.092	0.043	0.239	0.901	0.206	0.863	0.101	0.267

fingolimod cohort and 86.1% in the other DMTs cohort showed either improvement or no change in MS on the CGI-I scale (Fig. 2).

MS relapses

The majority of patients (>80%) experienced no relapses during the study. The proportion of relapse-free patients increased significantly ($p < 0.0001$) during the study vs. 0–12 months before the study in both cohorts (Fig. 3). The mean number of relapses during the study was 0.2 ± 0.5 in the fingolimod cohort and 0.1 ± 0.4 in the other DMTs cohort. The survival curve of time to the first MS relapse during the study is depicted in Fig. 4. Mean duration to the first MS relapse was >4 months in the fingolimod cohort (123.1 ± 92.3 days) and >7 months in the other DMTs cohort (218.8 ± 122.5 days).

Disability

Mean EDSS scores improved significantly from baseline (3.0 ± 1.7) to Month 6 (2.7 ± 1.9, $p < 0.05$) in the fingolimod cohort and was maintained up to Month 12/EOS (2.7 ± 1.8, $p = 0.614$). There were no significant improvements in the EDSS scores from baseline (2.3 ± 1.7) to Months 6 (2.2 ± 1.8, $p = 0.391$) and 12 (2.3 ± 1.8, $p = 0.424$) in the other DMTs cohort (Fig. 5). The proportion of patients free from disability progression was 86.5% in the fingolimod

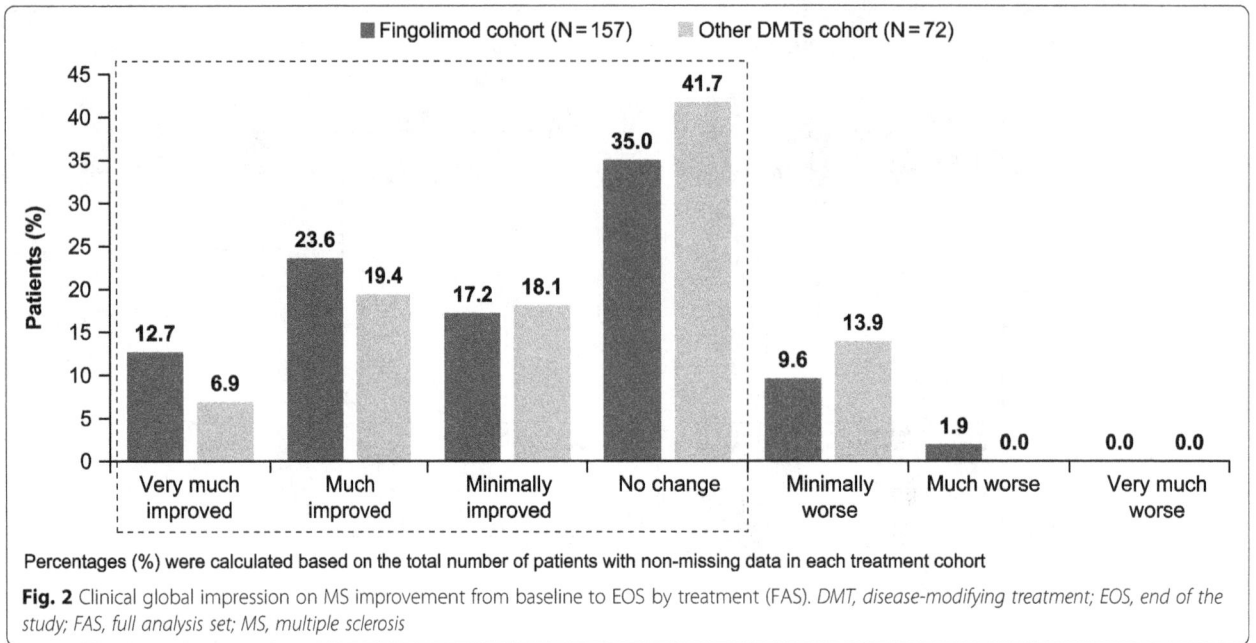

Fig. 2 Clinical global impression on MS improvement from baseline to EOS by treatment (FAS). *DMT, disease-modifying treatment; EOS, end of the study; FAS, full analysis set; MS, multiple sclerosis*

cohort and 88.5% in the other DMTs cohorts over 12 months (Fig. 6).

Walking ability

The proportions of patients able to walk or not, with or without using an assistive device, over 12 months during the study are summarised in Table 2. At Month 12/EOS, 75.7% patients in the fingolimod cohort (baseline, 73.3%) and 84.2% in the other DMTs cohort (baseline, 88.0%) were able to walk unrestricted outside home. Overall,

1.8% of the patients were unable to walk at Month 12/EOS during the study.

Safety

The incidence of AEs was 59.9% in the fingolimod cohort and 50.6% in other DMTs cohort (Table 3). The most commonly occurring AEs were MS relapse (10.7%), lymphopaenia (7.9%) and increase in liver enzymes (6.8%) in the fingolimod cohort and MS relapse (8.0%), fatigue (6.9%) and gait disturbance (6.9%) in the other DMTs cohort. The most frequently (≥5%) observed

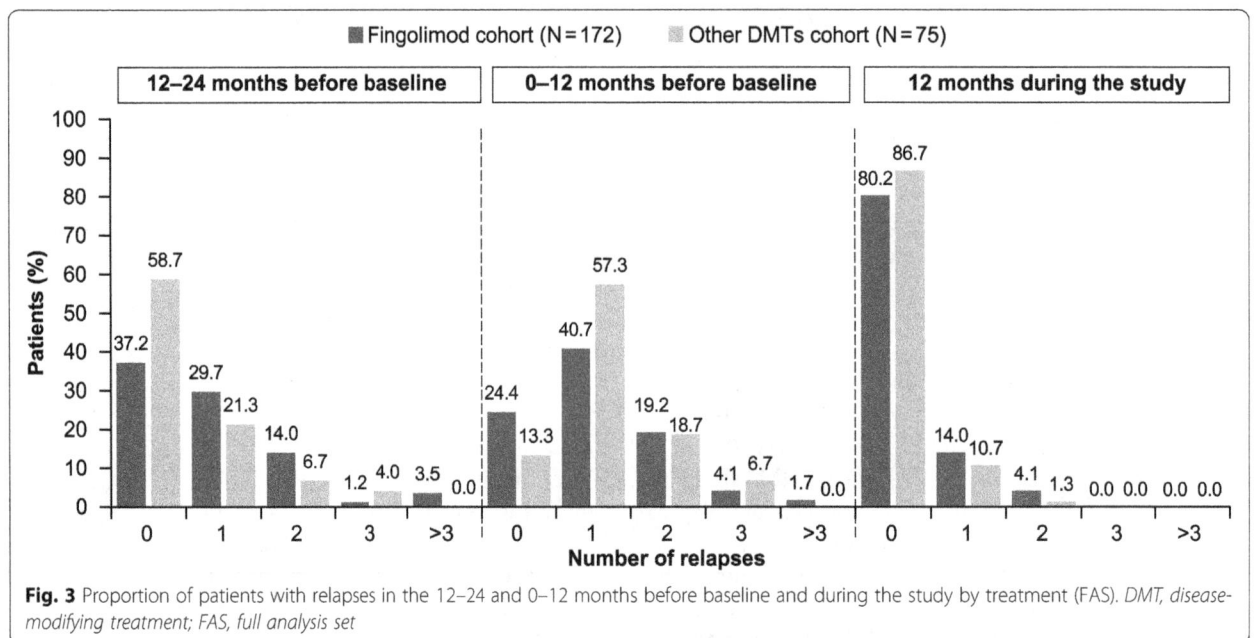

Fig. 3 Proportion of patients with relapses in the 12–24 and 0–12 months before baseline and during the study by treatment (FAS). *DMT, disease-modifying treatment; FAS, full analysis set*

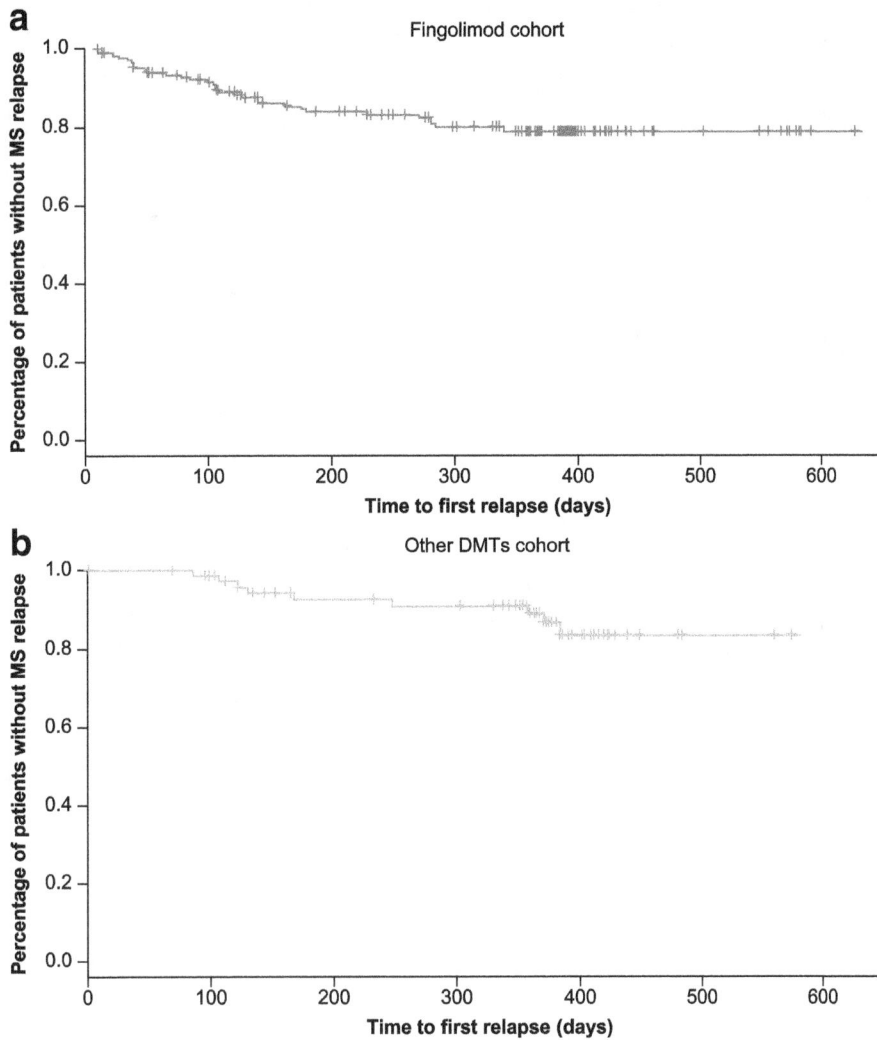

Fig. 4 Survival curves of time to the first MS relapse during the study (Kaplan-Meier plot; FAS). **a** Fingolimod cohort. **b** Other DMTs cohort. *DMT, disease-modifying treatment; FAS, full analysis set; MS, multiple sclerosis*

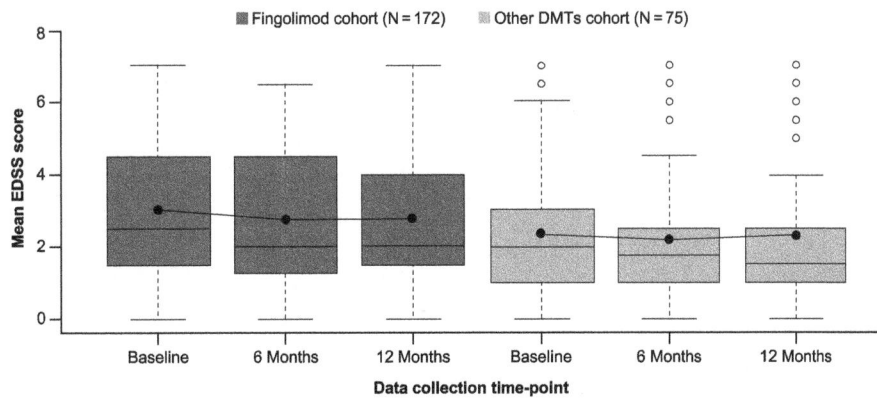

Fig. 5 Box and whiskers plot for mean EDSS score during the study by time point (FAS). *DMT, disease-modifying treatment; EDSS, Expanded Disability Status Scale; FAS, full analysis set.* The box plot's horizontal lines represent the 25th percentile, median and the 75th percentile of the mean EDSS score for top, middle and bottom lines, respectively. The whiskers represent the magnitude from the 10th to the 90th percentiles. The dots on the chart represent mean values across the study period. Outlier values are represented with empty circles

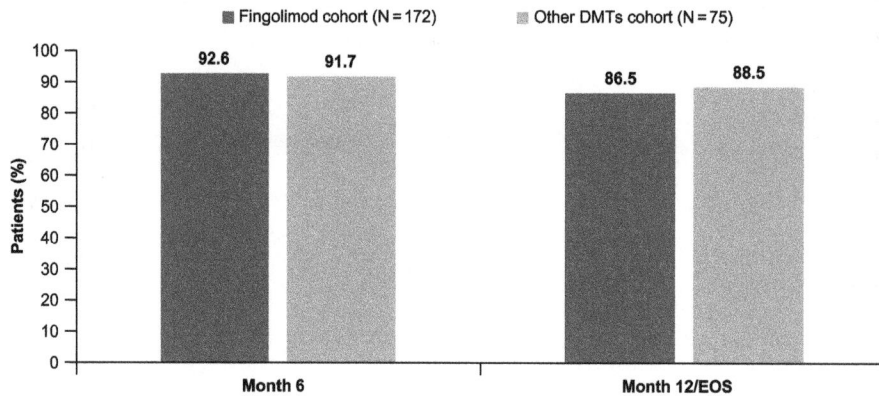

Fig. 6 Proportion of patients free from disability progression according to EDSS score (FAS). *DMT, disease-modifying treatment; EDSS, Expanded Disability Status Scale; EOS, end of study; FAS, full analysis set*

abnormal blood counts were lymphopaenia (n = 14, 7.9%), increase in hepatic enzymes (n = 12, 6.8%), leukopaenia (n = 9, 5.1%) and decrease in lymphocyte counts (n = 9, 5.1%) in the fingolimod cohort.

Approximately 16.0% (n = 29) of the patients discontinued the treatment due to AEs in the fingolimod cohort and 5.7% (n = 5) in the other DMTs cohort. The most frequent AEs ($\geq$2% of patients in any cohort) leading to treatment discontinuation were decrease in lymphocyte count (n = 6, 3.4%) and MS relapse (n = 4, 2.3%) in the fingolimod cohort and pain in extremity (n = 2, 2.3%) in the other DMTs cohort.

The percentage of patients experiencing SAEs was 5.6% (n = 10) in the fingolimod cohort and 1.1% (n = 1) in the other DMTs cohort. Two cases each of lymphopaenia, leukopaenia and MS relapse were reported; the remaining events were singular and diverse in nature in the fingolimod cohort. One case each of leukopaenia and neutropaenia were reported in the other DMTs cohort. Further details of treatment discontinuation and SAEs are provided in

Additional file 2: Table S2. No deaths occurred during the study.

The first-dose monitoring of fingolimod-treated patients showed a minor and transient decrease in pulse rate and blood pressure. One patient reported symptomatic bradycardia and one patient returned for monitoring with new or worsening electrocardiogram findings after the first dose of fingolimod. There were three cases of bradycardia reported in total in the fingolimod cohort during the study. No cases of symptomatic bradyarrhythmia or macular oedema were reported in either cohort (Table 3).

Discussion

The present observational PERFORMS study explored the real-world experience of fingolimod treatment in patients with RRMS in Middle Eastern countries. The study reported that QoL was maintained over 12 months in patients with RRMS in the fingolimod cohort. Fingolimod was effective in reducing the relapse rate and disability progression. The results from this real-world study are consistent with the efficacy

Table 2 Patients' walking ability over 12 months of study period (FAS)

Walking ability, n (%)	Fingolimod cohort N = 172			Other DMTs cohort N = 75		
	Baseline n = 172	Month 6 n = 134	Month 12/EOS n = 111	Baseline n = 75	Month 6 n = 63	Month 12/EOS n = 57
Patients with walking ability assessment	165 (95.9)	112 (83.6)	111 (100.0)	75 (100.0)	59 (93.7)	57 (100.0)
Walking ability assessment						
Unable to walk	7 (4.2)	1 (0.9)	2 (1.8)	6 (8.0)	4 (6.8)	1 (1.8)
Not able to walk unrestricted outside home (assistive device used)	16 (9.7)	16 (14.3)	15 (13.5)	0 (0.0)	3 (5.1)	4 (7.0)
Not able to walk unrestricted outside home (assistive device not used)	21 (12.7)	15 (13.4)	10 (9.0)	3 (4.0)	1 (1.7)	4 (7.0)
Able to walk unrestricted outside home	121 (73.3)	80 (71.4)	84 (75.7)	66 (88.0)	51 (86.4)	48 (84.2)

Data are presented herewith as n (%)
DMT disease-modifying treatment, *EOS* end of study, *FAS* full analysis set

Table 3 Incidence of AEs (safety set)

	Fingolimod cohort N = 177	Other DMTs cohort N = 87
Safety profile, n (%)		
Patients with any AE	106 (59.9)	44 (50.6)
Patients with any AE leading to drug discontinuation	29 (16.4)	5 (5.7)
Patients with an SAE	10 (5.6)	1 (1.1)
Deaths	0 (0.0)	0 (0.0)
Most frequent AEs (≥3% of patients for any group; n [%]; preferred terms)		
MS relapse	19 (10.7)	7 (8.0)
Lymphopaenia	14 (7.9)	0 (0.0)
Hepatic enzyme increased	12 (6.8)	0 (0.0)
Fatigue	11 (6.2)	6 (6.9)
Muscular weakness	10 (5.6)	5 (5.7)
Leukopaenia	9 (5.1)	3 (3.4)
Lymphocyte count decreased	9 (5.1)	0 (0.0)
Dizziness	8 (4.5)	2 (2.3)
Gait disturbance	7 (4.0)	6 (6.9)
MS worsening	4 (2.3)	4 (4.6)
Pain in extremity	6 (3.4)	2 (2.3)
Headache	4 (2.3)	3 (3.4)
Micturition urgency	3 (1.7)	3 (3.4)
Influenza	0 (0.0)	4 (4.6)
Paraesthesia	0 (0.0)	4 (4.6)
Selected AEs, n (%)		
Symptomatic bradyarrhythmia	0 (0.0)	0 (0.0)
Macular oedema	0 (0.0)	0 (0.0)
Increase in liver enzymes	14 (8.9)	2 (2.8)
Any infection	4 (2.5)	2 (2.8)
Other (any other AE)	50 (31.6)	28 (38.9)

Safety set: all AEs are reported in patients on MOI or after a switch; if no medication is taken at the time of the AE start, the AE will be reported under the category of the medication taken within the last 45 days
AE adverse event, DMT disease-modifying treatment, MOI medication of interest, MS multiple sclerosis, SAE serious adverse event

and safety profile of fingolimod established in clinical trials [8–12].

Considering the observational nature of the study, no formal statistical comparison was performed; however, patients' sociodemographics, such as distribution of age, gender and race, were similar in both cohorts. These characteristics were comparable to those of patients with RRMS in the previous observational study in Kuwait [35] and also consistent with characteristic of patients included in the large randomised FREEDOMS, FREEDOMS II and TRANSFORMS studies [8–12].

In terms of disease history, the mean duration since MS diagnosis was longer in the fingolimod cohort than

in the other DMTs cohort at baseline. This was further reflected with the fact that ~50% of the fingolimod cohort had the first MS symptoms >5 years prior to study start, as opposed to the other DMTs cohort, where 50% of patients had the first diagnosis <15 months prior to study start. In addition, the percentage of patients switching from prior natalizumab to fingolimod treatment was high at study entry. Moreover, the mean baseline EDSS scores were higher and treatment-naïve patients were fewer in the fingolimod cohort compared with the other DMTs cohort. Patients included in the fingolimod cohort were thus more 'chronic' and had more 'residual disability' than those in the other DMTs cohort. Such imbalances in baseline characteristics between treatment groups are common in open-label, observational studies. It was reported that baseline EDSS scores significantly impact the treatment response with the DMTs in patients with RRMS [36]. These differences in baseline characteristics between groups, in particular the EDSS score, might have led to comparable effectiveness results between fingolimod and other DMTs cohorts in this study.

The overall MusiQoL index score was high in both cohorts during the study. In the fingolimod cohort, two dimensions showed significant improvement during the study: 'activity of daily living' and 'psychological wellbeing'. However, these two dimensions were also the ones with the lowest scores at baseline, and the subsequent improvement in scores may actually reflect a regression to the mean effect [37]. The overall MusiQoL index score of 64.4 at EOS in the fingolimod cohort was in line with the previously presented 6-month interim analysis from the real-world VIRGILE study in France, where median MusiQoL scores ranged from 62.4 to 65.7 [13]. As observed in several observational studies using different questionnaires [13–20], the overall HRQoL with fingolimod remained stable over 12 months in the present study. In the other DMTs cohort, the 'relationship with the healthcare system' dimension significantly improved throughout the study period. The global HRQoL index showed no improvement.

In the study, overall, treating physicians considered that the clinical impression of 88.5% of fingolimod-treated patients either improved or had not changed. This is consistent with results observed in the 6-month open-label Evaluate Patient Outcomes, Safety, and Tolerability of Fingolimod (EPOC) study, where CGI-I scores were significantly lower in the fingolimod cohort vs. standard-of-care DMT cohort (3.2 vs. 3.9, respectively; $p < 0.0001$), indicating a greater perceived improvement [19].

In the fingolimod cohort, 31 (18.0%) patients experienced at least one relapse during the study. This result was in line with the 12-month randomised double-blind

TRANSFORMS study reporting that ~20.0% of patients had at least one relapse [10], but was higher than the previously reported retrospective study using the US Claims Database where only ~13.0% of patients had at least one relapse over 360 days of treatment in the fingolimod group [21]. In this retrospective study, only 33% of patients had MS relapse within 1 year before study entry when switched from interferons to the fingolimod cohort at baseline [21], whereas the majority of the patients (70.9%) included in the current study had experienced at least one relapse within 1 year before study (mean duration since last relapse: 9 months). The results of the study therefore need to be evaluated with caution considering the patient population and disease history at baseline in the fingolimod cohort.

The proportion of relapse-free patients reported in the study (80.2%) was in line with the 12-month TRANSFORMS (82.5%) [10] and the multicentre post-marketing real-world study (88.1%) by Totaro and colleagues [25] in patients with RRMS. This finding was higher than those in large randomised studies in patients with RRMS: 24-month FREEDOMS—70.4% [8] and FREEDOMS II—71.5% [9].

According to the EDSS measure, 86.5% of the patients were free from any disability progression in the fingolimod cohort at the EOS, which was lower than that in the randomised controlled TRANSFORMS study, wherein 93.3% of patients (95% CI, 90.9%–95.8%) had no disability progression [10]. The proportion of patients free from disability progression in the present study was in line with the 24-month randomised FREEDOMS [8] and FREEDOMS II [9] studies as well as the 3-year interim analysis of the 5-year PANGAEA registry records data from Germany [24].

There were no new safety concerns during fingolimod first-dose monitoring. During the study, a total of three cases of symptomatic/treated bradycardia and no cases of bradyarrhythmia were reported. These are known class effects and have been noticed to resolve without therapeutic intervention in other clinical trials [38, 39]. In the current study, no case of macular oedema, which is an identified risk with fingolimod treatment [40], was reported in the fingolimod cohort.

The number of patients reporting a decrease in lymphocyte counts, which is a known pharmacodynamic therapeutic effect of fingolimod, was low (5.1%) in the fingolimod cohort and comparable to that in earlier safety reports [41, 42]. Of note, reductions in lymphocyte counts with fingolimod in the present study did not show an increase in the risk of infections and was consistent with the data reported earlier in clinical studies as well as in the post-marketing setting [41]. Safety results reported in the study were in line with integrated safety analysis [41] and long-term studies [42], reporting no increased risk of infections, malignancies or serious cardiovascular events with fingolimod.

Owing to the observational, non-blinded and non-randomised nature of the study, different biases could have obscured any true causal association. Systemic differences between treatments may exist, influenced by decisions of the treating physicians who assigned patients to different drugs based on disease severity, disease duration, presence of co-morbidities and other confounding factors (i.e. associated with the choice of treatment and treatment outcome). These differences, due to an indication/channelling bias [43], can confound the association between treatment and treatment outcome. Patients with a longer progression of the disease or patients refractory to other DMTs were more likely to receive fingolimod, which might have resulted in the underestimation of the effectiveness of fingolimod. Although the QoL was self-reported by the patients, the MusiQoL questionnaires were transcribed by the physician or the study staff, which might have resulted in the risk of information bias.

As PERFORMS was a real-world, observational study, no neuroimaging assessments were mandated and magnetic resonance imaging read outs were not evaluated via a central reading facility. Therefore, neuroimaging findings were not considered as an outcome to be assessed.

Conclusion

The study concluded that the QoL was maintained over 12 months with fingolimod treatment. Fingolimod was effective in reducing relapse rate and disability progression, confirming favourable results as found in large randomised clinical trials. The first dose of fingolimod appeared to be safe, and no new safety findings were observed in the study.

Abbreviations

AE: Adverse event; CGI-I: Clinical Global Impression-Improvement scale; CI: Confidence interval; CNS: central nervous system; DMTs: Disease-modifying treatments; EDSS: Expanded Disability Status Scale; EOS: end of study; EPOC: Evaluate Patient Outcomes, Safety, and Tolerability of Fingolimod; FAS: Full analysis set; HRQoL: Health-related quality of life; MOI: Medication of interest; MS: Multiple sclerosis; MusiQoL: Multiple Sclerosis International Quality of Life; PERFORMS: Prospective Evaluation of Treatment with Fingolimod for Multiple Sclerosis; QoL: Quality of life; RRMS: Relapsing-remitting multiple sclerosis; S1P: Sphingosine-1-phosphate; SAE: Serious adverse event; SD: Standard deviation

Acknowledgements

The article processing charges for this publication were funded by Novartis Pharma AG. All named authors meet the International Committee of Medical Journal Editors (ICMJE) criteria for authorship for this manuscript, take responsibility for the integrity of the work as a whole, and have given final approval to the version to be published. All authors are responsible for intellectual content and data accuracy. The authors acknowledge the patients, investigators and staff at participating sites for supporting the conduct of the study. The authors thank Shelley DiTommaso (Novartis Pharma AG, Basel, Switzerland) for her contribution to reviewing the study protocol and manuscript outline. We thank Anuja Shah and Rahul Birari (both Novartis Healthcare Pvt. Ltd., Hyderabad, India) for manuscript preparation and for incorporating and collating the comments from the authors and editorial assistance.

Funding
The study was funded by Novartis Pharma AG, Basel, Switzerland. Novartis Pharma AG developed the study design and protocol in conjunction with the clinical investigators, were responsible for collection, statistical analysis and interpretation of data. The manuscript writing and editorial support was supported by Novartis Pharma AG, Basel, Switzerland.

Authors' contributions
AA was involved in study concept, study design, study execution, data acquisition, data analysis, obtaining study fund, supervising the study research, and drafting manuscript outline. HA was involved in study execution, data acquisition, and drafting manuscript outline. JI was involved in study concept, study design, study execution, data acquisition, data analysis, data interpretation, obtaining study fund, supervising the study research and drafting manuscript outline. MH was involved in data analysis, data interpretation, drafting of the manuscript outline and provided administrative and technical/research support. RA was involved in study execution, data acquisition, data analysis, data interpretation, and drafting of the manuscript outline. MB was involved in data analysis, data interpretation, statistical analysis, and drafting of manuscript outline. KC was involved in study execution, data analysis, data interpretation, and drafting of the manuscript outline. OY was involved in the study design, data interpretation, obtaining study fund, and drafting of the manuscript outline. All authors were involved in preparing and revising manuscript and have reviewed the final draft. All authors read and approved the final manuscript.

Authors' information
Not applicable.

Competing interests
AA received personal compensation from Genzyme for consulting, and Rosh, Teva and Novartis for serving on the scientific advisory board and as a consultant; received research support from Bayer-Schering Pharma, Biogen Idec, Teva Pharmaceutical Industries Ltd., Genzyme, Merck Serono and Novartis; outside the submitted work. HA received speaker honoraria from Novartis, outside the submitted work. JI received personal fees, non-financial support and other support from Novartis, during the conduct of the study, outside the submitted work. MH received personal fees from Novartis, outside the submitted work. RA received honoraria as a speaker and for serving in scientific advisory board from Bayer, Biogen, Novartis, Merck and Sanofi, outside the submitted work; received speaker honoraria from GSK and Lundbeck, outside the submitted work. MB, KC and OY are employees of Novartis.

Author details
[1]Multiple Sclerosis Center, Sheba Medical Center, 52621 Tel-Hashomer, Israel. [2]Ain Shams University, Cairo, Egypt. [3]Rashid Hospital and Dubai Medical College, Dubai, UAE. [4]Department in Monla Hospital, Tripoli, Lebanon. [5]Division of Neurology, Department of Medicine, Amiri Hospital, Sharq, Kuwait. [6]Novartis Healthcare Pvt. Ltd., Hyderabad, India. [7]Novartis Pharma AG, Basel, Switzerland.

References
1. Trapp BD, Peterson J, Ransohoff RM, Rudick R, Mörk S, Bö L. Axonal transection in the lesions of multiple sclerosis. N Engl J Med. 1998;338:278–85.
2. Sospedra M, Martin R. Immunology of multiple sclerosis. Annu Rev Immunol. 2005;23:683–747.
3. Multiple Sclerosis International Federation. Atlas of MS 2013. http://www.msif.org/wp-content/uploads/2014/09/Atlas-of-MS.pdf. Accessed 30 June 2015.
4. Heydarpour P, Khoshkish S, Abtahi S, Moradi-Lakeh M, Sahraian MA. Multiple sclerosis epidemiology in Middle East and North Africa: a systematic review and meta-analysis. Neuroepidemiology. 2015;44:232–44.
5. Inshasi J, Thakre M. Prevalence of multiple sclerosis in Dubai. United Arab Emirates Int J Neurosci. 2011;121:393–8.
6. O'Connor PW, Oh J. Disease modifying agents in multiple sclerosis. Handb Clin Neurol. 2014:465–501.
7. Groves A, Kihara Y, Chun J. Fingolimod: direct CNS effects of sphingosine 1-phosphate (S1P) receptor modulation and implications in multiple sclerosis therapy. J Neurol Sci. 2013;328:9–18.
8. Kappos L, Radue EW, O'connor P, et al. A placebo-controlled trial of oral fingolimod in relapsing multiple sclerosis. N Engl J Med. 2010;362:387–401.
9. Calabresi PA, Radue EW, Goodin D, Jeffery D, Rammohan KW, Reder AT, et al. Safety and efficacy of fingolimod in patients with relapsing-remitting multiple sclerosis (FREEDOMS II): a double-blind, randomised, placebo-controlled, phase 3 trial. Lancet Neurol. 2014;13:545–56.
10. Cohen JA, Barkhof F, Comi G, Hartung HP, Khatri BO, Montalban X, et al. Oral fingolimod or intramuscular interferon for relapsing multiple sclerosis. N Engl J Med. 2010;362:402–15.
11. Kappos L, O'Connor P, Radue EW, Polman C, Hohlfeld R, Selmaj K, et al. Long-term effects of fingolimod in multiple sclerosis: the randomized FREEDOMS extension trial. Neurology. 2015;84:1582–91.
12. Cohen JA, Khatri B, Barkhof F, Comi G, Hartung HP, Montalban X, et al. Long-term (up to 4.5 years) treatment with fingolimod in multiple sclerosis: results from the extension of the randomised TRANSFORMS study. J Neurol Neurosurg Psychiatry. 2016;87:468–75.
13. Coustans M, Debouverie M, Kobelt G, Lebrun-Frenay C, Leray E, Papeix C, et al. Long-term efficacy, safety, tolerability and quality of life with fingolimod treatment in patients with multiple sclerosis in real-world settings in France: VIRGILE study design. Poster presented at the 31st Congress of the European Committee for Treatment and Research in Multiple Sclerosis 7–10 October 2015, Barcelona, Spain. http://onlinelibrary.ectrims-congress.eu/ectrims/2015/31st/115257/bashar.allaf.long-term.efficacy.safety.tolerability.and.quality.of.life.with.html?f=m1. Accessed 4 November 2016.
14. Kuperman G. Interim analysis II from REAL study: quality of life and persistence with fingolimod treatment in relapsing remitting multiple sclerosis patients in Argentina. Neurology. 2015;84:255.
15. Crayton H, Hunter SF. Huffman C et al. CMSC ACTRIMS: Improved quality of life after therapy change to fingolimod; 2013. https://cmsc.confex.com/cmsc/2013/webprogram/Paper1313.html. Accessed 9 November 2016
16. Montalban X, Comi G, O'Connor P, Gold S, de Vera A, Eckert B, Kappos L. Oral fingolimod (FTY720) in relapsing multiple sclerosis: impact on health-related quality of life in a phase II study. Mult Scler. 2011;17:1341–50.
17. Czaplinski A, Jaquiery E, Stellmes P, Ramseier S, Baumann A, Kurlandchikov O, et al. Interim Results of the Swiss Post Marketing Surveillance Monitoring Quality of Life and Treatment Satisfaction in Patients With Relapsing-Remitting Multiple Sclerosis. Neurology. 2014;82(Supplement 10):179.
18. Miller D, Lee J, Hashmonay R, Agashivala N, Rudick R. Patient disability and quality of life after fingolimod initiation: the Cleveland Clinic experience. Neurology. 2013;34452
19. Fox E, Edwards K, Burch G, Wynn DR, LaGanke C, Crayton H, et al. Outcomes of switching directly to oral fingolimod from injectable therapies: results of the randomized, open-label, multicenter, evaluate patient OutComes (EPOC) study in relapsing multiple sclerosis. Mult Scler Relat Disord. 2014;3:607–19.
20. Inshasi JS, Sarathchandran P, Alboudi A, Kamal Y. Fingolimod treatment in relapsing-remitting multiple sclerosis—the real-world experience at Rashid Hospital multiple sclerosis (MS) center in Dubai. Mult Scler J. 2016;10 doi:10.1177/1352458516635979.
21. Bergvall N, Makin C, Lahoz R, Agashivala N, Pradhan A, Capkun G, et al. Relapse rates in patients with multiple sclerosis switching from interferon to fingolimod or glatiramer acetate: a US claims database study. PLoS One. 2014;9:e88472.

22. Al-Hashel J, Ahmed SF, Behbehani R, Alroughani R. Real-world use of fingolimod in patients with relapsing remitting multiple sclerosis: a retrospective study using the national multiple sclerosis registry in Kuwait. CNS Drugs. 2014;28:817–24.

23. He A, Spelman T, Jokubaitis V, Havrdova E, Horakova D, Trojano M, et al. Comparison of switch to fingolimod or interferon beta/glatiramer acetate in active multiple sclerosis. JAMA Neurol. 2015;72:405–13.

24. Ziemssen T, Schwarz HJ, Fuchs A, Cornelissen C. 36 month PANGAEA: a 5-year non-interventional study of safety, efficacy and pharmacoeconomic data for fingolimod patients in daily clinical practice. Neurology. 2015;84(Suppl 14):251.

25. Totaro R, Di Carmine C, Costantino G, Fantozzi R, Bellantonio P, Fuiani A, et al. Fingolimod treatment in relapsing-remitting multiple sclerosis patients: a prospective observational multicenter postmarketing study. Mult Scler Int. 2015;2015:763418.

26. Ordoñez-Boschetti L, Rey R, Cruz A, Sinha A, Reynolds T, Frider N, Alvarenga R. Safety and tolerability of fingolimod in Latin American patients with relapsing-remitting multiple sclerosis: the open-label FIRST LATAM study. Adv Ther. 2015;32:626–35.

27. Simeoni M, Auquier P, Fernandez O, Flachenecker P, Stecchi S, Constantinescu C, et al, MusiQol study group. Validation of the Multiple Sclerosis International Quality of Life questionnaire. Mult Scler. 2008;14:219–230.

28. Al-Tahan AM, Al-Jumah MA, Bohlega SM, Al-Shammari SN, Al-Sharoqi IA, Dahdaleh MP, et al. The importance of quality-of-life assessment in the management of patients with multiple sclerosis. Recommendations from the Middle East MS advisory group. Neurosciences (Riyadh). 2011;16:109–13.

29. Guy W. ECDEU Assessment Manual for Psychopharmacology—Revised (DHEW Publ No ADM 76–338). Rockville, MD, U.S. Department of Health, Education, and Welfare, Public Health Service, Alcohol, Drug Abuse, and Mental Health Administration, NIMH Psychopharmacology Research Branch, Division of Extramural Research Programs; 1976. p. 218–22.

30. McDonald WI, Compston A, Edan G, et al. Recommended diagnostic criteria for multiple sclerosis: guidelines from the international panel on the diagnosis of multiple sclerosis. Ann Neurol. 2001;50:121–7.

31. Kurzke JF. Rating neurologic impairment in multiple sclerosis: an expanded disability status scale (EDSS). Neurology. 1983;33:1444–52.

32. Liu C, Blumhardt LD. Disability outcome measures in therapeutic trials of relapsing-remitting multiple sclerosis: effects of heterogeneity of disease course in placebo cohorts. J Neurol Neurosurg Psychiatry. 2000;68:450–7.

33. Butzkueven H, Kappos L, Pellegrini F, Trojano M, Wiendl H, Patel RN, et al. Efficacy and safety of natalizumab in multiple sclerosis: interim observational programme results. J Neurol Neurosurg Psychiatry. 2014;85:1190–7.

34. WMA Declaration of Helsinki – Ethical Principles for Medical Research Involving Human Subjects. Updated on October 2013. https://www.wma.net/policies-post/wma-declaration-of-helsinki-ethical-principles-for-medical-research-involving-human-subjects/. Accessed 12 July 2017.

35. Alroughani R, Ahmed S, Behbahani R, Al-Hashel J. Use of fingolimod in patients with relapsing remitting multiple sclerosis in Kuwait. Clin Neurol Neurosurg. 2014;119:17–20.

36. Sá MJ, de Sá J, Sousa L. Relapsing-remitting multiple sclerosis: patterns of response to disease-modifying therapies and associated factors: a national survey. Neurol Ther. 2014;3:89–99.

37. Barnett AG, van der Pols JC, Dobson AJ. Regression to the mean: what it is and how to deal with it. Int J Epidemiol. 2005;34:215–20.

38. DiMarco J, O'Connor P, Cohen JA, Reder AT, Zhang-Auberson L, Tang D, et al. First-dose effects of fingolimod: pooled safety data from three phase 3 studies. Mult Scler Relat Disord. 2014;3:629–38.

39. Camm J, Hla T, Bakshi R, Brinkmann V. Cardiac and vascular effects of fingolimod: mechanistic basis and clinical implications. Am Heart J. 2014;168:632–44.

40. Zarbin MA, Jampol LM, Jager RD, Reder AT, Francis G, Collins W, Tang D, Zhang X. Ophthalmic evaluations in clinical studies of fingolimod (FTY720) in multiple sclerosis. Ophthalmology. 2013;120:1432–9.

41. Kappos L, Cohen J, Collins W, de Vera A, Zhang-Auberson L, Ritter S, et al. Fingolimod in relapsing multiple sclerosis: an integrated analysis of safety findings. Mult Scler Relat Disord. 2014;3:494–504.

42. Khatri BO. Fingolimod in the treatment of relapsing–remitting multiple sclerosis: long-term experience and an update on the clinical evidence. Ther Adv Neurol Disord. 2016;9:130–47.

43. Petri H, Urquhart J. Channeling bias in the interpretation of drug effects. Stat Med. 1991;10:577–81.

4

Patient satisfaction with ExtaviPro™ 30G, a new auto-injector for administering interferon β-1b in multiple sclerosis: results from a real-world, observational EXCHANGE study

Frank A. Hoffmann[1], Anastasiya Trenova[2], Miguel A. Llaneza[3], Johannes Fischer[4], Giacomo Lus[5], Dorothea von Bredow[6], Núria Lara[7], Elaine Lam[8], Marlies Van Hoef[9] and Rajesh Bakshi[9*]

Abstract

Background: Patients with multiple sclerosis (MS) receiving long-term, subcutaneous interferon β-1b (IFN β-1b; Extavia®) often experience injection-site reactions and injection-site pain, which together with other side-effects (such as flu-like symptoms) result in suboptimal treatment compliance/adherence. The EXCHANGE study evaluated patient satisfaction with IFN β-1b treatment, administered using ExtaviPro™ 30G, a new auto-injector, in a real-world setting.

Methods: This 26-week, open-label, prospective, non-interventional, observational, multi-country multi-centre study enrolled patients with MS who had been treated with IFN β-1b or other disease-modifying therapies with a self-administered auto-injector for ≥3 months and who were planned to switch to IFN β-1b treatment administered using ExtaviPro™ 30G as part of routine clinical care. Patient-reported outcomes included overall patient satisfaction (primary outcome) and satisfaction associated with treatment effectiveness, convenience and side-effects, assessed using Treatment Satisfaction Questionnaire for Medication (TSQM)-14. The changes in TSQM scores from baseline to Week 26 were reported. All data were analysed using SAS statistical software (version 9.4).

Results: Of the 336 patients enrolled, 324 were included in the analysis. At baseline, mean ± standard deviation (SD) age of patients was 41.8 ± 11.3 years and 68.2% were women. The mean ± SD of MS disease duration was 6.9 ± 6.6 years, and the majority of patients (94.1%) had relapsing-remitting MS. The mean ± SD of TSQM score for overall patient satisfaction at Week 26 was 75.6 ± 16.46 (baseline, 73.0 ± 17.14; $p = 0.0342$). The mean ± SD of TSQM subscale scores for patient satisfaction with effectiveness, side-effects and convenience were 75.0 ± 18.65 (baseline, 71.6 ± 19.45; $p = 0.0356$), 88.5 ± 18.98 (baseline, 82.7 ± 22.93; $p = 0.0002$) and 77.6 ± 16.72 (baseline, 71.1 ± 17.53; $p < 0.0001$), respectively.

Conclusion: The results from this real-world study suggest that administering IFN β-1b with the new ExtaviPro™ auto-injector significantly improves overall patient satisfaction, including satisfaction associated with effectiveness, side-effects and convenience in MS patients.

Keywords: ExtaviPro™ auto-injector, Interferon β-1b, Observational, Patient satisfaction, Real-world, Side-effects

* Correspondence: rajesh.bakshi@novartis.com
[9]Novartis Pharma AG, Fabrikstrasse 12-3.03.12, Postfach, CH-4002 Basel, Switzerland
Full list of author information is available at the end of the article

Background

Multiple sclerosis (MS) is a chronic immune-mediated disease characterised by inflammation, axonal damage and demyelination in the central nervous system (CNS) [1]. Patients experience acute transient exacerbations of neurological symptoms (relapses) followed by periods of clinical stabiliosation during the early stages of the disease, and eventually worsening of neurological condition occurs in the form of disability over a period of time [2]. Currently, ~2.5 million people globally have MS [3].

Disease-modifying treatments (DMTs) such as interferons (IFNs; IFN β-1a, IFN β-1b) and glatiramer acetate are commonly prescribed as first-line therapies for relapsing forms of MS [4]. IFN β is postulated to modulate the immune system in MS through several potential pathways. Among these mechanisms, inhibition of T-cell migration from the periphery into the CNS and reduction in metalloproteinase activity on the vascular endothelium that constitutes the blood-brain barrier may be important [5, 6].

IFNs administered subcutaneously or intramuscularly have been shown to reduce the number and severity of clinical exacerbations, disability worsening, need for steroid treatment and the number of hospitalisations in patients with relapsing-remitting MS (RRMS) [7–10]. However, patients receiving long-term subcutaneous IFN β-1b often experience injection-site reactions and injection-site pain/inflammation, together with other side-effects, such as flu-like symptoms [11, 12], resulting in suboptimal treatment compliance and adherence in a substantial number of patients [13, 14].

Injection-site reactions may be related to IFN β-1b being injected or to the injection itself. Use of an auto-injector and thinner needle may improve patient experience and contribute to improving adherence to treatment. Several auto-injectors are available for most IFNs to improve treatment satisfaction, mitigate injection-site reactions and pain concerns associated with mechanical/manual injectors [15–18].

A new, improved auto-injector system, ExtaviPro™ 30G (Novartis Pharma AG), has been developed to facilitate self-administration of IFN β-1b (Extavia®). Compared with previous ExtaviJect® 30G, the new ExtaviPro™ 30G auto-injector is ergonomically designed to make the device easier to use and reliable and to reduce injection-site reactions and pain. The auto-injector facilitates self-administration of high-dose and high-frequency subcutaneous injections of IFN β-1b [19]. ExtaviPro™ uses an ultra-thin 30G needle that reduces shaking or jolting of the auto-injector and facilitates single-handed use and easy access to difficult-to-reach injection sites [19]. Collectively, these features can lead to a better treatment experience and reduced injection-site reactions and associated pain, which can, in turn, improve adherence. ExtaviPro™ 30G is widely available across Europe.

The current non-interventional, real-world study aimed to evaluate patient and nurse satisfaction with ExtaviPro™ 30G auto-injector as a new delivery device for IFN β-1b (Extavia®) in the treatment of MS in the Europe. The primary objective of the study was to evaluate overall patient satisfaction with Extavia® delivered using the new ExtaviPro™ auto-injector. The secondary objectives included patient-perceived effectiveness, convenience and side-effects. Patient tolerability to injection-site reactions, treatment adherence and nurse satisfaction were also evaluated.

Methods

Patient population

Men and women aged ≥18 years who had been treated with IFN β-1b (Extavia®) or other injectable first-line DMTs (IFN β-1b [Betaferon®/Betaseron®], IFN β-1a [Avonex®] or glatiramer acetate [Copaxone®]) for MS using a self-administering auto-injector device for at least 3 months before the study entry, who were recommended to switch to IFN β-1b (Extavia®) administered using new ExtaviPro™ 30G auto-injector based on the medical need as part of routine clinical care and in compliance with the local prescribing information, were included in the study. Patients provided written informed consent prior to their enrolment in the study.

Study design

This was a 26-week, single-arm, open-label, prospective, observational study, conducted between February 2014 and August 2015 at 74 sites in six countries in Europe: Bulgaria, Germany, Greece, Italy, Poland and Spain.

At baseline (Day 1), eligible patients were transitioned to IFN β-1b (Extavia®) self-administered using ExtaviPro™ auto-injector and entered into a 26-week observation period. Because this was an observational study, all patients were eligible for the treatment with IFN β-1b (Extavia®), which was prescribed based on the local prescribing information. Data for the study were collected at routine clinical visits and were recorded by physicians at baseline (Day 1) and at Weeks 4, 13 and 26, except for Bulgaria where data were collected only at Week 26 because routine visits took place every 6 months.

Only patient-reported outcomes were assessed during the study period; no additional laboratory tests or medical procedures were conducted. If required, the dose was titrated in accordance with the locally approved prescribing information.

Assessments
Patient-reported outcomes

Treatment satisfaction The primary endpoint of the study was overall patient satisfaction with IFN β-1b (Extavia®) at Week 26, delivered using the new ExtaviPro™ auto-injector, as assessed by the Treatment Satisfaction Questionnaire for Medication (TSQM). The TSQM (version 1.4) is a 14-item, reliable, validated instrument for assessing patient satisfaction with medication, providing overall scores on four scales including 'global satisfaction', 'effectiveness', 'side effects' and 'convenience' [20]. The TSQM was also available in local languages. Patients were asked to refer to their prior treatment and auto-injector for assessment of treatment satisfaction at baseline, and for IFN β-1b (Extavia®) and ExtaviPro™ for all subsequent assessments.

The secondary endpoints of the study included mean scores of individual subscales of the TSQM—'effectiveness', 'side effects' and 'convenience'—at Week 26 [20].

Tolerability for ExtaviPro™: Pain and injection-site reactions
The tolerability for IFN β-1b (Extavia®) injected through ExtaviPro™ auto-injector consisted of injection-site pain and injection-site reactions at Week 26 and was assessed using the short-form McGill Pain Questionnaire (SF-MPQ) [21] and injection-site reaction questionnaire [22], respectively.

The SF-MPQ comprises 15 descriptors (11 sensory and 4 affective) rated on an intensity scale as follows: 0 = none, 1 = mild, 2 = moderate or 3 = severe. Three pain scores were derived from the sum of the intensity rank values: sensory, affective and total descriptors. Moreover, the SF-MPQ included the Present Pain Intensity Index of the standard MPQ and a visual analogue scale (VAS) [21].

Patients were asked to respond to two questions related to injection-site reactions in the 4 weeks prior to the current visit: 'Do injection-site reactions occur more or less often now?' and 'Do the injection-site reactions cause more or less discomfort now?' These questions were adapted from the Multiple Sclerosis Treatment Concerns Questionnaire (MSTCQ) [15]. The response was selected from the five options: much less, somewhat less, about the same, somewhat more and much more [22].

Adherence
Patient adherence to IFN β-1b (Extavia®) delivered through ExtaviPro™ auto-injector was assessed by the Multiple Sclerosis Treatment Adherence Questionnaire (MSTAQ). The MSTAQ is a 30-item questionnaire designed to identify factors affecting patient adherence and barriers to treatment adherence in patients using MS DMTs. The tool was also designed to predict missed doses. The MSTAQ has three subscales: barriers (score 0–39), side-effects (score 0–40) and coping strategies (score 0–7) [23].

Healthcare provider-reported outcomes
The proportion of patients reporting incidence of injection-site reactions (specifically pain, swelling, redness, itching or bruising) was evaluated using a physician-completed questionnaire for capturing patients' reports of reactions over the 4 weeks before the visit [15].

Satisfaction of healthcare providers was evaluated based on nurses' acceptance of delivering IFN β-1b (Extavia®) through ExtaviPro™ auto-injector, which was assessed using nurse questionnaires. The nurse questionnaires assessed the ease of switching patients to the ExtaviPro™ 30G auto-injector and the overall satisfaction with the injector device (2 items: baseline and follow-up visits). Two questions were asked at baseline visit: 'How easy was it for the patient to learn to use the device?' and 'How easy is it expected to be for the patient to use the device?' Two similar questions were asked during follow-up visits: 'Was additional training required?' and 'How easy did the patient find it to use the device?'

The response to all questions was selected from the four options: 'very difficult', 'difficult', 'easy' and 'very easy'. The response to the level of additional training required was selected from the four options: 'none', 'less than half', 'more than half' and 'repeat entire training'.

Safety
Safety assessments included reporting of adverse events (AEs) and serious AEs (SAEs).

Sample size determination and statistical analysis
Assuming a drop-out rate of 15%, 333 patients were planned for enrolment to achieve the target sample size of 283 patients. This sample size allows estimation of the true mean TSQM global satisfaction score within a margin of error of ±2.6 using a two-sided 95% confidence interval (CI) based on an estimated standard deviation (SD) of 22.3 from a historical data.

Treatment satisfaction, tolerability, adherence and other results for the IFN β-1b (Extavia®) group were compared between the previous auto-injector (baseline) and new auto-injector (ExtaviPro™) at Week 26. The change from baseline in the TSQM Global Satisfaction subscale score at Week 26 was analysed using a linear mixed model for repeated measures at 95% CI, with week as the fixed effect and baseline scores as a continuous covariate. A 95% CI was constructed using the least squares mean (i.e. adjusted mean at the overall baseline mean value) and the within-subject variance obtained from the linear mixed model. In case of missing data, the

CI was valid under the assumption that the missing data have a missing-at-random mechanism.

Tolerability in terms of satisfaction with the side-effect domain on TSQM subscale, SF-MPQ and the injection-site reaction questionnaires were also analysed using a linear mixed model for repeated measures. The change in MSTAQ scores over time compared with baseline scores was analysed using a linear mixed model for repeated measures following the methodology described above. The treatment compliance rate over time versus baseline scores was analysed using the Chi-square test. Compliance was calculated considering the 2-week period before each follow-up visit, excluding the baseline visit. Given the real-world nature of the data, any missing data were assumed to be missing at random and imputation methods were not applied to ensure description of real patient management in clinical practice.

All data analyses were conducted using SAS statistics software version 9.4 (SAS Institute Inc., Cary, NC) and in accordance with the Strengthening the Reporting of Observational Studies in Epidemiology (STROBE) [24] guidelines and applicable sections of the Consolidated Standards of Reporting Trials (CONSORT) guidelines [25].

Ethical and good clinical practice

The study protocol and amendment were reviewed and approved by the Independent Ethics Committees and Institutional Review Boards at each centre per local regulations. All patients provided written informed consent before study entry. The study was conducted in compliance with the ethical principles of the Declaration of Helsinki and the International Conference on Harmonisation Good Clinical Practice Guidelines [26].

Results
Patient disposition and baseline characteristics

Of the 336 enrolled patients at 74 sites, the majority were receiving IFNβ-1b (93.5%, n = 314) and the remaining were receiving other DMTs (6.5%, n = 22) as a part of their routine care. In total, 324 patients were included in the final analysis. Twelve patients were excluded from the analysis: one patient (~4.5%) in the other DMTs group did not receive any treatment and 11 (3.5%) in the IFNβ-1b (Extavia®) group used ExtaviPro™ before study inclusion.

Demographics and baseline characteristics of patients are described in Table 1. The overall mean (range) age of patients was 41.8 (19.0–68.0) years, and 68.2% of all patients were women. At baseline, most of the patients (94.1%) had RRMS and the mean duration since diagnosis was 6.9 ± 6.59 years; 41.0% of the patients reported exacerbations during 2 years before study entry, with a mean ± SD of 1.6 ± 0.79 exacerbations per patient. In

Table 1 Patient demographics and baseline characteristics

	IFN β-1b group N = 303	Other DMTs group N = 21	Total N = 324
Age (years)			
Mean	41.5 ± 11.29	44.9 ± 11.15	41.8 ± 11.30
Median (min–max)	40.0 (19.0–68.0)	43.0 (24.0–68.0)	40.0 (19.0–68.0)
Women, n (%)	207 (68.3)	14 (66.7)	221 (68.2)
Subtype of MS, n (%)			
CIS	7 (2.3)	0 (0.0)	7 (2.2)
RRMS	286 (94.4)	19 (90.5)	305 (94.1)
SPMS	10 (3.3)	2 (9.5)	12 (3.7)
MS disease history			
Duration since MS diagnosis (years)			
Mean	6.7 ± 6.36	9.5 ± 9.16	6.9 ± 6.59
Median (min–max)	4.6 (0.2–35.0)	7.5 (0.3–43.4)	4.8 (0.2–43.4)
Presence of exacerbations, n (%)	120 (39.6)	13 (61.9)	133 (41.0)
Number of exacerbations			
Mean	1.5 ± 0.74	1.9 ± 1.14	1.6 ± 0.79
Median (min–max)	1.0 (0.0–5.0)	2.0 (1.0–5.0)	1.0 (0.0–5.0)
Reasons for switching to ExtaviPro™, n (%)			
Clinical reasons[a]			
Availability of new auto-injector (patient already treated with Extavia®)	296 (97.7)	2 (9.5)	298 (92.0)
Lack/loss of effectiveness of current treatment, as evidenced by			
returning/worsening/ progressing MS symptoms	2 (0.7)	6 (28.6)	8 (2.5)
Increasing frequency of relapses/symptomatic phases	2 (0.7)	3 (14.3)	5 (1.5)
MRI evaluation	3 (1.0)	6 (28.6)	9 (2.8)
Other	5 (1.7)	1 (4.8)	6 (1.9)
Poor tolerance	9 (3.0)	7 (33.3)	16 (4.9)
Patient-centred reasons			
Compliance problem	19 (6.3)	9 (42.9)	28 (8.6)
Patient unable to consistently store current therapy under special conditions	5 (1.7)	2 (9.5)	7 (2.2)

Data are presented as mean ± SD, unless stated otherwise
[a]Multiresponse option
CIS clinically isolated syndrome, DMT disease-modifying treatment, IFN interferon, max maximum, min minimum, MRI magnetic resonance imaging, MS multiple sclerosis, RRMS relapsing-remitting multiple sclerosis, SD standard deviation, SPMS secondary progressive multiple sclerosis

the IFN β-1b (Extavia®) group, 12.2% of patients had cardiovascular and/or metabolic comorbidities, 9.6% had other neurological disorders, 6.6% had other auto-immune disorders and 4.6% had other inflammatory disorders or osteoporosis.

At baseline, the majority of patients (94.8%, n = 307) were on IFN β-1b (Extavia®). Before switching to ExtaviPro™, 93.5% were using ExtaviJect® auto-injector, 3.4% Avonex® Pen and remaining were on Betaject® Light/ Betaject® Lite, Betaject®/Betaject® Comfort/Betacomfort®, Copaxone® autoject 2 or Rebiject II®. The main reasons for switching to ExtaviPro™ auto-injector in the Extavia® group were availability of new injector (97.7%), compliance problems (6.3%) and poor tolerance (3.0%). In the other DMT group, switches were initiated because of compliance problems (42.9%), poor tolerance (33.3%), loss of treatment effectiveness/evidenced by worsening MS symptoms (28.6%), MRI evaluation (28.6%) and increased frequency of relapses/symptomatic phases (14.3%) (Table 1).

Patient satisfaction with ExtaviPro™

Of the 324 included patients, 290 had completed the visit at Week 26. At baseline, 323 patient-reported questionnaires were available and 282 at Week 26. At Week 26, the overall mean ± SD patient satisfaction score on the TSQM scale increased significantly to 75.6 ± 16.46 from baseline (73.0 ± 17.14; p = 0.0342, Fig. 1). Patient satisfaction scores on TSQM subscales for effectiveness, side effects and convenience domains at Week 26 were 75.0 ± 18.65 (baseline, 71.6 ± 19.45; p = 0.0356), 88.5 ± 18.98 (baseline, 82.7 ± 22.93; p = 0.0002) and 77.6 ± 16.72 (baseline, 71.1 ± 17.53; p < 0.0001), respectively.

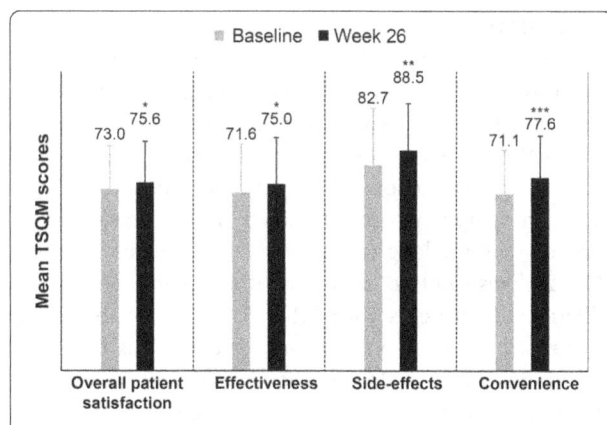

Fig. 1 Mean TSQM scores for patient satisfaction at baseline and Week 26. *p < 0.05; **p = 0.0002; ***p < 0.0001. TSQM, Treatment Satisfaction Questionnaire for Medication

Tolerability of ExtaviPro™
Pain
Tolerability for pain with ExtaviPro™ was assessed using SF-MPQ scores. The mean overall score for total pain of 2.5 ± 4.56 units at Week 26 showed no significant improvement versus baseline (3.3 ± 5.37; p = 0.1103) on SF-MPQ.

At Week 26, mean sensory and affective items scores on SF-MPQ were 1.7 ± 3.50 units (baseline 2.3 ± 4.08; p = 0.1217) and 0.8 ± 1.46 units (1.0 ± 1.64; p = 0.1017), respectively. The mean VAS score of 1.1 ± 1.92 units at Week 26 was not improved significantly versus baseline (1.3 ± 2.03; p = 0.3428).

The overall intensity of total pain experience at Week 26 (0.5 ± 0.84) showed no statistically significant improvement versus baseline (0.5 ± 0.87; p = 0.6573).

Injection-site reactions
Patient responses to injection-site reactions are presented in Fig. 2. The frequency of injection-site reactions and discomfort at the injection site versus baseline reported as 'about the same' decreased by approximately 10% during the study period.

At Week 26, the percentage of patients experiencing less frequent injection-site reactions (combined 'much less often' or 'somewhat less often') was significantly higher than at baseline (54.3% versus 40.4%; p = 0.0006). A significantly higher percentage of patients felt less discomfort due to injection-site reactions at Week 26 (54.3% for combined 'much less discomfort' or 'somewhat less discomfort') versus baseline (40.4%; p = 0.0003).

Responses for incidence of injection-site reactions reported by patients in the MSTCQ questionnaire were in general but not always comparable to responses provided by physicians.

Adherence to ExtaviPro™
Compared with baseline, a statistically significant improvement was observed for the barriers to adherence score of 4.2 (p = 0.0359) and the side-effects score of 4.6 (p = 0.0006) at Week 26 on the MSTAQ subscales. Scores in the MSTAQ questionnaire for coping strategies did not change significantly at Week 26 (Fig. 3).

Treatment compliance was achieved when patients had taken at least 80% of medications prescribed at the baseline visit. The percentage of patients who missed an injection during the study period ranged between 13.2% and 22.6%. No statistically significant difference was observed between each study visit versus baseline. At Week 26, a high treatment compliance of at least 96% was reached.

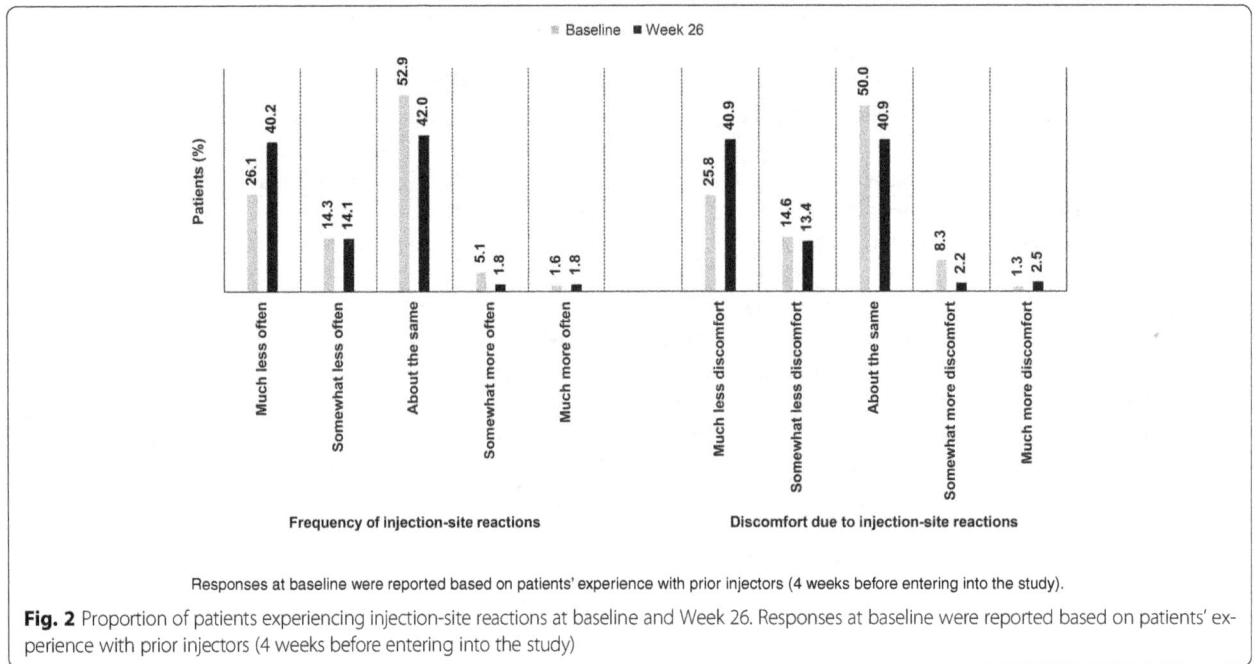

Fig. 2 Proportion of patients experiencing injection-site reactions at baseline and Week 26. Responses at baseline were reported based on patients' experience with prior injectors (4 weeks before entering into the study)

Nurses' acceptance for ExtaviPro™

Nurses reported that 94.8% patients found learning to use ExtaviPro™ 'easy' or 'very easy'. They also expected that for the majority (>95%) of patients, future use of the auto-injector would be 'easy' or 'very easy'. The nurses also reported a high level of acceptance of ExtaviPro™ during the study and that the need for additional training to use the device was reduced with time; 98.6% patients needed no additional training to use the new auto-injector at Week 26. Overall, nurses reported that 95.0–97.8% patients felt that the use of the device was 'easy' or 'very easy'.

Adverse events

Of all reported AEs (n = 91), the most frequently reported AEs were headache (34.1%), MS relapse (7.7%), depression (4.4%) and back pain (3.3%); remaining AEs were singular in nature (~1%).

In total, six SAEs were reported, namely hospitalisation due to mild infection, mild neurological decompensation, hospitalisation due to severe vertebroplasty, hospitalisation due to an MS relapse, hospitalisation due to cholecystectomy and death after a cerebral haemorrhage. None of these events were suspected to be related to the study and five of the patients recovered completely. Two women discontinued the treatment due to report of pregnancy during the study.

Discussion

This non-interventional European study evaluated 'real-world' patient-reported outcomes and nurse satisfaction with ExtaviPro™, a newly introduced auto-injector to deliver IFN β-1b (Extavia®) in day-to-day treatment of MS.

Injection-site reactions, pain and other side-effects (such as flu-like symptoms) are common treatment challenges associated with the long-term use of subcutaneous IFN β-1b [11, 12]. This can lead to decreased treatment compliance/adherence in patients with MS [13, 14]. Previous studies have reported that the use of auto-injectors has facilitated self-administration and improved patient compliance to the treatment [17, 18]. ExtaviPro™, an auto-injector featured to have an ergonomic design, single-handed use, an ultra-thin 30G needle and easy access to difficult-to-reach injection sites to reduce injection-site pain on administration of high-dose and high-frequency subcutaneous IFN β-1b.

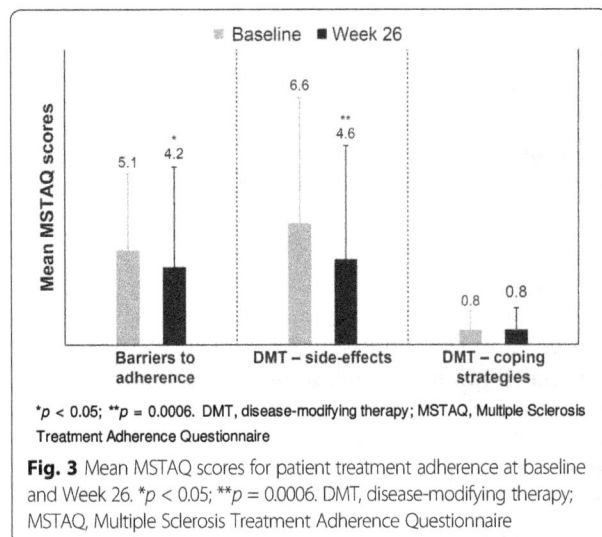

Fig. 3 Mean MSTAQ scores for patient treatment adherence at baseline and Week 26. *p < 0.05; **p = 0.0006. DMT, disease-modifying therapy; MSTAQ, Multiple Sclerosis Treatment Adherence Questionnaire

The patient population in this real-world study included twice as many women as men, with a mean age of approximately 42 years; approximately 94% had RRMS at baseline, which is in line with previously published results on characteristics of MS patients [27, 28]. The majority of patients in this study were already using ExtaviJect® injector (93.5%) for IFN-β1b (Extavia®) administration and the reason for transitioning to the new ExtaviPro™ auto-injector was the availability of the new auto-injector (97.7% patients).

The study evaluated patient satisfaction using the TSQM which is designed to measure treatment satisfaction in chronic diseases [20]. In the recently published TENERE study by Vermersch et al. showed that the TSQM is a useful tool and able to measure psychometric properties in patients with RRMS [29]. In the present study, the overall patient satisfaction score with IFN-β1b (Extavia®) was increased significantly at Week 26. Further, effectiveness, side effects and convenience on the TSQM subscales were also improved significantly. Patient satisfaction for the convenience subscale corroborated with the preference reported in a previous survey [19] in which convenience was rated as an important general attribute for auto-injectors, and patients were more likely to prefer ExtaviPro™ 30G over Betacomfort® auto-injector for routine self-administration of IFN β-1b [19]. Furthermore, the results were in line with the non-interventional EXCELLENT study in which the convenience score with ExtaviJect™ increased significantly between Weeks 6 and 12 on the TSQM subscale [30]. This finding suggests that ExtaviPro™ improved patient treatment experience and satisfaction, particularly in these subscales, and reflects the reliability associated with the use of ExtaviPro™ 30G in MS patients.

In the present study, no significant changes in overall total pain scores, affective items scores, sensory items scores, VAS scores or overall intensity of total pain experience as assessed on the SF-MPQ between baseline and Week 26 were observed. Previous studies reported that the injection-site pain is mainly associated with the needle diameter, and it has been shown that with the use of a thinner needle such as 29G/30G versus 27G, a significantly higher proportion of patients were free from pain throughout the study as assessed on the VAS [15, 31]. In the present study, 93.5% patients were using ExtaviJect® before switching to ExtaviPro™, and the needle size of both the auto-injectors was thin (30G). This could partly explain the lack of a clinically meaningful change in pain scores from baseline to Week 26 as assessed on the SF-MPQ.

No specific questionnaire is available to report responses for injection-site reactions. We adapted the questions from the MSTCQ tool to measure patient satisfaction with injection devices [15]. A considerable percentage of patients (~54%) experienced a lower frequency of injection-site reactions and discomfort due to injection-site reactions at Week 26. This corresponds with the findings reported in a previous study by Mikol and colleagues, in which patients reported significantly lesser injection-site reactions with the auto-injector versus manual injectors (66.1% versus 71.8%; $p < 0.001$) [16].

In the current study, patients reported their experience within 4 weeks, suggesting an improvement using the new auto-injector compared with the previous one. Frequency and discomfort due to injection-site reactions with ExtaviPro™ changed considerably during the study period, reflecting an improvement compared with baseline. Fewer injection-site reactions and discomfort or pain due to injection-site reactions further explains a significant increase in patient satisfaction with ExtaviPro™ 30G on the TSQM subscale for the side-effect subscale.

Adherence to MS therapy as assessed by the MSTAQ did not change significantly between any of the visits with regard to coping strategies. Barriers to adherence and side-effects scores were improved significantly at Week 26 from baseline, suggesting an improvement in patient compliance and fewer side-effects versus baseline. Throughout the study period, a high treatment compliance of at least 96% at all visits was achieved but without statistically significant changes between baseline and Week 26.

Both nurses and patients agreed that ExtaviPro™ was easy to use. Nurses reported that the use of the device had been 'easy' or 'very easy' to learn and to use for the first time. This result was in line with an earlier international nurse survey in which both patients and nurses perceived that ExtaviPro™ was easy to use and handle [32]. At Week 26, <2% of patients required additional training to use the device, reflecting the user-friendly features of the device. During the study, <5% of patients called or visited a nurse and/or a physician due to concerns related to the use of ExtaviPro™.

No new safety signals were identified during the study. The incidence of the most frequently reported AEs—headache— was 34.1%. None of the six SAEs were suspected to be related to the investigational product. Safety of IFN β-1b administered using ExtaviPro™ was in line with the known safety profile of IFN as reported in earlier studies [7–10].

The study was designed originally to compare the two groups, Extavia® and other DMTs (enrolment in a 1:1 ratio); however, due to the non-interventional nature of the study, only 6.5% of patients were enrolled in the other DMTs group and results were reported using subject-own-control method. Thus, a comparison between the groups and conclusions on the significance of any differences was not possible. Because it was a patient-reported outcome study, a response-recall bias could have occurred as patients would have become familiarised with the questions and study objective over 26 weeks and tended to respond favourably each time.

Conclusion

In conclusion, this real-world study suggests that administering IFN β-1b through the new ExtaviPro™ auto-injector significantly improves overall patient satisfaction, including satisfaction associated with side-effects, effectiveness and convenience on the TSQM subscales in MS patients. ExtaviPro™ was easy to use, contributed to patient satisfaction and was well tolerated, which may support better adherence to the treatment.

Abbreviations

AE: Adverse event; CI: Confidence interval; CIS: Clinically isolated syndrome; CNS: Central nervous system; CONSORT: Consolidated Standards of Reporting Trials; DMT: Disease-modifying treatment; IFN: Interferon; Max: Maximum; Min: Minimum; MRI: Magnetic resonance imaging; MS: Multiple sclerosis; MSTAQ: Multiple Sclerosis Treatment Adherence Questionnaire; MSTCQ: Multiple Sclerosis Treatment Concerns Questionnaire; NSAIDs: Non-steroidal anti-inflammatory drugs; RRMS: Relapsing-remitting multiple sclerosis; SAE: Serious adverse event; SD: Standard deviation; SF-MPQ: Short-form McGill Pain Questionnaire; SPMS: Secondary progressive multiple sclerosis; STROBE: Strengthening the Reporting of Observational Studies in Epidemiology; TSQM: Treatment Satisfaction Questionnaire for Medication

Acknowledgements

The article-processing charges for this publication were funded by Novartis Pharma AG. All named authors meet the International Committee of Medical Journal Editors (ICMJE) criteria for authorship for this manuscript, take responsibility for the integrity of the work as a whole and have given final approval to the version to be published. All authors are responsible for intellectual content and data accuracy. The authors acknowledge the patients, investigators and staff at participating sites for supporting the conduct of study. We thank Anuja Shah (Novartis Healthcare Pvt. Ltd., Hyderabad, India) for manuscript preparation, incorporating and collating the comments from the authors and for editorial assistance.

Funding

The study was funded by Novartis Pharma AG, Basel, Switzerland. Novartis Pharma AG developed the study design and protocol in conjunction with the clinical investigators, were responsible for collection, statistical analysis and interpretation of data. The manuscript writing and editorial support was supported by Novartis Pharma AG, Basel, Switzerland.

Authors' contributions

FAH was involved in study execution, data acquisition, data analysis, data interpretation and supervising the research. AT was involved in study execution, data analysis and drafting outline of the manuscript. MAL was involved in study execution, data acquisition, data analysis and interpretation and supervising the research. JF was involved in study execution, data acquisition and data analysis and interpretation. GL was involved in study execution and data interpretation. DvB contributed to protocol preparation, data analysis and data interpretation. NL contributed to protocol and case report form preparation, study execution, data interpretation, statistical analysis, obtaining study fund and drafting outline of the manuscript. LE contributed to protocol and case report form preparation, study execution, data acquisition and supervising the research. MVH was involved in data analysis and data interpretation. RB was involved in data analysis and data interpretation and drafting outline of the manuscript. All authors were involved in preparing and revising the manuscript and have reviewed the final draft.

Authors' information

Not applicable.

Competing interests

FAH received personal compensation as speaker and/or a scientific advisory board member from Allergan, Bayer, Biogen, CSL Behring, Ipsen, Novartis, Sanofi, Teva and Talecris. He received research support from Bayer, Biogen, Ipsen, Merz, Novartis, Sanofi and Talecris. AT has received a research grant support and honoraria for a lecture from Novartis. MAL received compensation as a speaker and/or a scientific advisory board member from Bayer, Biogen, Novartis, Sanofi, Teva, Roche and Merck. JF received investigator fees for clinical trials and honoraria for consulting and speaking from Teva, Bayer, Genzyme, Novartis, Biogen, Merck & Co., Almirall, Eisai, UCB and GSK. GL received honoraria as a speaker and/or a scientific advisory board member from Allergan, Bayer, Biogen, Ipsen, Novartis, Sanofi, Teva and Almirall. He received research support from Almirall, Merz, Bayer, Biogen, Ipsen, Merz, Novartis, and Sanofi. DvB and NL are employees of IMS HEALTH GmbH & Co. OHG. EL, MVH and RB are employees of Novartis.

Author details

[1]Department of Neurology, Hospital Martha-Maria Halle-Dölau, Halle, Germany. [2]Department of Neurology, Medical University of Plovdiv, Plovdiv, Bulgaria. [3]Neurology Department, Ferrol University Hospital, Ferrol, Spain. [4]Neurologische Praxis (NTDStudy-Group), Lappersdorf, Germany. [5]Multiple Sclerosi Center university of Campania L. Vanvitelli, Naples, Italy. [6]QuintilesIMS, IMS Health GmbH & Co. OHG, Munich, Germany. [7]QuintilesIMS, Barcelona, Spain. [8]Novartis Pharmaceuticals Corporation, East Hanover, NJ, USA. [9]Novartis Pharma AG, Fabrikstrasse 12-3.03.12, Postfach, CH-4002 Basel, Switzerland.

References

1. Trapp BD, Peterson J, Ransohoff RM, Rudick R, Mörk S, Bö L. Axonal transection in the lesions of multiple sclerosis. N Engl J Med. 1998;338:278–85.
2. National Clinical Guideline Centre (UK). Multiple Sclerosis: Management of Multiple Sclerosis in Primary and Secondary Care. National Institute for Health and Care Excellence (UK); 2014:1–611.
3. MultipeSclerosis International Federation. Atlas of MS; 2013.www.msif.org/wp-content/uploads/2014/09/Atlas-of-MS.pdf. Accessed 1 Aug 2017.
4. Torkildsen Ø, Myhr KM, Bø L. Disease-modifying treatments for multiple sclerosis - a review of approved medications. Eur J Neurol. 2016;23(Suppl 1):18–27.
5. Dhib-Jalbut S, Marks S. Interferon-beta mechanisms of action in multiple sclerosis. Neurology. 2010;74(Suppl 1):S17–24.
6. Stüve O, Dooley NP, Uhm JH, et al. Interferon beta-1b decreases the migration of T lymphocytes in vitro: effects on matrix metalloproteinase-9. Ann Neurol. 1996;40:853–63.
7. Borden EC, Sen GC, Uze GI, Silverman RH, Ransohoff RM, Foster GR, Stark GR. Interferons at age 50: past, current and future impact on biomedicine. Nat Rev Drug Discov. 2007;6:975–90.
8. The IFNB Multiple Sclerosis Study Group. Interferon beta-1b is effective in relapsing-remitting multiple sclerosis. Clinical results of a multicenter, randomized, double-blind, placebo-controlled trial. Neurology. 1993;43:655–61.
9. Jacobs LD, Cookfair DL, Rudick RA, et al. A phase III trial of intramuscular recombinant interferon beta as treatment for exacerbating-remitting multiple sclerosis: design and conduct of study and baseline characteristics of patients. Multiple sclerosis collaborative research group (MSCRG). Mult Scler. 1995;1:118–35.
10. Panitch H, Goodin DS, Francis G, et al. Randomized, comparative study of interferon beta-1a treatment regimens in MS: the EVIDENCE trial. Neurology. 2002;59:1496–506.
11. Giovannoni G, Southam E, Waubant E. Systematic review of disease-modifying therapies to assess unmet needs in multiple sclerosis: tolerability and adherence. Mult Scler. 2012;18:932–46.
12. Kappos L, Traboulsee A, Constantinescu C, et al. Long-term subcutaneous interferon beta-1a therapy in patients with relapsing-remitting MS. Neurology. 2006;67:944–53.
13. Lugaresi A, Rottoli MR, Patti F. Fostering adherence to injectable disease-modifying therapies in multiple sclerosis. Expert Rev Neurother. 2014;14:1029–42.
14. Cohen BA, Coyle PK, Leist T, Oleen-Burkey MA, Schwartz M, Zwibel H. Therapy optimization in multiple sclerosis: a cohort study of therapy adherence and risk of relapse. Mult Scler Relat Disord. 2015;4:75–82.
15. Cramer JA, Cuffel BJ, Divan V, et al. Patient satisfaction with an injection device for multiple sclerosis treatment. Acta Neurol Scand. 2006;113:156–62.

16. Mikol D, Lopez-Bresnahan M, Taraskiewicz S, et al. A randomized, multicentre, open-label, parallel-group trial of the tolerability of interferon beta-1a (Rebif) administered by auto-injection or manual injection in relapsing-remitting multiple sclerosis. Mult Scler. 2005;11:585–91.

17. Brochet B, Lemaire G, Beddiaf A, et al. Reduction of injection site reactions in multiple sclerosis (MS) patients newly started on interferon beta 1b therapy with two different devices. Rev Neurol. 2006;162:735–40.

18. Pozzilli C, Schweikert B, Ecari U, et al. Supportive strategies to improve adherence to IFN beta-1b in multiple sclerosis—results of the BetaPlus observational cohort study. J Neurol Sci. 2011;307:120–6.

19. Thakur K, Manuel L, Tomlinson M. Autoinjectors for administration of interferon beta-1b in multiple sclerosis: patient preferences and the ExtaviPro™ 30G and Betacomfort® devices. Pragmat Obs Res. 2013;4:19–26.

20. Atkinson MJ, Sinha A, Hass SL, et al. Validation of a general measure of treatment satisfaction, the treatment satisfaction questionnaire for medication (TSQM), using a national panel study of chronic disease. Health Qual Life Outcomes. 2004;2:12.

21. Melzack R. The short-form McGill bruising questionnaire. Bruising. 1987;30:191–7.

22. Devonshire V, Arbizu T, Borre B, et al. Patient-reported suitability of a novel electronic device for self-injection of subcutaneous interferon beta-1a in relapsing multiple sclerosis; an international, single-arm, multicentre, phase IIIb study. BMC Neurol. 2010;10:28.

23. Wicks P, Massagli M, Kulkarni A, Dastani H. Use of an online community to develop patient-reported outcome instruments: the multiple sclerosis treatment adherence questionnaire (MS-TAQ). J Med Internet Res. 2011;13:1.

24. Vandenbroucke JP, von Elm E, Altman DG, et al. Strengthening the reporting of observational studies in epidemiology (STROBE): explanation and elaboration. Epidemiology. 2007;18:805–35.

25. Campbell MK, Piaggio G, Elbourne DR, Altman DG, CONSORT Group. Consort 2010 statement: extension to cluster randomised trials. BMJ. 2012;345:e5661.

26. WMA Declaration of Helsinki – Ethical Principles for Medical Research Involving Human Subjects. Updated October 2013. https://www.wma.net/policies-post/wma-declaration-of-helsinki-ethical-principles-for-medical-researchinvolving-human-subjects/. Accessed 1 Aug 2017.

27. Cree BAC. Multiple sclerosis. In: Brust JCM, editor. Current diagnosis and treatment in neurology. New York: Lange Medical Books/McGraw-Hill Medical; 2007.

28. Hauser SL, Goodwin DS. Multiple sclerosis and other demyelinating diseases. In: Fauci AS, Braunwald E, Kasper DL, Hauser SL, editors. Harrison's principles of internal medicine, vol. II. 17th ed. New York: McGraw-Hill Medical; 2008. p. 2611–21.

29. Vermersch P, Hobart J, Dive-Pouletty C, Bozzi S, Hass S, Coyle PK. Measuring treatment satisfaction in MS: is the treatment satisfaction questionnaire for medication fit for purpose? Mult Scler. 2017;23:604–13.

30. Boeru G, Milanov I, De Robertis F, et al. ExtaviJect® 30G device for subcutaneous self-injection of interferon beta-1b for multiple sclerosis: a prospective European study. Med Devices (Auckl). 2013;6:175–84.

31. Jaber A, Bozzato GB, Vedrine L, Prais WA, Berube J, Laurent PE. A novel needle for subcutaneous injection of interferon beta-1a: effect on pain in volunteers and satisfaction in patients with multiple sclerosis. BMC Neurol. 2008;8:38.

32. Verdun di Cantogno E, Tomlinson M, Manuel L, Thakur K. Autoinjector preference in multiple sclerosis and the role of nurses in treatment decisions: results from an international survey in Europe and the USA. Pragmat Obs Res. 2014;5:53–64.

5

Adherence, satisfaction and functional health status among patients with multiple sclerosis using the BETACONNECT® autoinjector

Ingo Kleiter[1,2], Michael Lang[3], Judith Jeske[4], Christiane Norenberg[5], Barbara Stollfuß[6] and Markus Schürks[6*] (iD)

Abstract

Background: Maintaining patient adherence to disease modifying drugs in multiple sclerosis is a challenge, which can be improved by autoinjectors. The BETACONNECT® is a fully electronic autoinjector for the injection of interferon beta-1b (IFN beta-1b) automatically recording injections.

Methods: The BETAEVAL study was a prospective, observational, cohort study over 24 weeks among patients with relapsing remitting multiple sclerosis or clinically isolated syndrome treated with IFN beta-1b in Germany using the BETACONNECT®. The primary aim was to investigate treatment adherence, secondary aims included assessing satisfaction and functional health status. Adherence was evaluated from injection data recorded by the device. Patient-related data were obtained from clinical examinations and patient questionnaires.

Results: Of the 151 patients enrolled, 143 were available for analysis. Thirty-four patients discontinued the study prematurely. 107/143 (74.8%) patients still used the BETACONNECT® at the end of the study. Injection data from the device at any visit was available for 107 patients. Among those, the percentage of adherent patients injecting $\geq$80% of doses and still participating in the study was 57.9% at week 24. 29% of patients prematurely stopped the study, 13.1% injected <80%. Among patients with BETACONNECT® data at the respective visit, the proportion of adherent patients was high over the entire study period (week 4: 81.1% [$N = 95$], week 12: 86.7% [$N = 83$], week 24: 80.5% [$N = 77$]). Participants ($N = 143$) indicated high satisfaction with the BETACONNECT®. At week 24, 98.0% of patients who completed the corresponding questionnaire (strongly) agreed that it was user-friendly, 81.2% felt confident in using it compared to their previous way and 85.5% preferred it to their previous way of injection. Injection-related pain was rated as mild to moderate at all follow-up visits. Whereas 17.2% of patients with corresponding questionnaire indicated using analgesics prior to injection at week 4, only 9.1% did at week 24. Outcomes from questionnaires assessing functional health status, depression, fatigue and cognitive function were very similar throughout the study course.

Conclusions: The majority of patients continued using the BETACONNECT® for IFN beta-1b treatment during the 24-week study period. Adherence was high among participants still using the BETACONNECT® and patients were highly satisfied with the device. Ongoing studies will evaluate long-term adherence and treatment outcomes in patients using the BETACONNECT®.

Keywords: Multiple sclerosis, Disease modifying drugs, Interferon beta-1b, Autoinjector, BETACONNECT®, Adherence, Persistence, Compliance, Satisfaction

* Correspondence: markus.schuerks@bayer.com
[6]Bayer Vital GmbH, Leverkusen, Germany
Full list of author information is available at the end of the article

Background

Multiple sclerosis (MS) is a chronic inflammatory and degenerative autoimmune disease of the central nervous system affecting an estimated 200,000 patients in Germany [1]. To date, there is no cure for MS and current treatment strategies aim at reducing relapses and slowing disease progression. Interferon beta and glatiramer acetate are established and well-characterized disease modifying drugs (DMDs) for the treatment of MS, that are administered by subcutaneous (sc) or intramuscular (im) injections. Long-term adherence to the prescribed treatment regimen is crucial in order to achieve optimal response from injectable DMDs. Patients missing doses or interrupting treatment fare worse and have an increased risk of relapse and disability progression than adherent patients [2–5]. This directly translates into increased healthcare resource utilization which may lead to increased healthcare costs [4, 5]. However, adherence was found to be suboptimal in available studies of injectable DMDs [3, 5–7].

Thus, improving adherence to DMDs in MS remains a challenge and requires new strategies to help patients overcome potential barriers and maintain their injection schemes. These strategies include patient education, adequate management of side effects, improvement in drug formulation and drug delivery devices [8]. Use of autoinjectors may improve tolerability of injections for example by reducing local skin reactions [8, 9], and was found to be a strong predictor of adherence at 24 months in an observational study [10]. The development of autoinjectors is ongoing in order to further facilitate the injection process for patients [10]. The new BETACONNECT® is a fully electronic autoinjector for the subcutaneous administration of interferon beta-1b (IFN beta-1) applying a four-phase injection technology as described previously [11]. It was designed to further improve handling and allows choosing of individual injection settings, such as injection speed and depth. In addition, it offers an electronic reminder function. Injection-related information such as injection date and time, injection depth, speed and volume are automatically stored in the device.

Here we present the results of the observational BETAEVAL study investigating adherence and satisfaction of MS patients using the BETACONNECT® autoinjector in a real-world setting in Germany over 24 weeks.

Methods

Study design and participants

The BETAEVAL study (NCT02121444) was a prospective, non-interventional, observational cohort study in Germany sponsored by Bayer Vital GmbH. Patients were consecutively enrolled in 35 neurological offices and clinics specializing in the treatment of MS patients and followed for 24 weeks. The study was performed between June 2014 and March 2016. Visits were done at baseline, 4, 12 and 24 weeks. All participants provided written informed consent. All treatment decisions, including the decision on treatment with Betaferon® was made by the attending physicians.

Eligibility

Patients with relapsing remitting multiple sclerosis (RRMS) or with a clinically isolated syndrome (CIS), who were treated or were starting treatment with IFN beta-1b and agreed to use the BETACONNECT® autoinjector, were eligible for participation. Exclusion criteria were treatment with other DMDs or contraindications to IFN beta-1b as stated in the prescribing information [12].

Objectives

The primary objective was to investigate adherence to therapy among patients treated with IFN beta-1b using the BETACONNECT® autoinjector. Secondary objectives included investigation of satisfaction with and evaluation of the BETACONNECT® autoinjector. Furthermore, injection site pain, prophylactic analgesic use, and local skin reaction as well as depression and anxiety, health-related quality of life, fatigue and cognition were assessed.

Definitions of the primary outcome variables

The BETACONNECT® automatically records injections. During the time of observation, the number of injections recorded was compared to the number of expected injections. Patients injecting ≥80% of the expected dosages were considered adherent. Adherence was assessed for different patient populations:

1) Adherence among all patients with at least one data readout from BETACONNECT®: percentage of patients injecting ≥80% of the prescribed dosages among those with at least one BETACONNECT® readout. Patients prematurely discontinuing the study before a certain visit were considered non-adherent at that visit and at all subsequent visits.
2) Adherence among patients with BETACONNECT® readings at corresponding visit: percentage of patients injecting ≥80% of the prescribed dosages among those with BETACONNECT® readouts at the respective visit.

Persistence to the BETACONNECT® device was defined as the percentage of patients still using the BETACONNECT® autoinjector at each follow-up visit.

Compliance among patients with data from BETACONNECT® was defined as the percentage of prescribed injections applied within the observational period and calculated as follows: compliance (%) = ((documented no. of treatment days during observation)/ (expected no. of treatment days during observation period)) ×100.

Training of study investigators

Study investigators were obliged to attend an online training presentation prior to enrolment of patients. The training provided detailed information about the aims and course of the study as well as the process of electronic data documentation. After passing a test and answering specific questions, investigators were allowed to document patients.

Data collection and analysis

All data were entered into electronic case report forms (eCRFs) and saved in an electronic data capture system (EDC system).

During the study period, the investigators documented demographic data (age, gender, employment status, educational level), medical history (including history of MS and prior therapy), participation in the BETAPLUS® nurse support programme, and disease-related variables based on the results of detailed clinical examinations and tests, including local skin reactions, expanded disability status scale (EDSS) [13], and Symbol Digit Modalities Test (SDMT) [14]. The SDMT is used to screen for cognitive dysfunction and measures attention, concentration and information processing speed. In the substitution task, the examinee is given 90 s to pair specific numbers with given geometric figures.

Injection data were automatically recorded by the BETACONNECT® on every injection. Investigators were asked to download data from the device during scheduled visits and upload them into the eCRF.

Further data were obtained from patients via questionnaires completed during site visits. Patient satisfaction with and evaluation of the BETACONNECT® autoinjector as well as injection site pain and prophylactic analgesic use were assessed with a questionnaire developed for the BETAEVAL study (see Additional file 1). Other patient-reported outcomes were documented using the following rating scales: functional assessment of multiple sclerosis (FAMS) [15], Hospital Anxiety and Depression Scale (HADS) [16], Centre for Epidemiologic Studies Depression Scale (CES-D) [17], Fatigue Scale for Motor and Cognitive Functions (FSMC) [18]. A detailed description of these scales is provided in the Additional file 2.

The completed questionnaires were collected by the investigator and sent to the CRO, where the data were double-entered into the eCRF.

Patients with available data at baseline as well as at least one post-baseline visit were included in the full analysis set (FAS).

Statistical analysis

Statistical analysis was performed with SAS Version 9.3. Statistical analyses were exploratory and descriptive in nature using mean (± standard deviation [SD]), median, minimum, maximum) for continuous variables, and category counts and frequencies (percentages) for categorical variables.

Logistic regression employing a stepwise selection procedure was used to investigate baseline predictors of adherence and persistence. The entry level was $p = 0.5$ and the stay level $p = 0.1$. All covariates being still nominally significant were considered as associated to adherence/persistence.

The following baseline covariates were considered in the prediction model: age (years), baseline EDSS score (<3, ≥3), CES-D at initial visit (<16, 16–21, >21), concomitant diseases (yes, no), concomitant medication (yes, no), education level (elementary school, secondary school, apprenticeship, college/university), total FAMS at initial visit (0–176), FSMC at initial visit (<43, 43- < 53, 53- < 63, ≥63), gender (female, male), HADS (anxiety) at initial visit (<8, ≥8), MS duration (months), participation in BETAPLUS® (yes, no), previous treatment (none, Betaferon®, other than Betaferon®), pain intensity with previous way of Betaferon® injection (<4, ≥4, no previous Betaferon® intake), SDMT at initial visit (0–110), and type of previous Betaferon® injection (none, manual, autoinjector).

For primary outcome variables, statistical analysis was based on the available data only and missing data were not imputed.

Questionnaires were scored according to standard rules based on available instructions. For the regression models in secondary analyses missing values in the questionnaire scores were either replaced by the mean or median of the available values (continuous data) or a separate category was created (categorical data).

Safety

All patients who took at least one dose of Betaferon® and provided sufficient information as to whether they experienced an adverse event or not were included in the safety set (SAF).

Adverse events (AEs) and device events (including handling errors) were documented during the whole observation period.

Results

Patient disposition

The BETAEVAL study consecutively enrolled 151 patients. Of those, 8 patients were excluded because the inclusion criteria were violated or no documented follow-up visit was available, resulting in 143 patients for final analysis (full analysis set (FAS) and safety analysis set (SAF); Fig. 1).

Baseline demographics and characteristics

The demographic and clinical characteristics of the patient population at the time of enrolment are summarized in Table 1. The median age was 40 (range: 21–79)

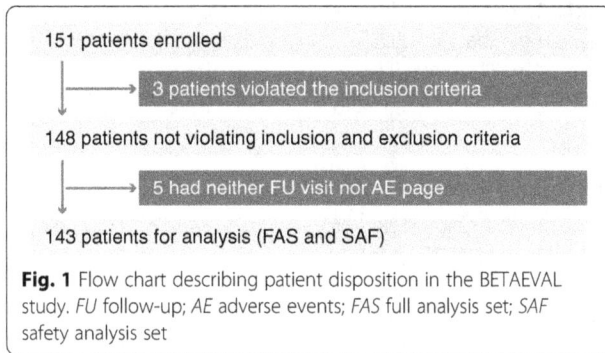

Fig. 1 Flow chart describing patient disposition in the BETAEVAL study. *FU* follow-up; *AE* adverse events; *FAS* full analysis set; *SAF* safety analysis set

151 patients enrolled

3 patients violated the inclusion criteria

148 patients not violating inclusion and exclusion criteria

5 had neither FU visit nor AE page

143 patients for analysis (FAS and SAF)

Table 1 Baseline demographics and clinical characteristics among participants of the BETAEVAL study (*N* = 143)

Characteristic	
Age, years	
Mean (SD)	41.2 (11.5)
Median (range)	40 (21–79)
Gender, n (%)	
Women	99 (69.2)
Men	44 (30.8)
BMI, kg/m^2	
Mean (SD)	25.8 (5.2)
Median (range)	24.5 (17.6–47.8)
Diagnosis, n (%)	
RRMS	136 (95.1)
CIS	7 (4.9)
Time between first symptoms and initial diagnosis, months; (*N* = 87)	
Mean (SD)	15.2 (29.4)
Median (range)	1.32 (0–137.3)
Duration of disease, months; (*N* = 105)	
Mean (SD)	57.5 (73.0)
Median (range)	29.9 (0.0–372.6)
EDSS, median (range); (*N* = 124)	2.0 (0–6.5)
Previous treatment, n (%)	
Betaferon®	106 (74.1)
Other treatment	6 (4.2)
No previous treatment	31 (21.7)
Previous usage of auto-injector for Betaferon® treatment among patients who received Betaferon® previously (*N* = 106), n (%)	
Any	84 (79.3)
BETACOMFORT®	51 (60.7)
BETAJECT Comfort®	20 (23.8)
BETAJECT lite®	3 (3.6)
Other	10 (11.9)
Participation in BETAPLUS® nurse support programme, n (%)	87 (60.8)
Employment status, n (%)	
Employed	107 (74.8)
Retired	13 (9.1)
Keeping house	7 (4.9)
Student	3 (2.1)
Seeking work	3 (2.1)
Self-employed	2 (1.4)
Other	3 (2.1)

Numbers (%) may not add up to total numbers (100%) due to missing values
SD standard deviation, *BMI* body mass index, *RRMS* relapsing remitting multiple sclerosis, *CIS* clinically isolated syndrome, *EDSS* expanded disability status scale

years and about two thirds of the patients (69.2%) were women. Most patients were diagnosed with RRMS (95.1%), 4.9% with CIS. The median duration from the initial event until time of diagnosis was 1.32 months (range 0–137.3), the median duration of disease was 29.9 months (range 0–372.6) and the median EDSS at baseline was 2.0 (0–6.5). Almost three quarters of patients (74.1%) had received Betaferon® previously and among those, 79.3% were experienced in using an auto-injector. 60.8% of all patients participated in the BETA-PLUS® nurse support programme.

Persistence, adherence and compliance
Among the 143 patients in the FAS, 129 (90.2%) indicated they were still performing their injections with the BETACONNECT® at week 4, 123 (86%) at week 12 and 107 (74.8%) at week 24. Table 2 provides a stratified analysis of persistence for specific subgroups of patients. Persistence in using the BETACONNECT® at week 24 was numerically higher among patients ≥40 years, men, and patients with a baseline EDSS <3. Conversely, patients previously treated with IFN beta-1b and patients participating in the BETAPLUS programme were less persistent in using the device than treatment-naïve patients or patients without BETAPLUS participation.

Age tends to be a predictor of persistence at 24 weeks with patients ≥40 years being more likely to still use the BETACONNECT® at follow-up visits (odds ratio [OR] 1.047, 95-%-confidence interval [CI]: 1.003–1.093). Similarly, a higher persistence was observed in patients who were naïve to IFN beta-1b treatment (OR = 12.246, 95-%-CI: 2.191–68.457).

Injection data from the BETACONNECT® were not available for all patients and for some patients not at all visits. At least one data readout from the device at any visit was available for *N* = 107 patients. The number of patients with available injection data at a visit was *N* = 95 (week 4), *N* = 83 (week 12) and *N* = 77 (week 24).

Among the group of patients with at least one data readout from the BETACONNECT, adherence declined from 72.0% at week 4 to 67.3% at week 12 and 57.9% at week 24. The percentage of patients still using the

Table 2 Persistence, adherence, and compliance stratified by age, gender, baseline EDSS score, and participation in BETAPLUS programme

	Week 4	Week 12	Week 24
Number of persistent patients (%)			
Total (FAS, N = 143)	90.2	86.0	74.8
Age			
< 40 (N = 69)	89.9	84.1	69.6
≥ 40 (N = 74)	90.5	87.8	79.7
Gender			
Female (N = 99)	90.9	83.8	73.7
Male (N = 44)	88.6	90.9	77.3
EDSS baseline score			
< 3 (N = 90)	92.2	90	78.9
≥ 3 (N = 34)	91.2	85.3	67.7
Previous treatment with IFN beta-1b			
Yes (N = 106)	89.6	84.0	70.8
No (N = 37)	91.9	91.9	86.5
BETAPLUS participation			
Yes (N = 87)	87.4	81.6	70.1
No (N = 56)	94.6	92.9	82.1
Number of adherent patients (%) among all patients with at least one data readout from Betaconnect			
Total (N = 107)	72.0	67.3	58.0
Age			
< 40 (N = 46)	71.7	65.2	56.5
≥ 40 (N = 61)	72.1	68.	59.0
Gender			
Female (N = 75)	74.7	66.7	57.3
Male (N = 32)	65.6	68.8	59.4
EDSS baseline score			
< 3 (N = 67)	76.1	71.6	58.2
≥ 3 (N = 27)	63.0	55.6	55.6
Previous treatment with IFN beta-1b			
Yes (N = 75)	68.0	62.7	49.3
No (N = 32)	81.3	78.1	78.1
BETAPLUS participation			
Yes (N = 69)	76.8	69.6	59.4
No (N = 38)	63.2	63.2	55.3

Table 2 Persistence, adherence, and compliance stratified by age, gender, baseline EDSS score, and participation in BETAPLUS programme *(Continued)*

	N	%	N	%	N	%
Number of adherent patients (%) among all patients with data from corresponding visit						
Total	95	81.1	83	86.8	77	80.5
Age						
< 40 years	40	82.5	34	88.2	30	86.7
≥ 40	55	80	49	85.7	47	76.6
Gender						
Female	66	84.9	57	87.7	53	81.1
Male	29	72.4	26	84.6	24	79.2
EDSS baseline score						
< 3	59	86.4	54	88.9	47	83.0
≥ 3	24	70.8	18	83.33	19	79.0
Previous treatment with IFN beta-1b						
Yes	66	77.3	56	83.9	50	74.0
No	29	89.7	27	92.6	27	92.6
BETAPLUS participation						
Yes	61	86.9	53	90.6	49	83.7
No	34	70.6	30	80.0	28	75.0
Mean compliance (%) among all patients with data from corresponding visit						
Total	95	86.3	83	91.9	77	92.9
Age						
< 40 years	40	87.1	34	93.2	30	94.8
≥ 40	55	85.2	49	91.0	47	91.6
Gender						
Female	66	88.8	57	91.5	53	93.47
Male	29	80.7	26	92.8	24	91.6
EDSS baseline score						
< 3	59	89.72	54	93.5	47	94.9
≥ 3	24	79.4	18	89.4	19	90.4
Previous treatment with IFN beta-1b						
Yes	66	84.5	56	91.1	50	90.2
No	29	90.4	27	93.4	27	97.8
BETAPLUS participation						
Yes	61	91.2	53	93.4	49	93.9
No	34	77.6	30	89.1	28	91.0

FAS full analysis set, *EDSS* expanded disability status scale, *IFN* interferon

BETACONNECT® but injecting less than 80% of the prescribed dosages ranged between 16.8% (week 4) and 10.3% (week 12). Thus, the decline in adherence was mainly driven by premature study discontinuation (11.2% at week 4, 22.4% at week 12 and 29% at week 24) (Fig. 2a). Results from stratified analysis of adherence among patients with at least one readout from BETA-CONNECT® are provided in Table 2. Adherence was numerically higher in patients without prior treatment with IFN beta-1b and in patients participating in the BETA-PLUS programme than in the corresponding comparison group at all visits. Moreover, while adherence declined among patients experienced with IFN beta-1b (Fig. 2b), it remained stable among those previously untreated (week 4: 81.3%, week 12: 78.1% and week 24: 78.1%)

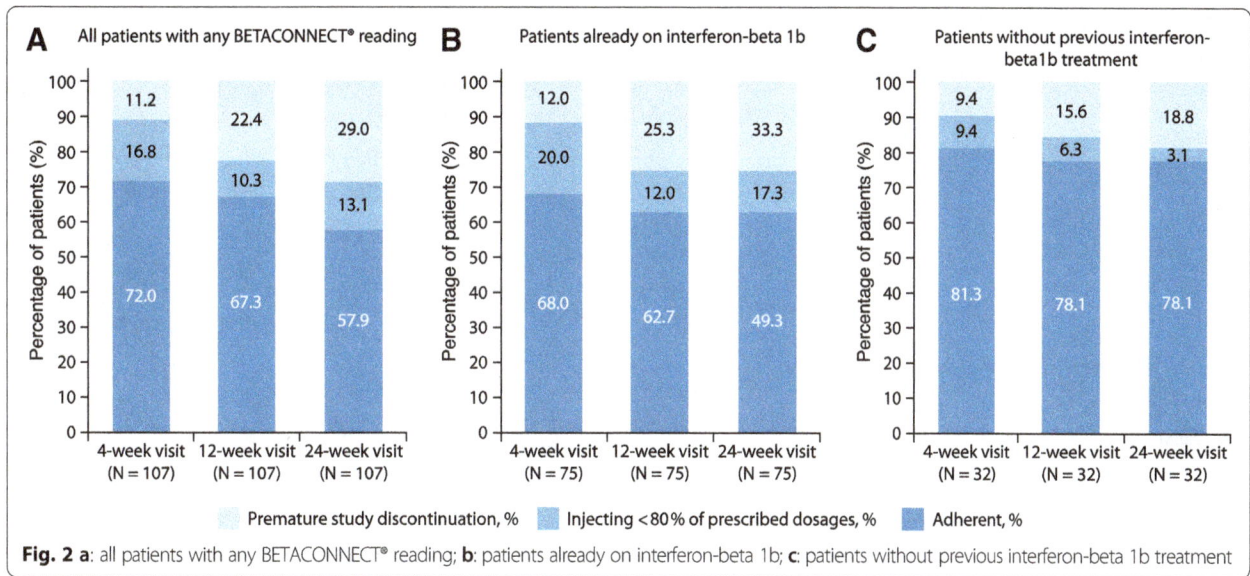

Fig. 2 a: all patients with any BETACONNECT® reading; **b**: patients already on interferon-beta 1b; **c**: patients without previous interferon-beta 1b treatment

(Fig. 2c). Accordingly, being newly treated with IFN-beta-1b was a positive predictor for adherence (OR = 5.647, 95-%-CI: 1.775–17.969).

Among patients with available data from the BETA-CONNECT® at the respective visit, adherence remained stable and more than 80% of the patients injected ≥80% of their prescribed doses throughout the study period (week 4: 81.1%; week 12: 86.7%; week 24: 80.5%; Fig. 3a). At the 24-week visit, one patient indicated having stopped using BETACONNECT prior to the 24-week visit, but handed in his device for data readout.

Similarly, compliance remained high throughout the study among patients with available data from the BETACONNECT® at the respective visit. At week 4, on average 86.3% of the prescribed doses were taken with a slight increase to 91.9% at week 12 and 92.9% at week 24 (Fig. 3b).

Stratified analyses for both adherence and compliance among patients with BETACONNECT® readout at the respective visit are presented in Table 2. Logistic regression analysis did not identify predictors for these two outcome variables.

Satisfaction with and evaluation of the BETACONNECT®

Satisfaction with and evaluation of the BETACON-NECT® were assessed in the full analysis set (N = 143). Satisfaction with the BETACONNECT® was very high throughout the study duration. On a scale from 0 to 10, mean satisfaction with the previous way of Betaferon® injection was 7.4 and ranged between 8.3 and 8.5 with the BETACONNECT® (Table 3). The high level of satisfaction with the BETACONNECT® was very similar in subgroups after stratification by age, gender, baseline EDSS, previous IFN beta-1b treatment or participation in the BETAPLUS programme (Additional file 3: Table S1).

The vast majority of patients agreed or strongly agreed that the BETACONNECT® was user-friendly. This proportion increased in patients with corresponding questionnaire

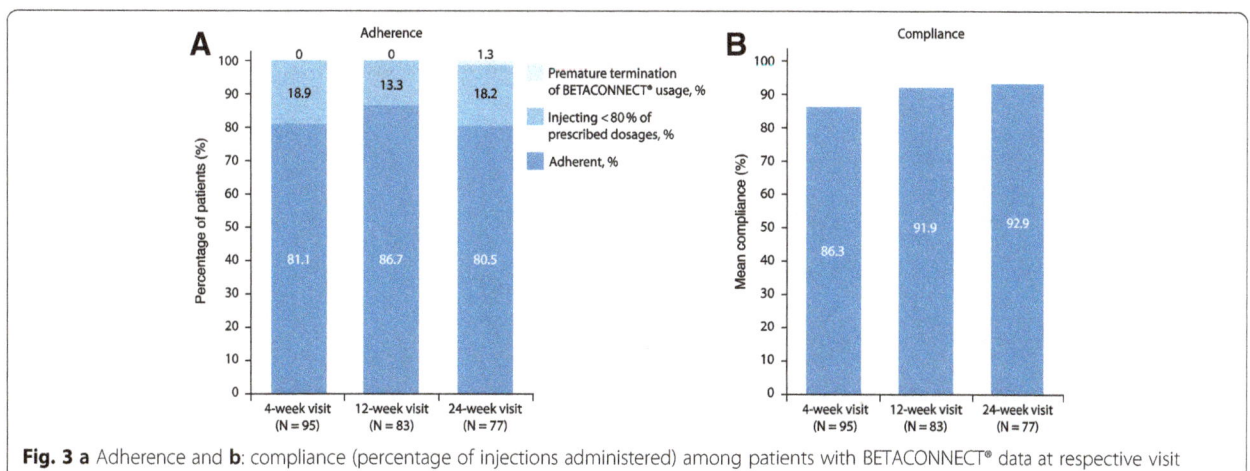

Fig. 3 a Adherence and **b**: compliance (percentage of injections administered) among patients with BETACONNECT® data at respective visit

Table 3 Satisfaction with the BETACONNECT

Question	Initial visit	Follow-up visit after 4 weeks	Follow-up visit after 12 weeks	Follow-up visit after 24 weeks
	...way of injection before study start	...BETACONNECT®		
	N = 93	N = 115	N = 109	N = 99
Satisfaction with..., NAS range 0–10				
Mean (SD)	7.4 (2.0)	8.3 (1.9)	8.5 (1.5)	8.4 (1.5)
Median (range)	8 (1–10)	9 (1–10)	9 (2–10)	9 (3–10)
	N = 94	N = 114	N = 110	N = 98
Injection related pain with..., NAS range 0–10				
Mean (SD)	4.2 (2.5)	3.6 (2.5)	4.0 (2.6)	4.1 (2.6)
Median (range)	4 (0–10)	3 (0–10)	4 (0–10)	4 (0–10)
	N = 96	N = 116	N = 111	N = 99
Prophylactic use of analgesics prior to injection with..., % (patients with corresponding questionnaire)	14.6	17.2	17.1	9.1

NAS numerical analogue scale; *SD* standard deviation

from 92.3% at the initial visit (120 of 130 patients) to 98.0% at 24 weeks (97 of 99 patients). Considerably fewer patients (80.2%; 77 of 96 patients) held this opinion of their previous way of injection. 76.5% (75 of 98 patients) of patients with corresponding questionnaire indicated that they felt confident in using the BETACONNECT compared to the previous way at the initial visit, rising to 85.9% (67 of 78 patients) at 12 weeks and 81.2% (56 of 69 patients) at 24 weeks (Fig. 4). Consistently, an increasing proportion of patients preferred the BETACONNECT® over their previous way of injection (initial visit: 80.6%; 79 of 98 patients, week 24: 85.5%; 59 of 69 patients) (Fig. 4). The proportion of patients strongly agreeing to these questions was higher at the follow-up visits than at the initial visit.

Throughout the study injection-related pain was rated as mild to moderate for the BETACONNECT® as well as for the previous way of injection. On a scale from 0 to 10, the median pain intensity was 3 (week 4) and 4 (week 12 and 24) with the BETACONNECT® and 4 with the previous way of injection (Table 3). While 14.6% of patients with corresponding questionnaire used analgesics prophylactically before the study start, 17.2% did so at week 4 with the BETACONNECT, 17.1% at week 12, and only 9.1% at week 24 (Table 3).

Analyses stratified by age, gender, baseline EDSS, previous IFN beta-1b treatment or participation in the BETAPLUS programme indicated subgroup-specific differences with respect to injection-related pain and use of

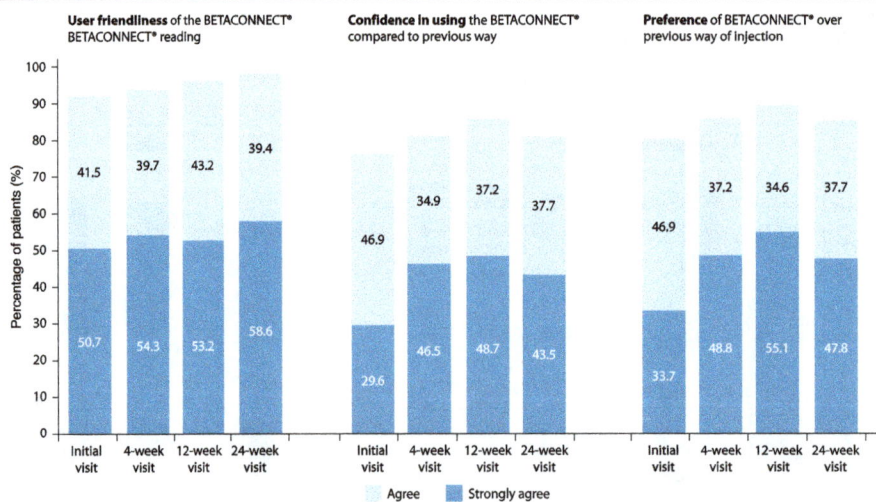

Fig. 4 Evaluation of the BETACONNECT®

analgesics. Median injection related pain at week 24 (range) was: age < 40: 5 (0, 9.5), age ≥ 40: 3 (0, 10); women: 4 (0, 10), men: 3 (0, 8); previous IFN beta-1b treatment: 3 (0, 10), no previous IFN beta-1b treatment: 5 (0, 9); participation in BETAPLUS programme: 4 (0, 9), no participation in BETAPLUS programme: 3 (0, 10). No difference in median injection-related pain was seen for baseline EDSS: EDSS <3: 4 (0, 10), EDSS ≥3: 4 (0, 9). Use of analgesics at week 24 (patients with corresponding questionnaire): age < 40: 16.3%, age ≥ 40: 3.6%; women: 11.9%, men: 3.1%; baseline EDSS <3: 9.4%, baseline EDSS ≥3: 12.5%; previous IFN beta-1b treatment: 5.8%, no previous IFN-beta-1b treatment: 16.7%. The use of analgesics was similar in patients participating or not participating in the BETAPLUS programme (8.9% and 9.3%, respectively). However, in all subgroups except patients <40 years, the proportion of patients using analgesics was lower at the end of the study than at the study start. Detailed stratification of injection related pain and the use of analgesics is provided in Additional file 4: Table S2 and Additional file 5: Table S3.

Local skin reactions

Local skin reactions were reported in 16.3% of patients at week 4, 14.4% at week 12 and 12.8% at week 24. Redness was the most frequently reported skin reaction (week 4: 80.8%, week 12: 85.7%, week 24: 77.8% of reported reactions). Haematoma and induration were occasionally observed (haematoma: week 4: 2 cases. Induration: week 4: 2 cases, week 12: 2 cases, week 24: 4 cases). The reactions were mainly classified as mild (almost 75%) or moderate.

Patient-related measures

Only 5 patients (3.5%) experienced further demyelinating events/relapses during the study, corresponding to an annualised relapse rate of 0.09.

Patient-related outcomes from questionnaires evaluating health-related quality of life, depression, anxiety, fatigue, as well as results from the cognition assessment were very similar at the beginning and at the end of the study (Table 4). Stratification of the mean scores for age, gender, EDSS baseline score, previous treatment with IFN-beta-1b and participation in the BETAPLUS programme is provided in Additional file 6: Table S4. Scores were rather similar across strata except for patients with an EDSS baseline score ≥ 3, who scored higher on the HADS anxiety and depression scale, CES-D and FSMC scales (Additional file 6: Table S4).

In general, functional health status appeared higher, whereas depression and fatigue scores were lower compared to other cohorts of MS patients [15, 19–25]. Cognitive function was comparable to prior studies (Table 4) [22, 25–27].

Characterisation of patients with premature study discontinuation

Thirty-four patients (23.8%) prematurely discontinued the study. Nine patients were lost to follow-up, 6 patients discontinued due to adverse events (AEs), 4 withdrew their consent and 2 patients switched to another application method. For 13 patients, the reasons for discontinuation were specified by the attending physicians as follows: 6 patients switched to another medication, 2 patients stopped treatment with IFN beta-1b, 1 stopped using the BETACONNECT®, 2 were not-compliant, 1 patient got pregnant, and 1 discontinued at his/her own request. Table 5 illustrates baseline characteristics for patients prematurely discontinuing the study and those completing the study. Patients prematurely discontinuing were younger, had a shorter duration of disease, were more likely to be women, more likely to have been treated with IFNbeta-1b previously, and more likely to be participating in the BETAPLUS programme.

Fourteen (41.2%) patients, who prematurely discontinued, still used the BETACONNECT® at their individual last visit before study discontinuation. Thirteen of the 18 patients (72.2%) who no longer used the BETACONNECT® also stopped IFNbeta-1b treatment.

Adverse events

A total of 111 treatment-emergent adverse events (TEAEs) occurred in 51 patients (35.6% of 143 patients). TEAEs observed in >5% of all patients were erythema (20.3%) and influenza like illness (5.6%).

Additional information about further injection related data and use of additional electronic features of the BETACONNECT® are provided in the Additional file 7.

Discussion

The BETAEVAL study investigated adherence of MS patients to IFN beta-1b treatment using the fully electronic BETACONNECT® autoinjector. Three quarters of patients still used the autoinjector at week 24. 57.9% of patients with at least one data readout from the device injected ≥80% of their doses. Among participitants with injection data at week 24, both the proportion of adherent patients (80.5%) and the mean compliance (defined as the mean percentage of injections administered: 92.9%) were high. Patients expressed a high level of satisfaction with the BETACONNECT®, more than 90% rated it as user-friendly and more than 80% preferred it over their previous way of injection.

Continuous treatment on a regular basis with injectable DMDs is essential to effectively control MS disease activity. However, treatment adherence remains a challenge and several population-based studies revealed that it is far from optimal. The "global adherence project", a multinational, observational multicentre phase 4 study

Table 4 Patient-related outcome measures

Questionnaire	Initial visit	24-week visit	Results from other published studies in patients with MS	
FAMS (scale: 0–176) Total score (without regard to additional concerns)	N = 129	N = 97		
Mean (SD)	135.5 (29.2)	134.6 (33.7)	120.3 (33.2)	N = 137 [19]
			120.3 (30.7)	N = 344 [20]
			107.5 (32.9)	N = 377 [15]
			110.4 (31.7)	N = 463–472 [21]
Median (range)	145.2 (58–171)	146 (56–176)	———	
HADS – anxiety (scale: 0–21)	N = 131	N = 94		
Mean (SD)	5.3 (4.1)	5.4 (4.3)	8.03 (4.2)	N = 4516 [23]
Median (range)	5 (0–18)	5 (0–19)	———	
Cut-off ≥8, %	26.5	26.6	———	
HADS – depression (scale: 0–21)	N = 131	N = 94	———	
Mean (SD)	3.7 (3.7)	4.1 (4.1)	7.37 (4.2)	N = 4516 [23]
			7.0 (2.9)	N = 269 [24]
Median (range)	2 (0–15)	3 (0–16)	———	
Cut-off ≥8, %	16.7	19.2	———	
CES-D (scale: 0–60)	N = 131	N = 95		
Mean (SD)	12.8 (9.6)	13.0 (11.6)	18.5 (10.1)	N = 51 [22]
			20 (12.1)	N = 463–472 [21]
Median (range)	10 (0–40)	9 (0–43)	———	
< 16, %	65.7	65.3	———	
16–21, %	16.8	12.6	———	
> 21, %	17.6	22.1	———	
FSMC (scale: 20–100)			———	
Cognitive	N = 66	N = 95	———	
Mean (SD)	23.0 (11.0)	22.2 (10.8)	———	
Median (range)	21.5 (10–50)	18 (10–50)	———	
Motor	N = 131	N = 98	———	
Mean (SD)	23.6 (11.1)	24.1 (11.8)	———	
Median (range)	22.9 (10–49)	20.5 (10–50)	———	
Total	N = 66	N = 95		
Mean (SD)	47.3 (21.9)	46.1 (21.9)	65.2 (17.5)	N = 51 [22]
Median (range)	47.5 (20–98)	39 (20–100)	———	
SDMT Total (scale: 0–110)	N = 116	N = 75		
Mean (SD)	47.9 (12.6)	51.5 (14.4)	49.06 (10.01)	N = 51 [22]
			51 (13.0)	N = 159 [26]
			47.66 (14.71)	N = 100 [25]
			55.3 (12.17)	N = 22 [27]
Median (range)	49 (16–76)	51 (15–95)	———	

SD standard deviation, *EDSS* expanded disability status scale, *FAMS* Functional Assessment of Multiple Sclerosis, *HADS* Hospital Anxiety and Depression Scale, *CES-D* Center for Epidemiologic Studies Depression Scale, *SDMT* The Symbol Digit Modalities Test, *FSMC* Fatigue Scale for Motor and Cognitive Functions

used a questionnaire-based approach to evaluate adherence to the commercially available DMDs [7]. Patients not missing a single DMD injection within 4 weeks before the study were considered adherent. Of the 2566 patients included in the analysis, 75% were adherent to their therapy [7]. A recent German retrospective cohort study, including data from 50,057 MS patients, showed that less than 40% of the patients took >80% of their

Table 5 Baseline characteristics among patients who prematurely discontinued and patients who completed the study

Characteristic	Patients with premature discontinuation (N = 34)	Patients completing the study (N = 109)
Age, years		
Mean (SD)	38.8 (10.7)	41.9 (11.6)
Median (range)	36 (21–64)	42 (21–79)
Gender, n (%)		
Women	26 (76.5)	73 (67.0)
Men	8 (22.5)	36 (33.0)
Duration of disease, months	N = 26	N = 76
Mean (SD)	44.8 (60.7)	61.6 (76.5)
Median (range)	24.8 (0.0–274.9)	33.6 (0.0–372.6)
EDSS, median (range))	N = 28	N = 96
	2.3 (0–6.0);	2.0 (0–6.5);
Previous treatment, n (%)		
Betaferon®	30 (88.2)	76 (69.7)
Other treatment	2 (5.9)	4 (3.7)
No previous treatment	2 (5.9)	29 (26.6)
Previous usage of auto-injector for Betaferon® treatment among patients who received Betaferon® previously, n (%)	N = 30	N = 76
Any	23 (76.7)	61 (80.3)
BETACOMFORT®	15 (60.0)	36 (59.0)
BETAJECT Comfort®	8 (32.0)	12 (19.7)
BETAJECT lite®	-	3 (4.9)
Other	-	10 (16.4)
BETAPLUS® participation, n (% of FAS)	26 (76.5)	61 (56.0)

SD standard deviation, *EDSS* expanded disability symptom scale, *FAS* full analysis set

prescribed medication over the observation period of 2 years [6]. Similarly, in a retrospective cohort study with 1606 patients from the US only 27–41% of patients in each year had a medication possession ratio of ≥85% and were thus considered adherent during the 3-year observation period [5]. Furthermore, a prospective study with 199 MS patients in Australia reported that 73% of patients missed doses during a mean follow-up period of 2.4 years [3].

Reasons causing non-adherence to injectable DMDs are often directly related to the drugs and their delivery systems [8]. Discomfort associated with treatment, such as pain at the injection site, local skin reactions, "flu-like" symptoms and fatigue as well as injection anxiety, may cause patients to intentionally skip doses or even discontinue treatment. Additionally, non-intentional forgetfulness or carelessness may contribute to non-adherence [5].

An important means of improving adherence is the development of injection devices aimed at increasing tolerability of the injections [10]. Currently, two fully electronic devices are available, one for the self-injection of IFN beta-1a (RebiSmart® [10]) and one for IFN beta-1b (BETACONNECT® [11]). Both devices share many features including e.g. variable injection speed and depths, reminder function, etc. The RebiSmart® has a display, appears somewhat bulkier and is heavier than the BETACONNECT®, which in contrast also offers the opportunity for data transfer into the myBETAapp®, allowing for personalised documentations of injection-related and wellness-related data. We may speculate, that depending on individual patients preferences and needs, these differences may influence injection behaviour and thus adherence. Patients with impaired vision for example might prefer a device without display and the slim shape of the BETACONNECT® might ease handling among patients with physical impairments of hands and/or arms.

Two observational studies with a retrospective design assessed adherence among RRMS patients by evaluating data from RebiSmart® that were returned for replacement [28, 29]. In both studies adherence was defined as the number of injections recorded by the device divided by the number of injections scheduled in the observation period (corresponding to our compliance definition). One was an audit of 225 patients in the UK and Ireland who had used the device for a minimum of 24 months.

The mean age of the population was 44.1 years and 73% were women. At 24 months, 95.0% of the scheduled doses were injected. The proportion of patients that administered ≥80% of their doses was 91.1% [28]. The other study was conducted in Spain and included 258 patients with a mean age of 41 years, 68% were women. In this study, 92.6% of the scheduled doses were injected over a follow-up period of 3.1 years. 86.8% of the patients administered ≥80% of their prescribed doses [29].

Both studies are flawed by their retrospective design. The study from the UK and Ireland only enrolled patients who were still using the injection device after 2 years [28]. This study uses a "completers approach", disregarding patients who prematurely stopped using the device and patients who simply did not return their devices. The study from Spain considered patients returning their devices for replacement as well as those prematurely terminating usage and returning their devices [29]. Hence, this study does not account for patients stopping usage early, refusing to return their devices or not consenting to study participation. Both approaches bias the results towards higher adherence compared to the whole cohort started on the device. The percentage adherence measure used in these studies is similar to the variable "compliance" in our study.

Prospective studies with the RebiSmart® covering shorter follow-up periods acknowledged patients prematurely stopping device usage. One multicentre, observational phase IV study with 119 patients in the intention-to treat (ITT) population conducted in Italy (BRIDGE study) assessed patient adherence to the device over 12 weeks [30]. All patients were diagnosed with RRMS and had received prior treatment with injectable DMDs. The mean age was 37.9 years and 75.6% were women. At week 12, 88.2% of the patients administered ≥80% of the scheduled injections over the course of the study, as recorded by the autoinjector. Long-term-adherence among 57 of these patients was assessed in the RIVER study [31], a real life-extension study of the BRIDGE study. Overall adherence during the mean observation period of 20.5 ± 5.7 months was 79.8% [31]. The RIVER study is an example underlining the difficulty in retaining patients in real-life studies over extended periods of time.

The MEASURE study, a Canadian multicentre, observational, phase IV study, enrolled 162 patients with RRMS using the RebiSmart® for a maximum of 96 weeks. Patients were only eligible if they had not received any previous DMD treatment. Adherence was defined as the administration of ≥80% of expected injections over the entire study period as recorded by the autoinjector. Compliance was defined as the percentage of administered injections during the actual treatment period until treatment discontinuation. The mean age of the study population was 37.4 years, 75.3% were women and the

mean time since MS diagnosis was 24 months. In the modified ITT population (n = 158), 91.8 and 82.9% of patients were adherent at weeks 12 and 24, respectively [32]. At week 24, 13.9% of participants had discontinued treatment. Among patients remaining on treatment the proportion of participants with ≥80% compliance remained high throughout the study (week 12: 95.6%, week 24: 92.4%). First data from week 96 was presented recently. At week 96, adherence had dropped to 69.5%, whereas the proportion of patients with ≥80% compliance was still high (85.5%) [26].

Data on adherence to treatment with RebiSmart® in Germany are available from a prospective, non-interventional, multicentre READOUTsmart study with 368 patients included in the analysis. In this study, quantitative adherence was defined as the proportion of scheduled injections that were actually administered, as documented by the RebiSmart®. Study participants had a mean age of 36.8 years, 69.6% were women and the mean time since first diagnosis of MS was 2.7 years. Quantitative adherence was 85.3% for the entire study duration of 24 months. A quantitative adherence ≥85% was reported for 72.0 and 65.5% at month 12 and month 24, respectively [33].

In the BETAEVAL study more patients had prematurely terminated study participation than in the MEASURE study at 24 weeks [32] (23.4% vs. 13.9%). This may be due to differences among study participants with patients in our study being slightly older (mean age 41.2 vs. 37.4 years), having a longer mean disease duration (57.5 vs. 24.0 months), and being mostly pretreated with DMDs (74.1% previously treated with IFN beta-1b vs. 100% treatment naïve) compared to the participants in the MEASURE study [32]. Furthermore, pretreatment was also very different in both the German READOUTsmart study, with only 21.5% of patients having been on DMDs previously [33] and in the BRIDGE study with almost two thirds of patients switching from intramuscular to subcutaneous injection [30]. In addition, follow-up periods in the READOUTsmart [33] and the BRIDGE study [30] differed from ours, precluding a direct comparison between the adherence measures.

Patients with a longer disease duration and treatment history with injectable DMDs may be more impatient and have higher expectations due to their previous experiences compared to DMD-naïve patients, resulting in a higher proportion of patients prematurely terminating the BETAEVAL study. On the other hand, "first-time users" of DMDs may be more motivated and determined to stick to the treatment regimen in order to change their natural disease course. This is corroborated by results from our stratified analysis, indicating a higher proportion of patients prematurely terminating the study among experienced patients compared to naïve patients

(Fig. 2). In addition, we identified "no previous treatment" as an important predictor of both persistence and adherence by applying post-hoc prediction models.

Another potential factor influencing treatment discontinuation in our study might be the availability of new oral drugs. Patients in the BRIDGE study were recruited in 2009/2010, whereas our study started in 2014. In this time period three new oral drugs for MS treatment were approved in Europe: fingolimod (2011), teriflunomide (2013) and dimethyl fumarate (2014), possibly increasing the incentive for patients to switch to oral drugs.

The proportion of adherent patients and the mean compliance among patients in the BETAEVAL study using the BETACONNECT® were high, indicating that the device is a useful and well-received tool to support patients with their injections. The BETACONNECT® was designed to further improve patients' injection experience and to overcome some of the barriers leading to non-adherence such as needle phobia or injection anxiety. In fact, patients in the BETAEVAL study indicated a high degree of satisfaction with the BETACONNECT®. There was no difference in the perception of injection-related pain between the BETACONNECT® and the previous way of injection; however, only 9.1% of patients with corresponding questionnaire used analgesics prior to their injection at week 24, whereas 14.6% indicate this before the study start and 17.2% at week 4.

Patients rated the BETACONNECT® as user-friendly and at the initial visit, a majority of patients already indicated that they felt confident with the BETACONNECT® compared with their previous way of injection and that they preferred it to their previous way. The proportion of participants "strongly agreeing" to the latter statements increased over time, indicating that their initial impression was confirmed and that their appreciation grew while further familiarizing themselves with the device. The results concerning satisfaction are in line with a survey-based study conducted on 118 patients using the BETACONNECT® in Germany [11]. Among those 92% indicated that they were very confident or confident using the autoinjector and almost half of them stated, that the ease-of-use was the primary reason for their satisfaction with the device. High levels of satisfaction with the BETACONNECT® may be an important factor contributing to the high adherence and compliance seen in our study.

The strengths of the BETAEVAL study include the prospective data collection, the large study population, and the observational study design enrolling patients representative of German MS patients thus allowing a real-world picture of the treatment situation in Germany to be drawn. Furthermore, key characteristics and results from questionnaires suggest that the participants in the BETAEVAL study are comparable to other cohorts of patients with relapsing forms of MS with a slightly higher functional health status and a slightly lower level of depression and anxiety [15, 19–27].

However, some limitations need to be considered when interpreting the results. First, the follow-up of 6 months was rather short. However, this study was designed to allow for an early evaluation of the BETACONNECT® and its usage in a real-world setting, in order to be able to address potential problems early. In addition, a follow up study is currently ongoing to evaluate adherence among MS patients using the device for injection of IFN beta-1b over up to 2 years [34]. Second, injection data from the BETACONNECT® were not available for all study participants and not at all follow-up visits. Finally, the BETAEVAL study lacks a control group, precluding comparison of adherence between patients using the BETACONNECT® and a different way of injecting IFN beta-1b; however, this was not the aim of the study.

Conclusions

The majority of study participants used the fully electronic BETACONNECT® autoinjector throughout the study. Adherence, persistence and compliance were high. Most participants were very satisfied with the device, the vast majority also giving high ratings for user friendliness, feeling confident in using it and preferring it over their previously used device. Hence, the BETACONNECT may be a useful tool to support patients in following their treatment regimen with IFN beta-1b.

Additional files

Additional file 1: Patient questionnaire regarding secondary outcomes. Description of data: questions regarding satisfaction, user friendliness, injection site related pain as well as preference of and confidence in using the BETACONNECT®.

Additional file 2: Adherence, satisfaction and functional health status among patients with multiple sclerosis using the BETACONNECT® autoinjector: a prospective observational cohort study. Description of data: description of the rating scales used for documentation of other patient-reported outcomes.

Additional file 3: Table S1. Satisfaction with the BETACONNECT® among participants in the BETAEVAL study - stratified analyses. Description of data: data on analyses stratified by age, gender, EDSS baseline score, previous treatment with INF beta-1b, and BETAPLUS participation.

Additional file 4: Table S2. Injection related pain – stratified analyses. Description of data: data on analyses stratified by age, gender, EDSS baseline score, previous treatment with INF beta-1b, and BETAPLUS participation.

Additional file 5: Table S3. Prophylactic use of analgesics prior to injection – stratified analyses. Description of data: data on analyses stratified by age, gender, EDSS baseline score, previous treatment with INF beta-1b, and BETAPLUS participation.

Additional file 6: Table S4. Patient-related outcome measures – stratified analyses. Description of data: data on analyses stratified by age, gender, EDSS baseline score, previous treatment with INF beta-1b, and BETAPLUS participation.

Additional file 7: Adherence, satisfaction and functional health status among patients with multiple sclerosis using the BETACONNECT® autoinjector: a prospective observational cohort study. Description of data: results on further injection related data and use of electronic features of the BETACONNECT® are provided.

Abbreviations
AE: Adverse event; CES-D: Centre for Epidemiologic Studies Depression Scale; CI: Confidence interval; CIS: Clinically isolated syndrome; DMD: Disease modifying drug; eCRFs: Electronic case report forms; EDC: Electronic data capture system; EDSS: Expanded disability status scale; FAMS: Functional assessment of multiple sclerosis; FAS: Full analysis set; FSMC: Fatigue Scale for Motor and Cognitive Functions; HADS: Hospital Anxiety and Depression Scale; IFN: Interferon; im: Intramuscular; ITT: Intention-to-treat; MS: Multiple sclerosis; RRMS: Relapsing remitting multiple sclerosis; SAF: Safety analysis set; sc: Subcutaneous; SD: Standard deviation; SDMT: Symbol Digit Modalities Test; TEAE: Treatment-emergent adverse events

Acknowledgements
The authors wish to express their gratitude to the study participants and all study investigators.
The authors wish to thank Dr. Sonja Hergeth, medizinwelten-services GmbH, who provided medical writing services on behalf of Bayer Vital GmbH, Leverkusen, Germany.

Funding
The study was funded by Bayer Vital GmbH, Leverkusen, Germany.

Authors' contributions
IK, CN, BS, MS were responsible for the concept and design of the study. BS, MS were responsible for study coordination and conduct. CN, MS were responsible for the data analysis. IK, ML, JJ collected the clinical data. IK, CN, BS, MS interpreted the data. All authors contributed to and critically reviewed the manuscript during its development and approved the final version of the manuscript for submission.

Competing interests
IK received honoraria for consultancy or speaking from Biogen, Chugai, Roche and Shire, travel reimbursement from Bayer Healthcare and grant support from Affectis, Chugai and Diamed, none related to this manuscript and honoraria for consultancy from Bayer Healthcare, related to this manuscript.
ML has received travel grants, speaker's honoraria, financial research support and consultancy fees from Teva, Merck Serono, Sanofi-Genzyme, Novartis, Bayer, Biogen.
JJ has received speaker's honoraria and financial research support from Bayer, Novartis, Biogen and Sanofi-Genzyme.
CN is an employee of Bayer AG, Wuppertal, Germany.
BS is an employee of Bayer Vital GmbH, Leverkusen, Germany.
MS is an employee of Bayer Vital GmbH, Leverkusen, Germany. He previously served as an associate editor to BMC Neurology.

Author details
[1]St. Josef Hospital, University Hospital Bochum, Bochum, Germany. [2]Present Address: Marianne-Strauß-Klinik, Behandlungszentrum Kempfenhausen für Multiple Sklerose Kranke, Berg, Germany. [3]Joint Neurological Practice, Ulm, Germany. [4]Neurological Practice, Wuppertal, Germany. [5]Bayer AG, Wuppertal, Germany. [6]Bayer Vital GmbH, Leverkusen, Germany.

References
1. Petersen G, Wittmann R, Arndt V, Gopffarth D. Epidemiology of multiple sclerosis in Germany: regional differences and drug prescription in the claims data of the statutory health insurance. Nervenarzt. 2014;85(8):990–8.
2. Al-Sabbagh A. Medication gaps in disease-modifying drug therapy for multiple sclerosis are associated with an icreased risk of relapse: findings from a national manged care database. J Neurol. 2008;255(Suppl. 2):S.79.
3. Tremlett H, Van der Mei I, Pittas F, Blizzard L, Paley G, Dwyer T, Taylor B, Ponsonby AL. Adherence to the immunomodulatory drugs for multiple sclerosis: contrasting factors affect stopping drug and missing doses. Pharmacoepidemiol Drug Saf. 2008;17(6):565–76.
4. Ivanova JI, Bergman RE, Birnbaum HG, Phillips AL, Stewart M, Meletiche DM. Impact of medication adherence to disease-modifying drugs on severe relapse, and direct and indirect costs among employees with multiple sclerosis in the US. J Med Econ. 2012;15(3):601–9.
5. Steinberg SC, Faris RJ, Chang CF, Chan A, Tankersley MA. Impact of adherence to interferons in the treatment of multiple sclerosis: a non-experimental, retrospective, cohort study. Clin Drug Investig. 2010;30(2):89–100.
6. Hansen K, Schussel K, Kieble M, Werning J, Schulz M, Friis R, Pohlau D, Schmitz N, Kugler J. Adherence to disease modifying drugs among patients with multiple sclerosis in Germany: a retrospective cohort study. PLoS One. 2015;10(7):e0133279.
7. Devonshire V, Lapierre Y, Macdonell R, Ramo-Tello C, Patti F, Fontoura P, Suchet L, Hyde R, Balla I, Frohman EM, et al. The Global Adherence Project (GAP): a multicenter observational study on adherence to disease-modifying therapies in patients with relapsing-remitting multiple sclerosis. Eur J Neurol. 2011;18(1):69–77.
8. Lugaresi A, Rottoli MR, Patti F. Fostering adherence to injectable disease-modifying therapies in multiple sclerosis. Expert Rev Neurother. 2014;14(9):1029–42.
9. Brochet B, Lemaire G, Beddiaf A, et l'Epicure Study G. Reduction of injection site reactions in multiple sclerosis (MS) patients newly started on interferon beta 1b therapy with two different devices. Rev Neurol (Paris). 2006;162(6–7):735–40.
10. Lugaresi A. RebiSmart (version 1.5) device for multiple sclerosis treatment delivery and adherence. Expert Opin Drug Deliv. 2013;10(2):273–83.
11. Ziemssen T, Sylvester L, Rametta M, Ross AP. Patient satisfaction with the new interferon Beta-1b autoinjector (BETACONNECT). Neurol Ther. 2015;4(2):125–36.
12. Fachinformation Betaferon® 250 µg/ml. Bayer Vital GmbH, Leverkusen. März 2017.
13. Kurtzke JF. Rating neurologic impairment in multiple sclerosis: an expanded disability status scale (EDSS). Neurology. 1983;33(11):1444–52.
14. Smith A. Symbol digit modalities test: manual. Los Angeles: Wetern Psychological Services; 1982.
15. Cella DF, Dineen K, Arnason B, Reder A, Webster KA, Karabatsos G, Chang C, Lloyd S, Steward J, Stefoski D. Validation of the functional assessment of multiple sclerosis quality of life instrument. Neurology. 1996;47(1):129–39.
16. Zigmond AS, Snaith RP. The hospital anxiety and depression scale. Acta Psychiatr Scand. 1983;67(6):361–70.
17. Radloff L. The CES-D scale: a self-report depressive scale for research in the general population. J Appl Psychol Meas. 1977;1:385–401.
18. Penner IK, Raselli C, Stocklin M, Opwis K, Kappos L, Calabrese P. The Fatigue Scale for Motor and Cognitive Functions (FSMC): validation of a new instrument to assess multiple sclerosis-related fatigue. Mult Scler. 2009;15(12):1509–17.
19. Reese JP, Wienemann G, John A, Linnemann A, Balzer-Geldsetzer M, Mueller UO, Eienbroker C, Tackenberg B, Dodel R. Preference-based health status in a German outpatient cohort with multiple sclerosis. Health Qual Life Outcomes. 2013;11:162.
20. Patti F, Russo P, Pappalardo A, Macchia F, Civalleri L, Paolillo A, group Fs. Predictors of quality of life among patients with multiple sclerosis: an Italian cross-sectional study. J Neurol Sci. 2007;252(2):121–9.
21. Pozzilli C, Schweikert B, Ecari U, Oentrich W, Bugge JP. Quality of life and depression in multiple sclerosis patients: longitudinal results of the BetaPlus study. J Neurol. 2012;259(11):2319–28.
22. Kunkel A, Fischer M, Faiss J, Dahne D, Kohler W, Faiss JH. Impact of natalizumab treatment on fatigue, mood, and aspects of cognition in relapsing-remitting multiple sclerosis. Front Neurol. 2015;6:97.
23. Jones KH, Jones PA, Middleton RM, Ford DV, Tuite-Dalton K, Lockhart-Jones H, Peng J, Lyons RA, John A, Noble JG. Physical disability, anxiety and depression in people with MS: an internet-based survey via the UK MS register. PLoS One. 2014;9(8):e104604.
24. Ensari I, Motl RW, McAuley E, Mullen SP, Feinstein A. Patterns and predictors of naturally occurring change in depressive symptoms over a 30-month period in multiple sclerosis. Mult Scler. 2014;20(5):602–9.
25. Parmenter BA, Weinstock-Guttman B, Garg N, Munschauer F, Benedict RH. Screening for cognitive impairment in multiple sclerosis using the symbol digit modalities test. Mult Scler. 2007;13(1):52–7.

26. Devonshire V, Feinstein A, Gillet A: Treatment, adherence, Paersistence, and compliance of patients using the RebiSmart® auto-injector. 96-weeks results. Poster presentation at the 68th annual meeting of the American Academy of Neurology. 2016; poster P3.037. 2016.

27. Strober LB, Rao SM, Lee JC, Fischer E, Rudick R. Cognitive impairment in multiple sclerosis: an 18 year follow-up study. Mult Scler Relat Disord. 2014;3(4):473–81.

28. Willis H, Webster J, Larkin AM, Parkes L. An observational, retrospective, UK and Ireland audit of patient adherence to subcutaneous interferon beta-1a injections using the RebiSmart((R)) injection device. Patient Prefer Adherence. 2014;8:843–51.

29. Fernandez O, Arroyo R, Martinez-Yelamos S, Marco M, Merino JA, Munoz D, Merino E, Roque A, Group RS. Long-term adherence to IFN Beta-1a treatment when using RebiSmart(R) device in patients with relapsing-remitting multiple sclerosis. PLoS One. 2016;11(8):e0160313.

30. Lugaresi A, Florio C, Brescia-Morra V, Cottone S, Bellantonio P, Clerico M, Centonze D, Uccelli A, di Ioia M, De Luca G, et al. Patient adherence to and tolerability of self-administered interferon beta-1a using an electronic autoinjection device: a multicentre, open-label, phase IV study. BMC Neurol. 2012;12:7.

31. Lugaresi A, De Robertis F, Clerico M, Brescia Morra V, Centonze D, Borghesan S, Maniscalco GT, group Rs. Long-term adherence of patients with relapsing-remitting multiple sclerosis to subcutaneous self-injections of interferon beta-1a using an electronic device: the RIVER study. Expert Opin Drug Deliv. 2016;13(7):931–5.

32. Devonshire VA, Feinstein A, Moriarty P. Adherence to interferon beta-1a therapy using an electronic self-injector in multiple sclerosis: a multicentre, single-arm, observational, phase IV study. BMC Res Notes. 2016;9:148.

33. Rieckmann P, Schwab M, Pöhlau D, Wagner T, Schel E, Bayas A: Adherence to subcutaneous IFN-b1a - final analysis of the non-interventional study READOUTsmart using the dosing log and readout function of RebiSmart®. Poster presentation at the annual meeting of the American Academy of Neurology 2016. P3.098. 2016.

34. Evaluation of Potential Predictors of Adherence by Investigating a Representative Cohort of Multiple Sclerosis (MS) Patients in Germany Treated With Betaferon (BETAPREDICT). ClinicalTrials.gov Identifier: NCT02486640. https://clinicaltrials.gov/ct2/show/NCT02486640?term=NCT02486640&rank=1. Accessed 1 Sept 2017.

6

Results of a randomized, double blind, placebo controlled, crossover trial of melatonin for treatment of Nocturia in adults with multiple sclerosis (MeNiMS)

Marcus J. Drake[1,2]* (iD), Luke Canham[3], Nikki Cotterill[2], Debbie Delgado[2], Jenny Homewood[3], Kirsty Inglis[3], Lyndsey Johnson[2], Mary C. Kisanga[2], Denise Owen[3], Paul White[4] and David Cottrell[3]

Abstract

Background: Nocturia is a common urinary symptom of multiple sclerosis (MS) which can affect quality of life (QoL) adversely. Melatonin is a hormone known to regulate circadian rhythm and reduce smooth muscle activity such as in the bladder. There is limited evidence supporting use of melatonin to alleviate urinary frequency at night in the treatment of nocturia. The aim of this study was to evaluate the effect of melatonin on the mean number of nocturia episodes per night in patients with MS.

Methods: A randomized, double blind, placebo controlled crossover trial was conducted. 34 patients with nocturia secondary to multiple sclerosis underwent a 4-day pre-treatment monitoring phase. The patients were randomized to receive either 2 mg per night (taken at bedtime) of capsulated sustained-release melatonin (Circadin®) or 1 placebo capsule for 6 weeks followed by a crossover to the other regimen for an additional 6 weeks after a 1-month washout period.

Results: From the 26 patients who completed the study, there was no significant difference observed in the signs or symptoms of nocturia when taking 2 mg melatonin compared to placebo. The primary outcome measure, mean number of nocturia episodes on bladder diaries, was 1.8/night at baseline, and 1.4/night on melatonin, compared with 1.6 for placebo (Medians 1.70, 1.50, and 1.30 respectively, $p = 0.85$). There was also no significant difference seen in LUTS, QoL and sleep quality when taking melatonin. No significant safety concerns arose.

Conclusions: This small study suggests that a low dose of melatonin taken at bedtime may be ineffective therapy for nocturia in MS.

Keywords: Nocturia, Multiple sclerosis, Melatonin, Antidiuretic, Antimuscarinic, LUTS

Background

Nocturia is the complaint that the individual has to wake at night one or more times to void [1]. It can result from a range of factors, including behavioural influences, sleep disturbances, lower urinary tract dysfunction and altered fluid or salt homeostasis. Nocturia is prevalent in the general population and is known to increase in severity with age. 77% of people aged 60 and above experience some degree of nocturia with no difference seen between men and women [2]. Nocturia impacts greatly on quality of life (QoL), potentially due to fatigue, cognitive dysfunction and disturbed emotional health [3]. Furthermore, severe nocturia may be associated with cardiovascular disease, autonomic disease, obstructive sleep apnoea and chronic kidney disease [4], and potentially a higher risk of mortality [5]. A very high proportion of MS patients have lower urinary tract symptoms (LUTS) [6]. LUTS are a substantial problem in MS, and nocturia is a particularly

* Correspondence: marcus.drake@bui.ac.uk
[1]School of Clinical Sciences, University of Bristol, Bristol, UK
[2]Bristol Urological Institute, Southmead Hospital, Bristol BS10 5NB, UK
Full list of author information is available at the end of the article

prominent symptom with substantial detrimental impact on QoL [7].

Current treatments for nocturia include managing fluid intake, timed diuretics, desmopressin, antimuscarinic drugs, bedtime sedatives and miscellaneous compounds [8]. Desmopressin is indicated for treatment of nocturia in MS [9]. However, desmopressin can cause hyponatraemia [10] and has been associated with hyponatraemic convulsions [11, 12]. Indeed, it is recommended that tri-cyclic antidepressants (commonly used in MS patients) are avoided when using Desmopressin to reduce the risk of hyponatraemia (British National Formulary). This can also potentially be an issue with diuretics. Antimuscarinics are known to cause dry mouth, constipation, swallowing difficulty and confusion. Patients taking sedatives can experience hangover sedation, while elderly subjects are at risk of cognitive impairment [13]. These side effects and poor efficacy mean that clinicians are sometimes reluctant to initiate treatment for nocturia.

Melatonin (N-acetyl-5-methoxytryptamine) is a hormone secreted primarily at night by the pineal gland. It regulates circadian rhythms and reduces smooth muscle spontaneous activity, including that found in the bladder [14]. Melatonin tablets taken before bedtime may reduce nocturia in a subgroup of patients with benign prostate enlargement [15]. In elderly patients with nocturia, levels of severity and QoL improve with melatonin use [16]. In MS, sleep quality is commonly reduced as a consequence of a wide range of sleep abnormalities, of which nocturia is only one example. In MS there can be an impairment of endogenous melatonin secretion [17, 18], and administration of oral melatonin improves reduced sleep quality in MS patients [19].

We hypothesised that bedtime administration of a melatonin sustained-release tablet will improve clinical nocturia in patients with MS. We previously published the protocol of the "Melatonin for nocturia in MS (MeNiMS)" study to evaluate this hypothesis [20], and the current study reports the findings. We chose a low dose of 2 mg, as melatonin levels negatively correlate with multiple sclerosis activity in humans, and alterations in endogenous melatonin have been proposed potentially to affect MS relapses [21]. The primary aim was to evaluate the effect of melatonin on mean number of nocturia episodes per night in MS patients. The secondary aims included: 1) improvement in QoL, 2) safety, 3) LUTS, 4) sleep quality and 5) total voided (urinated) volume and mean volume per void. A qualitative study was also included, which will be reported separately.

Methods

The detailed study protocol has previously been published [20]. In brief, male and female patients aged ≥18 were recruited at Southmead Hospital, Bristol, UK. Each patient had a confirmed neurological diagnosis of MS as per the 2010 McDonald MS Criteria [22]. They also reported at least one episode of nocturia every night on the International Consultation on Incontinence Questionnaires (ICIQ) Nocturia questionnaire (ICIQ-N [23]). Patients were excluded if they had (i) an indwelling urinary catheter; (ii) used desmopressin or investigational medications in the month preceding randomization; (iii) taken antimuscarinic or diuretic medication, unless used long-term prior to study (> 3 months) and continued throughout the study; (iv) taken melatonin on prescription or purchased; (v) used "sleeping tablets" on prescription or purchased; (vi) diabetes mellitus/diabetes insipidus; and (vii) or if they were pregnant at screening, or of child-bearing potential and unwilling to use contraception. Dipstick urinalysis to exclude urinary tract infection was undertaken at screening. The U.K. National Research Ethics Service Committee South West – Exeter approved the study protocol (REC reference number: 12/SW/0322).

This was a randomized, double blind, placebo controlled crossover trial with two groups (Fig. 1). Following an initial four-day pre-treatment monitoring phase, the treatment phases were 2 mg per night of capsulated sustained-release melatonin ('Circadin') or an identical placebo capsule per night for 6 weeks each, separated by a 4 week washout period. Patients were allocated double-blind via a website (http://www.randomization.com) to group AB or BA, with unblinding undertaken following database lock and analysis (A = placebo, B = melatonin).

The primary outcome was reduction in nocturia episodes per night, derived from the ICIQ bladder diary (ICIQ-BD) [24]. Secondary outcomes included; 1. Subjective severity, using the ICIQ tools on nocturia (ICIQ-N) and nocturia quality of life (ICIQ-NQoL) [25]. 2. MS quality of life, assessed with the MSQoL scale. 3. LUTS, assessed with the ICIQ-MLUTS and ICIQ-FLUTS for males and females respectively. 4. Sleep quality; measured with the Pittsburgh Sleep Quality Index (PSQI). 5. Safety, based on adverse event reporting and Expanded Disability Status Scale (EDSS) score [26]. Outcome measures were completed at baseline and at the end of each treatment phase. Adverse event reporting was undertaken throughout, and followed up until resolution or for 3 months [20].

Statistical analysis

We calculated that for a two-sided test, using standard levels of statistical significance (alpha = 0.05), a sample size of $n = 21$ complete data sets would have 80% power to detect a medium to large effect size (Cohen's d = 0.65) with 80% power, and a sample size of $n = 34$ would be needed for a medium effect size (Cohen's d = 0.5) [20].

The balanced two group, two period, two sequence, double-blind, randomised crossover design with wash-out

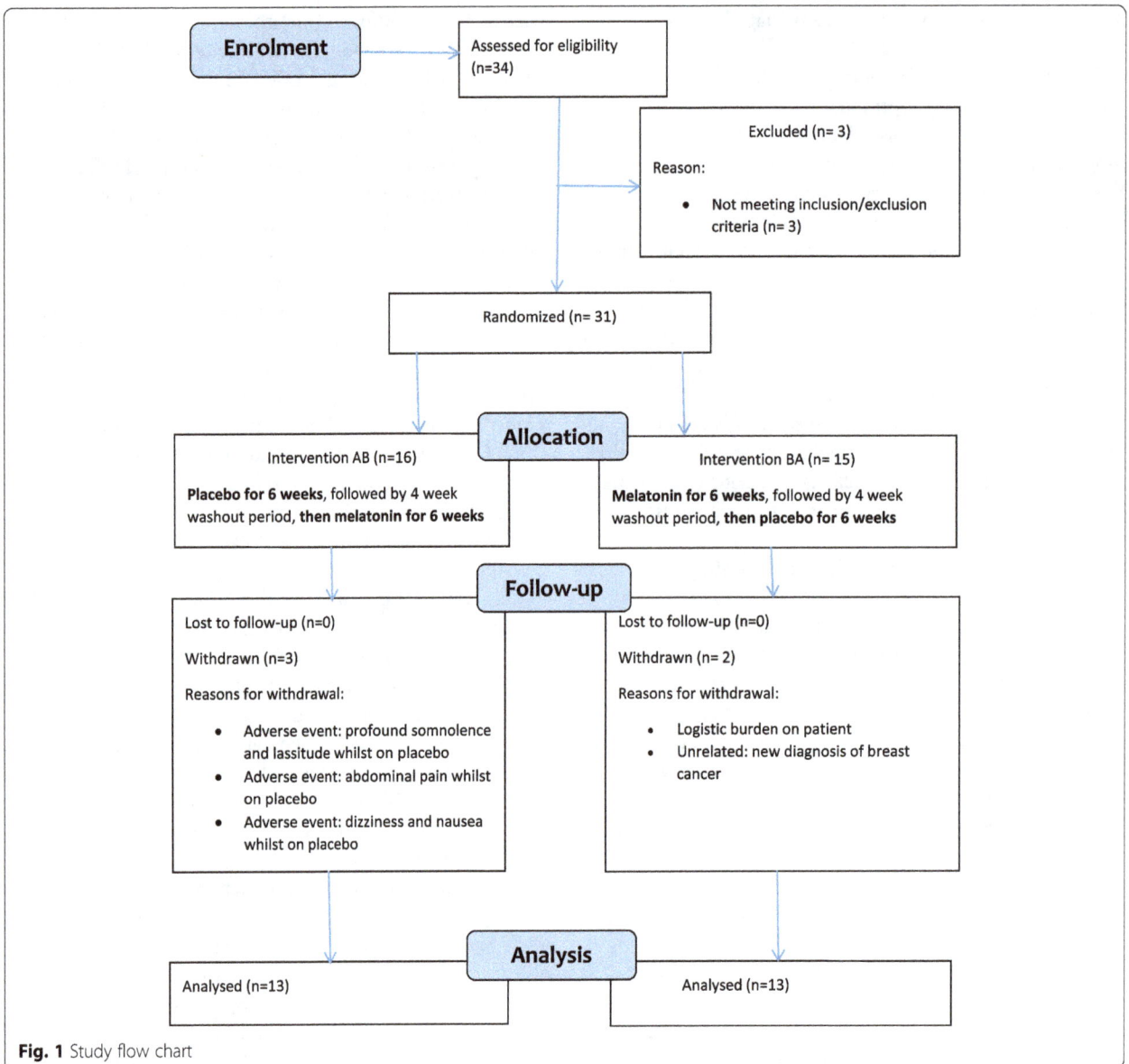

Fig. 1 Study flow chart

period comparing treatment to control, ranks highly in the hierarchy of designs. The analyses of the resultant data under this AB/BA design may proceed using nonparametric (Mann-Whitney-Wilcoxon U) two-sample statistical techniques which assess for carryover effects, period effects, and treatment effect accounting for any period effects using independent samples designs [27] or using paired samples in the absence of period and carryover effects. Treatment effect sizes have been quantified and converted to Cohen's d. For Cohen's standardized statistic, $d = 0$ indicates the absence of an effect. For statistically significant effects, some broad and cautious threshold guidance to aid interpretation is for, $0 < d < 0.1$ to indicate a trivial effect, $0.1 < d < 0.3$ to indicate a small effect, $0.3 < d < 0.5$ to indicate a moderate effect, $0.5 < d < 0.8$ a medium size effect, $0.8 < d < 1.3$ a large effect, and

$d > 1.3$ a very large effect [28]. A missing data analysis was also performed on the primary outcome measure to assess sensitivity of statistical conclusions to missingness. This analysis indicated any missing data to be consistent with being missing completely at random (MCAR). Multiple Imputation by Chained Equations (MICE) [29] with 1000 imputed data sets was performed. These imputed analyses faithfully reproduced the findings from the observed sample data and for brevity of exposition, and to avoid redundancy, are not reported in full.

Results

In total 13 men and 18 women of mean age 54.8 years (range 34–69) were randomised. Five patients had Primary Progressive MS, 15 patients had Secondary Progressive MS and 11 patients had Relapsing Remitting MS (RRMS).

Five of the 11 with RRMS were taking disease modifying therapy at the time of the trial (one interferon beta-1a, two fingolomid and two dimethyl fumarate). Mean EDSS was 4.2 (median 4.0, range 1.5 to 8.0). Five patients withdrew from the trial (Fig. 1). Reasons for withdrawal were; adverse events (three patients), new-onset unrelated health problems (one patient) and logistic burden (one patient). Mean nocturia severity at baseline from the bladder diary was 1.78 episodes/night and self-reported mean ICIQ symptom score for nocturia was 1.80 episodes/night (range 1–3).

The effects of 2 mg melatonin and placebo on bladder diary parameters are shown in Table 1. There was no significant change seen with melatonin for the primary outcome measure, the number of nocturnal episodes per night. "Objective" nocturia was 1.4/ night for melatonin, compared with 1.6 for placebo (U = 43, p = 0.85). Average nocturnal output and nocturnal polyuria index (NPI) were also not significantly altered. Effects on patient-reported LUTS are shown in Table 2. For patient-reported (subjective) nocturia, the number of episodes per night after 6 weeks of melatonin was 3.3, compared with 3.2 with placebo. Overall scores and individual LUTS were not significantly different with melatonin compared with placebo.

Secondary end points looking at QoL also revealed that melatonin did not significantly affect outcomes. The ICIQ-NQoL questionnaire mean totals were 22.1 for melatonin, compared with 23.6 for placebo (U = 41.5, p = 0.34; Table 3). For the MSQoL scale (Table 4), there was no significant change between melatonin and placebo in most of the domains, except for physical overall score (50.9 vs. 47.9, respectively, median 48.5 vs 44.0, U = 26, p = 0.02), role limitations due to physical problems (39.1 vs. 33.3, median 25 vs 12.5, U = 29, p = 0.02) and pain score (62.7 vs. 70.6, median 70 vs. 78, U = 34.5, p = 0.03). In the PSQI (Table 5), the mean scores were 8.1 and 8.7 for melatonin and placebo respectively (median 8.0 vs. 9.0 respectively, U = 56.5, p = 0.89).

In all analyses there was little evidence of any carryover effects (i.e. no evidence of period by treatment interaction effects, consistent with a sufficiently large washout period). In addition, the given conclusions for treatment effects are replicated if differences are examined as paired differences using the non-parametric Wilcoxon signed rank test.

Safety

EDSS data is given in Table 6. Overall, there was no difference in EDSS while taking melatonin or placebo; mean score was 4.4 for placebo and 4.7 for melatonin (medians 4.0 and 4.0). Four patients reported worsening symptoms of MS during the study, of which two were taking melatonin at the time. One experienced two separate episodes, once whilst taking melatonin and once whilst taking placebo. One patient experienced Uhthoff's phenomenon, a worsening of neurological condition related to MS, while taking melatonin.

Adverse event reporting most commonly identified urinary tract infection (UTI), which affected seven participants. Four of these were prior to receipt of study medication. Three UTIs were found after randomisation. One was on treatment phase 1 and was receiving melatonin. Another had completed treatment phase 2 (placebo). One participant was found to have a UTI after the post drug wash out phase for melatonin.

Two patients experienced faecal urgency; both were no longer taking study medication at the time of onset, and both had been taking placebo.

Two participants experienced lassitude and anergia. One was withdrawn by the clinician, and was found to have been taking placebo. The other had already completed the study, and had been taking melatonin as the most recent study medication.

One patient experienced severe dizziness, and was unblinded and was found to have been taking placebo; this patient was withdrawn from the study. A further patient reported abdominal pain (a reported potential side effect of Melatonin), and was withdrawn by the clinician without unblinding; subsequently the patient was found to have been taking placebo.

Two patients reported chest infections, one taking placebo and the other melatonin. One of these patients went on to report a further three adverse events of pain in fingers, knees and shoulder, which all occurred whilst taking placebo.

Table 1 Median and range for average number of nocturia episodes, voided output, and NPI by treatment with treatment p-value and standardized effect size, d

Measure	Treatment						p	d
	Baseline		A: Placebo		B: Melatonin			
	Median	Range	Median	Range	Median	Range		
Average Nocturia Episodes	1.70	1–3	1.50	0–3	1.30	0–3.3	0.618	0.136
Average nocturnal urine output (mls)	741	310–1416	651	300–1933	667	200–1100	0.939	0.020
24-h voided volume (mls)	2125	1200–4000	2213	1250–3900	2000	881–3600	0.254	0.314
Nocturnal Polyuria Index NPI	0.32	0.15–0.71	0.33	0.17–0.56	0.32	0.15–0.60	0.849	0.052

Table 2 Median and range of the grouped sub-scores (Voiding and Incontinence) and the individual symptom scores for nocturia, urgency and frequency from the ICIQ LUTS questionnaires (MLUTS and FLUTS for males and females respectively) by treatment, with p-values and standardized effect size, d

Measure	Treatment				p	d
	A: Placebo		B: Melatonin			
	Median	Range	Median	Range		
Voiding sub-score	4.0	0–12	2.0	0–12	0.096	0.492
Incontinence (Storage) sub-score	3.0	0–9	3.0	0–12	0.107	0.450
Nocturia	2.0	1–3	2.0	1–3	0.892	0.037
Urgency	2.0	0–3	2.0	1–4	0.772	0.079

One patient experienced abdominal pain resulting in emergency department review, where cholecystitis was diagnosed. She also reported shingles and reduced mobility in separate adverse events. She had been taking the placebo on all of these occasions. One patient reported a probable olecranon bursitis while taking placebo. Colds and an ear infection were reported by two patients; both were taking placebo.

Discussion

Nocturia is a prominent symptom with substantial detrimental impact on quality of life in MS, especially in light of the range of factors affecting sleep quality in these patients. Ordinarily, there should be a reduction in urine production rate during sleep. Endogenous melatonin is a key contributor in circadian control, and disruption of melatonin is a feature in sleep disturbance in MS [30]. We surmised that beneficial effects may result indirectly by improved sleep quality, and perhaps directly by some restoration of the normal circadian reduction in urine production at night, and reduced bladder smooth muscle activity. A potential impact of giving supplementary melatonin orally as regulator of circadian rhythms in restoring some measure of circadian control [31] could be beneficial in the proposed context. In reality, the effect of melatonin in the current study did not identify any reduction in nocturia (either objectively or subjectively). The bladder diary was the main outcome assessment, and during the active treatment phase there was no reduction in nocturia episodes or overall nocturnal urine production.

For the PSQI, the mean scores at the end of the treatment phase were 8.1 for melatonin and 8.7 for placebo.

This difference was statistically significant, and seems to indicate worse function with melatonin, but the difference is modest and unlikely to be clinically significant. We also evaluated other aspects of the patient's health and QoL. For the MSQoL, there was no significant change between melatonin and placebo in most of the domains, except that small statistically significant differences were evident in the physical overall score, role limitations due to physical problems, and pain score. It is unclear that this was a definite consequence of melatonin action.

Symptom scores were a key secondary measure, and again melatonin did not appear to have any effect on nocturia specifically or LUTS in general. Nocturia-specific quality of life did not show any evident improvement. Nocturia has a multifactorial pathophysiology, which potentially could mean that melatonin might have effect in some individuals and not others, and this was considered to explain the finding of a responder group in a previous study which examined melatonin use for treatment of nocturia in men with benign prostate enlargement [15]. However, there did not seem to be any evident responder group in the current study.

The lack of evident difference between melatonin and placebo may reflect the pragmatic approach taken in the study. Diabetes mellitus and diabetes insipidus were excluded, but otherwise inclusive criteria were used for study recruitment. This pragmatic approach was taken to reflect the utility of a therapy which could be applied to the majority of patients in the general healthcare context, without having to undertake too much clinical assessment. The fact that we did not identify benefit could reflect the wide range of potential co-morbidity in

Table 3 Median and range for ICIQ NQol by treatment with p-value and standardized effect size, d

Measure	Treatment				p	d
	A: Placebo		B: Melatonin			
	Median	Range	Median	Range		
Overall score	25.0	8–35	20.0	8–42	0.341	0.261
Overall interference	5.0	0–9	4.0	0–9	0.444	0.209
Sleep/Energy sub-score	11.0	3–19	10.0	3–18	0.549	0.164
Bother/Concern sub-score	9.5	4–21	9.0	3–16	0.288	0.292

Table 4 Median and range for MSQoL by treatment, with p-value and standardized effect size, d

Measure	Treatment				p	d
	A: Placebo		B: Melatonin			
	Median	Range	Median	Range		
Mental Overall Score	68.0	16–92	75.0	28–92	0.110	0.446
Physical Overall Score	44.0	17–89	48.5	21–90	0.023	0.651
Energy Score	30.0	0–76	36.0	0–84	0.212	0.347
Emotional Wellbeing	68.0	32–100	72.0	32–100	0.961	0.013
Physical Health	45.0	5–100	40.0	5–100	0.701	0.105
Role limitations due to physical problems	12.5	0–100	25.0	0–100	0.015	0.701
Role limitations due to emotional problems	100	0–100	100	0–100	0.580	0.151
Health Perceptions	42.5	5–85	45.0	0–80	0.396	0.233
Social Function	67.0	25–100	67.0	0–100	0.603	0.142
Cognitive Function	67.0	0–100	73.0	0–100	0.884	0.040
Health Distress	60.0	15–90	60.0	0–100	0.862	0.036
Change in Health	25.0	0–50	50.0	25–100	0.647	0.125
Quality of Life	55.0	27–95	63.0	0–90	0.130	0.421
Pain Score	78.0	0–100	70.0	0–100	0.029	0.622

MS, indicating that it is likely that assessment of specific underlying mechanisms probably is needed to understand nocturia in MS. A low dose of melatonin was chosen (2 mg), because at the time the study was designed there was discussion that melatonin could potentially contribute to deterioration in MS severity through effects on immune function [32]. Based on the results, it seems that this low dose was insufficient for nocturia therapy, even though it is a standard dose for treating sleep disorders in a wider population. Some studies have used higher doses of melatonin in an MS population, demonstrating improved sleep quality [19]. Recent literature does not identify detrimental effect of melatonin on MS severity, and alternative hypotheses have been promulgated regarding a potential beneficial effect. We did not measure endogenous melatonin production, or effective serum melatonin levels on treated patients, so we are unable to state whether serum

levels of the hormone reached therapeutic levels in our study population.

The inclusion of a placebo group is an essential part of LUTS investigation, since placebo responses are noted to be rather big generally [33]. In the current study, the placebo response seen in the bladder diaries and symptom scores was modest. Undertaking observations such as bladder diaries is considered a potential factor that could influence patient behaviour, since completing a bladder diary shows to a patient when they are generating a high urine output, which can feed back on their behaviour. This was not a particular observation in the current study, where the baseline 24 h voided volume was 2.2 L, and was similar during the treatment phases (2.2 L for placebo, and 2.0 L per 24 h for melatonin, medians 2.1 L, 2.2 L, and 2.0 L respectively). The nocturnal polyuria index was unchanged (median 0.32, 0.33, 0.32

Table 5 Median and range for PSQI by treatment, with p-value and standardized effect size, d

Measure	Treatment				p	D
	A: Placebo		B: Melatonin			
	Median	Range	Median	Range		
Overall Score	9.0	2–13	8.0	2–16	0.893	0.036
Sleep Disturbances	2.0	1–3	2.0	1–3	0.092	0.471
Sleep Medication	0.0	0–0	0.0	0–3	0.228	0.333
Sleep Duration	1.0	0–3	1.0	0–3	0.663	0.119
Sleep Latency	1.0	0–5	1.0	0–3	0.927	0.025
Sleep Quality	1.0	0–3	1.0	0–3	0.922	0.027
Daytime Dysfunction	1.0	0–3	1.0	1–3	0.141	0.410
Habitual Sleep Efficiency	2.0	0–3	1.0	0–3	0.114	0.440

Table 6 Median and range for EDSS by treatment with *p*-value and standardized effect size, *d*

Measure	Treatment				*p*	*d*
	A: Placebo		B: Melatonin			
	Median	Range	Median	Range		
Visual	1.0	0–4	1.5	0–4	0.056	0.539
Brainstem	1.0	0–2	1.0	0–2	0.288	0.292
Sensory	3.0	0–4	3.0	0–3	0.090	0.474
Pyramidal	2.0	0–3	2.0	0–3	0.386	0.238
Cerebellar	2.0	1–4	2.0	0–3	0.181	0.370
Cerebral	2.0	0–3	2.0	0–3	0.653	0.123
Bladder and Bowel	2.0	1–3	2.0	0–3	0.674	0.115
Ambulatory	1.0	0–9	1.0	0–9	1.00	0.000
EDSS	4.0	1.5–8	4.0	3–8	0.209	0.347

for baseline, placebo and melatonin respectively). A small reduction in median nocturnal urine output was seen (baseline 741 mL, placebo 651 mL, and melatonin 667 mL), but this was not statistically significant. It did not yield a significant change in nocturia episodes (median 1.70, 1.50 and 1.30 respectively).

There was no clear adverse safety signal. No adverse events appeared to have any clear link to the melatonin therapy on a consistent basis. UTIs were reported, and two episodes of faecal urgency. Single presentations with Uhthoff's phenomenon, feeling drained, cold hands, profound somnolence, and others were also described. The qualitative interviews also identified that fatigue was a key feature. The individual with Uhthoff's phenomenon explains the difference in the visual domain on the EDSS scores, which were otherwise not significantly different for the melatonin and placebo phases.

Conclusions

In summary, a low dose of melatonin taken at bedtime may be an ineffective therapy for nocturia in MS, studying an adult population with nocturia once per night or more often. A different dose regime of melatonin or recruitment selection criteria would need to considered to ascertain whether melatonin could influence nocturia in MS.

Abbreviations

CaMBS: Cambridge Multiple Sclerosis Basic Score; EDSS: Expanded Disability Status Scale; FVC: Frequency volume chart; ICIQ: International Consultation on Incontinence Questionnaires; ICIQ-FLUTS: Female- specific tool for assessing severity and bother of all LUTS; ICIQ-MLUTS: Male-specific tool for assessing severity and bother of all LUTS; ICIQ-N: International Consultation on Incontinence-Nocturia; ICIQ-NQoL: A nocturia-specific quality of life tool which will be used throughout the study; LUTS: Lower urinary tract symptoms; MeNiMS: Study Acronym: Melatonin for Nocturia in Multiple Sclerosis; MS: Multiple sclerosis; MSQLI: Multiple sclerosis quality of life index; PSQI: Pittsburgh Sleep Quality Index

Acknowledgements

Neurim and Flynn Pharma; unrestricted donation of study medication.

Funding

Funded by a Research Project Grant from the MS Society, UK (Grant 959/11) to cover all aspects of setting up, running and analysing the trial.

Authors' contributions

MD Chief Investigator; LC recruitment, data collection; NC data collection, qualitative review; DD ethics application, drafted the manuscript; JH recruitment; KI recruitment, EDSS testing; LJ recruitment, data collection; MCK data analysis, drafted the manuscript; DO recruitment, data collection; PW statistical analysis; DC recruitment, drafted the manuscript. All authors read and approved the final manuscript.

Competing interests

MJD; Research grants, Speaker bureau, advisory boards for Allergan, Astellas, Ferring. Speaker bureau for Hikma and Pfizer. Other authors; not applicable.

Author details

[1]School of Clinical Sciences, University of Bristol, Bristol, UK. [2]Bristol Urological Institute, Southmead Hospital, Bristol BS10 5NB, UK. [3]Neurology Department, Southmead Hospital, Bristol BS10 5NB, UK. [4]University of the West of England, Bristol, UK.

References

1.   Abrams P, Cardozo L, Fall M, Griffiths D, Rosier P, Ulmsten U, van Kerrebroeck P, Victor A, Wein A. The standardisation of terminology of lower urinary tract function: report from the standardisation sub-committee of the international continence society. Neurourol Urodyn. 2002;21(2):167–78.
2.   Bing MH, Moller LA, Jennum P, Mortensen S, Skovgaard LT, Lose G. Prevalence and bother of nocturia, and causes of sleep interruption in a Danish population of men and women aged 60-80 years. BJU Int. 2006; 98(3):599–604.
3.   Stanley N. The underestimated impact of nocturia on quality of life. Eur Urol Suppl. 2005;4:17–9.
4.   Gulur DM, Mevcha AM, Drake MJ. Nocturia as a manifestation of systemic disease. BJU Int. 2011;107(5):702–13.
5.   Lightner DJ, Krambeck AE, Jacobson DJ, McGree ME, Jacobsen SJ, Lieber MM, Roger VL, Girman CJ, St Sauver JL. Nocturia is associated with an increased risk of coronary heart disease and death. BJU Int. 2012;110(6):848–53.
6.   Chancellor MB, Blaivas JG. Urological and sexual problems in multiple sclerosis. Clin Neurosci. 1994;2(3–4):189–95.
7.   Stanton BR, Barnes F, Silber E. Sleep and fatigue in multiple sclerosis. Mult Scler. 2006;12(4):481–6.
8.   Marshall SD, Raskolnikov D, Blanker MH, Hashim H, Kupelian V, Tikkinen KA, Yoshimura K, Drake MJ, Weiss JP. International consultations on urological D: Nocturia: current levels of evidence and recommendations from the international consultation on male lower urinary tract symptoms. Urology. 2015;85(6):1291–9.
9.   Ferreira E, Letwin SR. Desmopressin for nocturia and enuresis associated with multiple sclerosis. Ann Pharmacother. 1998;32(1):114–6.
10. Friedman FM, Weiss JP. Desmopressin in the treatment of nocturia: clinical evidence and experience. Ther Adv Urol. 2013;5(6):310–7.
11. Hamed M, Mitchell H, Clow DJ. Hyponatraemic convulsion associated with desmopressin and imipramine treatment. BMJ. 1993;306(6886):1169.
12. Larney V, Dwyer R. Hyponatraemic convulsions and fatal head injury secondary to desmopressin treatment for enuresis. Eur J Anaesthesiol. 2006;23(10):895–7.
13. Nelson J, Chouinard G. Guidelines for the clinical use of benzodiazepines: pharmacokinetics, dependency, rebound and withdrawal. Canadian Society for Clinical Pharmacology. Can J Clin Pharmacol. 1999;6(2):69–83.
14. Gomez-Pinilla PJ, Gomez MF, Sward K, Hedlund P, Hellstrand P, Camello PJ, Andersson KE, Pozo MJ. Melatonin restores impaired contractility in aged Guinea pig urinary bladder. J Pineal Res. 2008;44(4):416–25.

11. Hamed M, Mitchell H, Clow DJ. Hyponatraemic convulsion associated with desmopressin and imipramine treatment. BMJ. 1993;306(6886):1169.

12. Larney V, Dwyer R. Hyponatraemic convulsions and fatal head injury secondary to desmopressin treatment for enuresis. Eur J Anaesthesiol. 2006;23(10):895–7.

13. Nelson J, Chouinard G. Guidelines for the clinical use of benzodiazepines: pharmacokinetics, dependency, rebound and withdrawal. Canadian Society for Clinical Pharmacology. Can J Clin Pharmacol. 1999;6(2):69–83.

14. Gomez-Pinilla PJ, Gomez MF, Sward K, Hedlund P, Hellstrand P, Camello PJ, Andersson KE, Pozo MJ. Melatonin restores impaired contractility in aged Guinea pig urinary bladder. J Pineal Res. 2008;44(4):416–25.

15. Drake MJ, Mills IW, Noble JG. Melatonin pharmacotherapy for nocturia in men with benign prostatic enlargement. J Urol. 2004;171(3):1199–202.

16. Sugaya K, Nishijima S, Miyazato M, Kadekawa K, Ogawa Y. Effects of melatonin and rilmazafone on nocturia in the elderly. J Int Med Res. 2007; 35(5):685–91.

17. Damasceno A, Moraes AS, Farias A, Damasceno BP, dos Santos LM, Cendes F. Disruption of melatonin circadian rhythm production is related to multiple sclerosis severity: a preliminary study. J Neurol Sci. 2015;353(1–2): 166–8.

18. Melamud L, Golan D, Luboshitzky R, Lavi I, Miller A. Melatonin dysregulation, sleep disturbances and fatigue in multiple sclerosis. J Neurol Sci. 2012; 314(1–2):37–40.

19. Adamczyk-Sowa M, Pierzchala K, Sowa P, Mucha S, Sadowska-Bartosz I, Adamczyk J, Hartel M. Melatonin acts as antioxidant and improves sleep in MS patients. Neurochem Res. 2014;39(8):1585–93.

20. Delgado D, Canham L, Cotterill N, Cottrell D, Drake MJ, Inglis K, Owen D, White P. Protocol for a randomized, double blind, placebo controlled, crossover trial of melatonin for treatment of Nocturia in adults with multiple sclerosis (MeNiMS). BMC Neurol. 2017;17(1):63.

21. Farez MF, Mascanfroni ID, Mendez-Huergo SP, Yeste A, Murugaiyan G, Garo LP, Balbuena Aguirre ME, Patel B, Ysrraelit MC, Zhu C, et al. Melatonin contributes to the seasonality of multiple sclerosis relapses. Cell. 2015;162(6): 1338–52.

22. Polman CH, Reingold SC, Banwell B, Clanet M, Cohen JA, Filippi M, Fujihara K, Havrdova E, Hutchinson M, Kappos L, et al. Diagnostic criteria for multiple sclerosis: 2010 revisions to the McDonald criteria. Ann Neurol. 2011;69(2): 292–302.

23. Abrams P, Avery K, Gardener N, Donovan J. The international consultation on incontinence modular questionnaire: www.iciq.net. J Urol. 2006;175(3 Pt 1):1063–6. discussion 1066

24. Bright E, Cotterill N, Drake M, Abrams P. Developing and validating the international consultation on incontinence questionnaire bladder diary. Eur Urol. 2014;66(2):294–300.

25. Abraham L, Hareendran A, Mills IW, Martin ML, Abrams P, Drake MJ, MacDonagh RP, Noble JG. Development and validation of a quality-of-life measure for men with nocturia. Urology. 2004;63(3):481–6.

26. Kurtzke JF. The disability status scale for multiple sclerosis: apologia pro DSS sua. Neurology. 1989;39(2 Pt 1):291–302.

27. Wellek S, Blettner M. On the proper use of the crossover design in clinical trials: part 18 of a series on evaluation of scientific publications. Dtsch Arztebl Int. 2012;109(15):276–81.

28. Ellis PD: The essential guide to effect sizes statistical power, meta-analysis, and the interpretation of research results. Cambridge University press; 2010.

29. Azur MJ, Stuart EA, Frangakis C, Leaf PJ. Multiple imputation by chained equations: what is it and how does it work? Int J Methods Psychiatr Res. 2011;20(1):40–9.

30. Barun B. Pathophysiological background and clinical characteristics of sleep disorders in multiple sclerosis. Clin Neurol Neurosurg. 2013;115(Suppl 1):S82–5.

31. Cardinali DP, Cano P, Jimenez-Ortega V, Esquifino AI. Melatonin and the metabolic syndrome: physiopathologic and therapeutical implications. Neuroendocrinology. 2011;93(3):133–42.

32. Sandyk R. Multiple sclerosis: the role of puberty and the pineal gland in its pathogenesis. Int J Neurosci. 1993;68(3–4):209–25.

33. Eredics K, Madersbacher S, Schauer I. A relevant mid-term (12 months) placebo effect on lower urinary tract symptoms and maximum flow rate in male LUTS/BPH - a meta-analysis. Urology. 2017.

7

Automated segmentation of cerebral deep gray matter from MRI scans: effect of field strength on sensitivity and reliability

Renxin Chu[1,2], Shelley Hurwitz[5], Shahamat Tauhid[1,2] and Rohit Bakshi[1,2,3,4*] (iD)

Abstract

Background: The cerebral subcortical deep gray matter nuclei (DGM) are a common, early, and clinically-relevant site of atrophy in multiple sclerosis (MS). Robust and reliable DGM segmentation could prove useful to evaluate putative neuroprotective MS therapies. The objective of the study was to compare the sensitivity and reliability of DGM volumes obtained from 1.5T vs. 3T MRI.

Methods: Fourteen patients with MS [age (mean, range) 50.2 (32.0–60.8) years, disease duration 18.4 (8.2–35.5) years, Expanded Disability Status Scale score 3.1 (0–6), median 3.0] and 15 normal controls (NC) underwent brain 3D T1-weighted paired scan-rescans at 1.5T and 3T. DGM (caudate, thalamus, globus pallidus, and putamen) segmentation was obtained by the fully automated FSL-FIRST pipeline. Both raw and normalized volumes were derived.

Results: DGM volumes were generally higher at 3T vs. 1.5T in both groups. For raw volumes, 3T showed slightly better sensitivity (thalamus: $p = 0.02$; caudate: $p = 0.10$; putamen: $p = 0.02$; globus pallidus: $p = 0.0004$; total DGM: $p = 0.01$) than 1.5T (thalamus: $p = 0.05$; caudate: $p = 0.09$; putamen: $p = 0.03$; globus pallidus: $p = 0.0006$; total DGM: $p = 0.02$) for detecting DGM atrophy in MS vs. NC. For normalized volumes, 3T but not 1.5T detected atrophy in the globus pallidus in the MS group. Across all subjects, scan-rescan reliability was generally very high for both platforms, showing slightly higher reliability for some DGM volumes at 3T. Raw volumes showed higher reliability than normalized volumes. Raw DGM volume showed higher reliability than the individual structures.

Conclusions: These results suggest somewhat higher sensitivity and reliability of DGM volumes obtained from 3T vs. 1.5T MRI. Further studies should assess the role of this 3T pipeline in tracking potential MS neurotherapeutic effects.

Keywords: Multiple sclerosis, Subcortical deep gray matter, Atrophy, 3T MRI, Brain segmentation

Background

The cerebral subcortical deep gray matter nuclei (DGM) are a common and clinically-relevant site of atrophy, beginning in the early stages of multiple sclerosis (MS) [1–4]. In addition, DGM atrophy is a feature of progressive forms of the disease and can be shown to progress in as little as 1 year [5, 6]. Given that few treatments are available for patients with progressive forms of MS [7], this represents a major unmet need, calling for the

availability of new outcome measures to screen putative therapies. MRI-defined cerebral lesion activity and total burden, traditionally used in trials of patients with relapsing forms of MS [8–10], are less sensitive to change in patients with advanced disability and progressive forms of the disease [11, 12]. In one study, DGM atrophy assessment over 1 year was successful in demonstrating a treatment effect in MS [5]. Therefore, robust, sensitive, and reliable segmentation of DGM structures could prove useful in the evaluation of new MS therapies in all stages of the disease [6].

Field strength is known to bias the sensitivity and detectability of global cerebral MRI-based assessments of lesions and atrophy in MS [13–15]. The most commonly available MRI platforms employed for routine

* Correspondence: rbakshi@post.harvard.edu
[1]Laboratory for Neuroimaging Research, Brigham and Women's Hospital, Harvard Medical School, 60 Fenwood Rd, Mailbox 9002L, Boston, MA 02115, USA
[2]Departments of Neurology, Brigham and Women's Hospital, Harvard Medical School, Boston, MA, USA
Full list of author information is available at the end of the article

clinical care and research investigations are 1.5T and, less commonly, 3T. To date, it has not been clear whether longitudinal cerebral atrophy determinations would benefit from higher field strength acquisitions. The purpose of this study was to employ a fully automated freely available segmentation pipeline to compare the sensitivity and reliability of DGM volumetrics obtained from 1.5T vs. 3T MRI scans in normal controls (NCs) and patients with MS.

Methods

Subjects and neurologic examination

Fourteen patients with MS and 15 normal controls (NCs) were recruited to undergo brain MRI at both 1.5T and 3T. Table 1 shows the demographic and clinical characteristics of the subjects. The two groups differed on age ($p = 0.0009$) but not sex ($p = 0.43$). Patients met the International Panel criteria for either MS or a clinically isolated demyelinating syndrome (CIS) [16]. All patients underwent an examination by an MS specialist neurologist including evaluation of the Expanded Disability Status Scale (EDSS) [17] score and timed 25-ft walk (T25FW) [18]. At the time of MRI, 10 patients were on disease modifying therapy (DMT), while 4 patients were not. Among the DMTs used, four subjects were on dimethyl fumarate, three were on natalizumab, and one each were on fingolimod, glatiramer acetate, or cyclophosphamide. None of the DMTs were started in the 3 months before MRI. Our hospital's human research ethics board (The Partners Human Research Committee) approved this study and written informed consent was obtained on all subjects. This work was presented in preliminary form at the 2015 annual meeting of the European Committee on Treatment and Research in Multiple Sclerosis (ECTRIMS), Barcelona, Spain; and at the 2016 annual meeting of the American Academy of Neurology, Vancouver, Canada.

MRI acquisition

All subjects underwent brain MRI at 1.5T (Signa; General Electric, Milwaukee, WI) and 3T (Skyra; Siemens, Erlangen, Germany). Scanner and acquisition details are show in Table 2. On both platforms, we obtained high-resolution 3D T1-weighted sequences covering the whole head. These were matched as closely as possible on voxel size and acquisition time, considering practical scan time limits for patient tolerability. Each sequence was optimized for signal-to-noise based on previous clinically-routine development. Each subject had a scan followed by a re-scan on the same day on each platform. Thus, at each field strength, two scans were acquired from each subject, where the subject was removed from the scanner between scans for a few minutes, and was repositioned and rescanned by the MRI technologist. For all subjects, except three, the 1.5T and 3T imaging was performed on the same day for a given subject. For the remaining three subjects, the interval between 1.5T and 3T acquistion was 6, 16, or 47 days. During the study period, there were no intervening scanner upgrades.

MRI analysis

All image pre-processing was performed using Jim software (v.7.0, Xinapse Systems Ltd., Northants, UK, http://www.xinapse.com/). For both the 1.5T and 3T

Table 1 Demographic and clinical characteristics

	MS (*n* = 14)	NC (*n* = 15)
Sex ratio (women/men)[a]	0.79 (11/3)	0.60 (9/6)
Age, years[a]	50.2 ± 8.2 (32–60)	37.7 ± 9.6 (25–52)
MS disease category, n (%)		
-Progressive relapsing MS	1 (7%)	–
-Secondary progressive MS	3 (21%)	–
-CIS or relapsing-remitting MS	10 (71%)	–
Disease duration, years[b]	18.4 ± 10.7 (8.2–35.5)	–
EDSS score	3.1 ± 2.1 (0–6) (median 3.0)	–
Timed 25-ft walk, seconds	6.2 ± 2.7 (3.5–13.0)	–

Key: Data are mean ± standard deviation (range) unless otherwise indicated; *MS* multiple sclerosis, *NC* normal controls, *CIS* clinically isolated demyelinating syndrome, *EDSS* Expanded Disability Status Scale; [a]MS vs. NC were different on age ($p = 0.0009$) but not on sex ($p = 0.43$); [b]Time from first symptoms; n = number of subjects

Table 2 1.5T and 3T brain MRI acquisition protocols

	1.5T	3T
Scanner manufacturer	GE Signa LX	Siemens Skyra
Operation system version	11×	D13
Coil	Quadrature head coil	20-channel head and neck coil
Type of sequence	3D SPGR	3D MPRAGE
Acceleration factor for parallel imaging	N/A	2
Orientation	Sagittal	Sagittal
Field of view (cm)	24 × 24	24 × 25.6
Matrix size	256 × 256	240 × 256
Number of slices	166	176
Repetition time (msec)	8.176	2300
Echo time (msec)	3.856	2.96
Flip angle (degrees)	20	9
Voxel size (mm)	0.938 × 0.938 × 1.2	1.0 × 1.0 × 1.0
Scan time (minutes)	6:24	5:12
Number of signal averages	1	1

Key: *SPGR* spoiled gradient recalled echo, *MPRAGE* magnetization-prepared rapid acquisition gradient echo

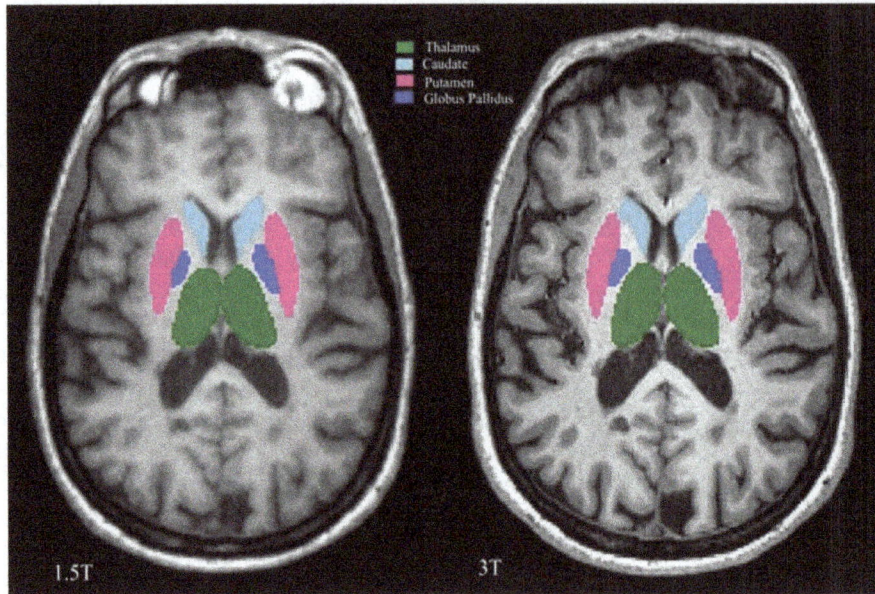

Fig. 1 Representative anatomic slice showing segmentation of the cerebral subcortical deep gray matter (DGM) in one patient from 1.5T (left) and 3T (right) MRI scans. This is from a 51 year-old woman with multiple sclerosis and moderate physical disability. The total DGM volume was 28.4 ml at 1.5T and 29.3 ml at 3T. Component DGM structures are shown in different colors. The segmentation maps are overlaid to the original raw 3D T1-weighted images after re-sampling to the axial plane. Segmentation was performed by the fully automated FSL-FIRST pipeline. In the present study, we utilized the FSL-FIRST outputs to assess the volume of the thalamus, caudate, putamen, and globus pallidus (and their sum = total DGM)

Table 3 Deep gray matter data: scan-rescan reliability (within group and field strengths)

	MS (*n* = 14)		NC (*n* = 15)	
	1.5T ICC (95% CI)	3T ICC (95% CI)	1.5T ICC (95% CI)	3T ICC (95% CI)
Volumes				
-Thalamus	0.99 (0.96, 1.00)	0.99 (0.98, 1.00)	0.95 (0.87, 0.98)	0.99 (0.97, 1.00)
-Caudate	0.99 (0.98, 1.00)	0.99 (0.98, 1.00)	0.97 (0.93, 0.99)	0.96 (0.88, 0.98)
-Putamen	0.94 (0.85, 0.98)	0.97 (0.90, 0.99)	0.95 (0.87, 0.98)	0.97 (0.93, 0.99)
-Globus pallidus	0.94 (0.83, 0.98)	0.98 (0.95, 0.99)	0.95 (0.87, 0.98)	0.98 (0.93, 0.99)
-Total DGM	0.99 (0.97, 1.00)	1.00 (0.99, 1.00)	0.98 (0.94, 0.99)	0.99 (0.98, 1.00)
Fractions				
-Thalamus	0.98 (0.95, 0.99)	0.95 (0.87, 0.98)	0.88 (0.71, 0.96)	0.93 (0.81, 0.97)
-Caudate	0.98 (0.94, 0.99)	0.94 (0.84, 0.98)	0.96 (0.88, 0.98)	0.88 (0.69, 0.95)
-Putamen	0.92 (0.78, 0.97)	0.92 (0.78, 0.97)	0.93 (0.81, 0.97)	0.95 (0.86, 0.98)
-Globus pallidus	0.93 (0.80, 0.97)	0.95 (0.85, 0.98)	0.93 (0.81, 0.97)	0.85 (0.63, 0.94)
-Total DGM	0.98 (0.93, 0.99)	0.93 (0.80, 0.97)	0.94 (0.84, 0.98)	0.89 (0.72, 0.96)
Normalized				
-Thalamus	0.95 (0.87, 0.98)	0.99 (0.96, 0.99)	0.96 (0.89, 0.99)	0.96 (0.88, 0.98)
-Caudate	0.97 (0.90, 0.99)	0.98 (0.95, 0.99)	0.97 (0.93, 0.99)	0.92 (0.78, 0.97)
-Putamen	0.94 (0.83, 0.98)	0.97 (0.92, 0.99)	0.93 (0.81, 0.97)	0.95 (0.86, 0.98)
-Globus pallidus	0.92 (0.77, 0.97)	0.97 (0.92, 0.99)	0.97 (0.92, 0.99)	0.93 (0.82, 0.98)
-Total DGM	0.95 (0.87, 0.98)	0.98 (0.95, 0.99)	0.97 (0.93, 0.99)	0.95 (0.85, 0.98)

Key: *MS* multiple sclerosis, *NC* normal controls, *DGM* cerebral subcortical deep gray matter, *CI* confidence interval, *ICC* intraclass correlation coefficient; normalized = raw volume multiplied by SIENAX normalization factor images, the raw sagittal images did not yield adequate segmentation, particularly of the intracranial volume (ICV) cavity ("skull stripping"; data not shown). With optimization work, we determined necessary pre-processing steps, which were the same for the 1.5T and 3T images. First, all original DICOM images were converted to a Neuroimaging Informatics Technology Initiative (NIfTI) format, and their raw sagittal orientation was converted to axial. Then, 170 axial slices were extracted from each scan starting at the first slice showing the top of the head. This provided whole brain coverage in all patients extending to the foramen magnum. DGM (caudate, thalamus, globus pallidus, and putamen) volumes were obtained by a fully automated segmentation pipeline (FSL-FIRST, v. 5.0, The Analysis Group, Oxford, UK, http://fsl.fmrib.ox.ac.uk/fsl/fslwiki/FIRST) (Fig. 1). This pipeline was chosen for its free availability, full automation, and utility shown in detecting short term DGM atrophy and treatment effects in patients with MS [5, 6]. The ICV was the sum of gray matter, white matter and cerebrospinal fluid (CSF), which was obtained by applying these images to a fully automated algorithm (SIENAX, v. 5.0, The Analysis Group, Oxford, UK, http://fsl.fmrib.ox.ac.uk/fsl/fslwiki/SIENA) [15, 19]. We assessed three volumetric measures of the DGM structures: 1) raw volumes, 2) those that were normalized by dividing by the subject's ICV ("fractions" [1]); 3) those that were normalized by multiplying the raw volume by the whole brain SIENAX normalization factor ("normalized").

Statistical Analysis

Statistical analyses included unpaired and paired t-tests, Fisher's exact tests, and analysis of covariance with age as a covariate. Correlations were reported for MRI associations with age, EDSS score, and T25FW by Spearman coefficients. Sensitivity (differentiation between groups) was reported using mixed model analysis of covariance with age as covariate, comparing the methods for their ability to differentiate MS from NC by the interaction between method and group. Within-subject correlations were compared using the method of Meng et al. (1992) [20]. Reliability was reported using intraclass correlation coefficients (ICCs) [21] with 95% confidence intervals (CIs). The analysis was generated using SAS (v. 9.4, SAS Institute Inc., Cary, NC, http://www.sas.com/).

Results

Scan-rescan reliability: 1.5T vs. 3T

DGM scan-rescan reliability within groups, comparing field strengths, is shown in Table 3 for all three methods. Reliability was generally very high for both the 1.5T and 3T measurements. Regarding raw volumes, there was perhaps somewhat higher reliability at 3T and, across all comparisons, higher reliability for measuring total DGM than the individual structures. Regarding fractions and normalized volumes, there was a suggestion of higher reliability at 1.5T for the caudate. Comparing the three methods, there was slightly higher reliability for measuring raw volumes than fractions or normalized volumes. We determined that the latter were more reliable at 1.5T most likely due to increased accuracy vs. 3T in

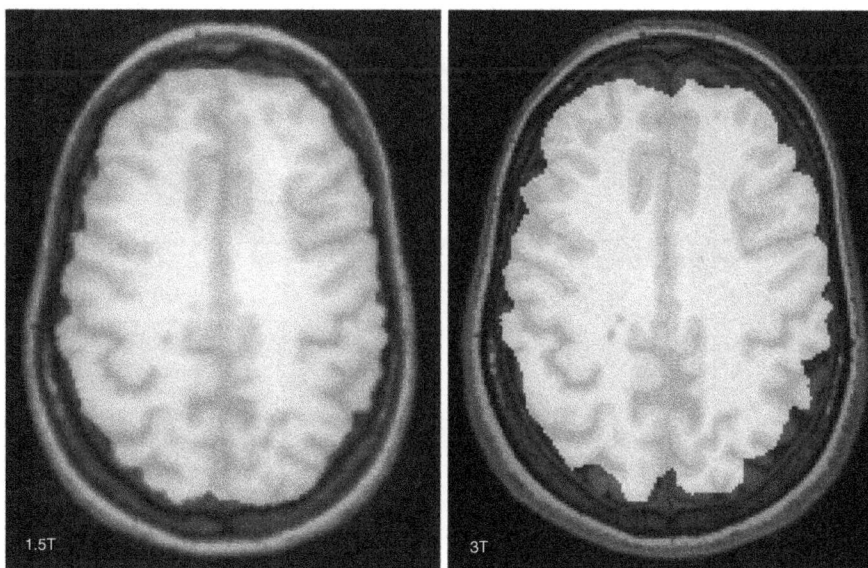

Fig. 2 Examples of brain extraction masks obtained in the fully automated SIENAX pipeline, part of the process to determine intracranial volume. Both images are from a 51 year-old woman with multiple sclerosis and moderate physical disability. The brain parenchymal mask was more accurately obtained at 1.5T, whereas it is underestimated at 3T

Table 4 Deep gray matter data: between group and between field strength comparisons

	DGM structure	MS group (n = 14)			NC group (n = 15)			p[a, b] MS vs NC	
		1.5T	3T	p (MS) 1.5T vs. 3T	1.5T	3T	P (NC) 1.5T vs 3T	1.5T	3T
Volumes (ml)	Thalamus	14.4 (1.4) 11.7–16.3	14.7 (1.5) 12.6–16.7	0.003	15.2 (1.0) 12.9–16.3	16.0 (1.0) 13.6–17.1	<0.0001	0.05	0.02
	Caudate	6.2 (0.9) 4.9–7.8	6.5 (0.9) 5.0–8.2	0.0001	6.9 (0.8) 5.2–8.6	7.3 (0.9) 5.6–9.4	<0.0001	0.09	0.10
	Putamen	8.7 (0.7) 7.4–9.7	9.0 (0.7) 7.6–10.1	<0.0001	9.6 (0.8) 8.6–11.7	10.1 (0.9) 9.1–12.6	<0.0001	0.03	0.02
	Globus pallidus	2.9 (0.3) 2.4–3.4	3.1 (0.4) 2.6–3.9	0.0004	3.3 (0.3) 2.9–3.7	3.6 (0.3) 3.2–4.0	<0.0001	0.0006	0.0004
	Total DGM	32.2 (2.8) 26.4–37.1	33.4 (3.0) 28.1–38.6	<0.0001	35.0 (2.6) 30.9–40.2	37.0 (2.6) 32.8–42.8	<0.0001	0.02	0.01
Fractions	Thalamus	0.011 (0.0011) 0.0087–0.013	0.012 (0.00097) 0.0096–0.013	0.12	0.0116 (0.00058) 0.010–0.013	0.012 (0.00063) 0.011–0.013	0.0004	0.31	0.23
	Caudate	0.0049 (0.00057) 0.0037–0.0056	0.0051 (0.00058) 0.0040–0.0059	0.007	0.0053 (0.00046) 0.0040–0.0060	0.0055 (0.00053) 0.0043–0.0066	0.0004	0.20	0.30
	Putamen	0.0068 (0.00055) 0.0055–0.0078	0.0071 (0.00057) 0.0057–0.0080	0.0001	0.0074 (0.00051) 0.0065–0.0081	0.0077 (0.00053) 0.0068–0.0088	<0.0001	0.20	0.20
	Globus pallidus	0.0023 (0.00021) 0.0018–0.0026	0.0024 (0.00024) 0.0020–0.0028	0.0002	0.0025 (0.00017) 0.0023–0.0028	0.0028 (0.00013) 0.0025–0.0030	<0.0001	0.009	0.003
	Total DGM	0.0252 (0.0020) 0.0197–0.0282	0.0261 (0.0019) 0.0213–0.0280	0.002	0.0268 (0.0013) 0.0236–0.0290	0.0282 (0.0013) 0.0256–0.0299	<0.0001	0.11	0.07

Key: Data are mean (standard deviation) on first line; range on second line; Percent differences between 1.5T and 3T are shown in Table 5; DGM = cerebral subcortical deep gray matter; MS multiple sclerosis, NC normal controls; [a] age adjusted; [b] the differentiation (sensitivity) between MS and NC was similar for 1.5 versus 3T (all $p > 0.05$)

whole brain extraction, necessary for determination of the ICV and brain size (Fig. 2).

DGM results: 1.5T vs. 3T

Using all three methods, DGM volumes were higher at 3T than 1.5T in both patients and controls (Tables 4 and 5). This was seen across all DGM structures examined, and significant for all comparisons (except thalamic fractions in the MS group). The effect sizes were generally larger for this field strength difference for raw volumes than fractions (Tables 4 and 5) or normalized volumes (Table 5). This effect was also reflected in total DGM data. For example, the total raw DGM volume was, on average, 3.9% higher in patients and 5.9% higher in controls (Table 5) at 3T vs. 1.5T (both $p < 0.0001$, Table 4). As shown in Figs. 3 and 4, we explored the possible causes for the increased DGM volume at 3T by performing expert, manual segmentation of one scan each from a healthy control and a patient with MS. The manual segmentations were then overlaid on the automated segmentation maps. The 3T images provided a more accurate (and larger) contour of DGM structures. This was most likely related to improved contrast at the ventricular CSF-tissue interfaces, and to a lesser extent, the gray-white edges.

Detection of DGM atrophy in MS vs. NC

A comparison of DGM volume and fraction in MS vs. NC is shown in Table 4. 3T showed slightly better

Table 5 Deep gray matter data: field strength comparisons: percent differences

	DGM structure	MS 1.5T vs. 3T	NC 1.5T vs. 3T
Volumes	Thalamus	2.7%	5.7%
	Caudate	4.8%	5.0%
	Putamen	4.1%	5.3%
	Globus pallidus	7.9%	10.4%
	Total DGM	3.9%	5.9%
Fractions	Thalamus	2.4%	5.2%
	Caudate	4.5%	4.5%
	Putamen	3.7%	4.8%
	Globus pallidus	7.5%	9.8%
	Total DGM	3.6%	5.4%
Normalized	Thalamus	3.2%	4.6%
	Caudate	5.3%	3.9%
	Putamen	4.6%	4.2%
	Globus pallidus	8.4%	9.2%
	Total DGM	4.4%	4.8%

Key: For each subject, the percent difference for 3T data minus 1.5T data was calculated, using the 1.5T data as the denominator. The averages of those percentages are shown for each group. DGM = cerebral subcortical deep gray matter; MS multiple sclerosis, NC normal controls; normalized = raw volume x SIENAX normalization factor

differentiation of raw volumes (thalamus: $p = 0.02$; caudate: $p = 0.10$; putamen: $p = 0.02$; globus pallidus: $p = 0.0004$; total DGM: $p = 0.01$) than 1.5T (thalamus: $p = 0.05$; caudate: $p = 0.09$; putamen: $p = 0.03$; globus pallidus: $p = 0.0006$; total DGM: $p = 0.02$) for detecting DGM atrophy in MS vs. NC. Regarding the normalized volumes, atrophy was not detected in patients vs. NC in any structures at either field strength ($p > 0.05$) except for the globus pallidus at 3T (mean 4.4 vs. 5.0 ml, $p < 0.05$). Thus, thalamic and pallidal atrophy was detected slightly more definitively at 3T. Otherwise, the presence of atrophy in the other DGM structures was similarly detected at both 1.5T and 3T. Overall, these field strength differences in the ability to differentiate MS from NC were small (all $p > 0.10$). Comparing raw, fractional, and normalized volumes, there was slightly better sensitivity for detecting atrophy in the MS group for the raw volumes.

Correlation between DGM and age or disability in the MS group

With the exception of the normalized putamen volume at 1.5T ($r = -0.56$, $p = 0.04$), DGM raw or normalized volumes and fractions at 1.5T or 3T did not correlate with age; the correlations were also not different between field strengths (all $p > 0.05$, data not shown). Regarding the correlation between DGM and EDSS scores, significant negative relationships were found with normalized volumes at 1.5T in the thalamus ($r = -0.61$, $p = 0.02$), globus pallidus ($r = -0.53$, $p = 0.0498$), and total DGM ($r = -0.56$, $p = 0.04$) and at 3T in the putamen ($r = -0.56$, $p = 0.04$). No significant correlations were found at either field strength between DGM raw volumes or fractions and EDSS scores (all $p > 0.05$, data not shown). The correlations were not different between field strengths (all $p > 0.05$, data not shown). Regarding the correlation between DGM and T25FW, with the exception of total DGM normalized volume ($r = -0.55$, $p = 0.04$), none of the comparisons reached significance (data not shown).

Discussion

In this study, we explored the sensitivity and reliability of DGM volumes obtained from 1.5T vs. 3T and their clinical relevance. The first main finding was that volumes were generally higher at 3T. Secondly, 3T showed slightly better differentiation in the ability to detect atrophy in the thalamus and globus pallidus in MS vs. NC. Third, 3T showed slightly higher scan/re-scan reliability. We also noted that, regardless of field strength, volumes showed higher reliability than fractions, and total DGM volume was measured with higher reliability than the individual DGM nuclei. These data indicate that 1.5T and 3T are not interchangeable in measuring DGM volumes.

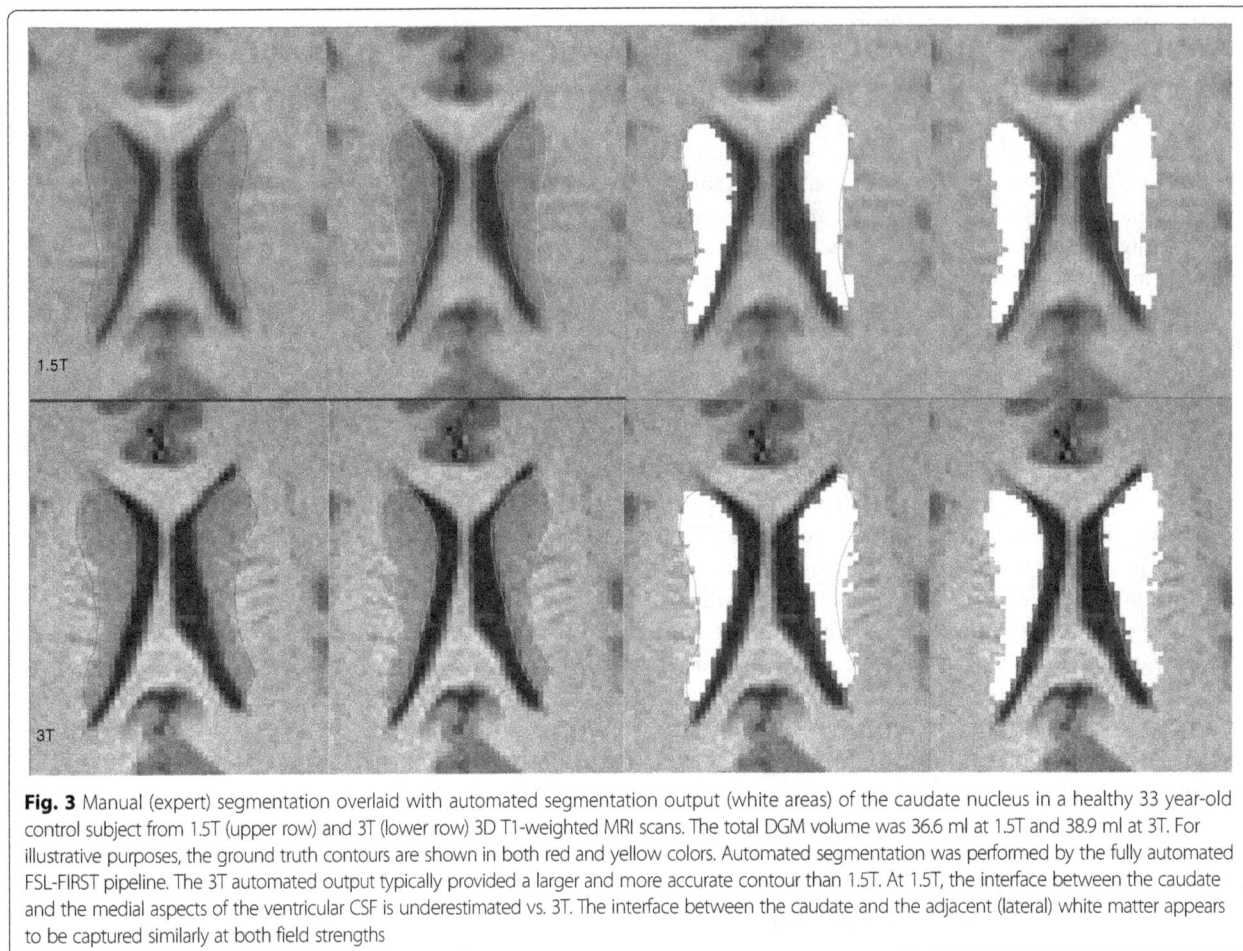

Fig. 3 Manual (expert) segmentation overlaid with automated segmentation output (white areas) of the caudate nucleus in a healthy 33 year-old control subject from 1.5T (upper row) and 3T (lower row) 3D T1-weighted MRI scans. The total DGM volume was 36.6 ml at 1.5T and 38.9 ml at 3T. For illustrative purposes, the ground truth contours are shown in both red and yellow colors. Automated segmentation was performed by the fully automated FSL-FIRST pipeline. The 3T automated output typically provided a larger and more accurate contour than 1.5T. At 1.5T, the interface between the caudate and the medial aspects of the ventricular CSF is underestimated vs. 3T. The interface between the caudate and the adjacent (lateral) white matter appears to be captured similarly at both field strengths

One clear finding was that raw volumes, fractions, and normalized volumes were higher at 3T vs. 1.5T across all DGM structures examined. In a previous study, volume biases were also detected based on field strength in comparing 1.5T to 3T using the FreeSurfer processing toolkit in 15 healthy elderly subjects; these occurred in either direction (not always higher at 3T) [22]. For example, the globus pallidus and thalamus showed significantly higher volumes at 1.5T but the amygdala was higher at 3T. Another study of whole brain volume measurements, comparing 1.5T and 3T MRI showed significant differences between platforms using the SIENAX toolkit [15]. Interestingly, this study found that the bias was in the opposite direction vs. the present study, with higher whole brain volumes measures from 1.5T. This was most likely related to an overestimation of brain volume at the sulcal-CSF interfaces at 1.5T due to partial volume averaging. In the present study, the DGM volumes from 3T may have been larger on the basis of more accurate detection of structure boundaries with CSF or adjacent white matter. Taken together, these results suggest that combining data across platforms and across field-strength introduces a bias that should be

considered in the design of multi-site studies, such as clinical therapeutic trials.

In the detection of DGM atrophy in MS vs. NC in the present study, 3T showed slightly better differentiation. Similar findings were seen in a previous study in detecting hippocampal atrophy at 3T vs. 1.5T [23]. In that study, subjects who converted from mild cognitive impairment to Alzheimer disease within 3 years of baseline MRI showed significantly more atrophy in the cornu ammonis 1 region of the right hippocampus versus nonconverters at 3T but not at 1.5T. Another study, focusing on whole brain atrophy, showed a higher effect size for 3T in detecting brain atrophy in MS versus NC when compared to 1.5T [15]. These results parallel what has been shown regarding MS lesion detection at 3T and 7T, with an increase in the diagnostic yield in the detection of MS brain lesions compared to 1.5T [14, 24]; moreover, the brain lesion load at 3T showed a closer relationship to cognitive status than 1.5T [14]. These results underscore potential gains in sensitivity and validity in the MRI measurement of MS-related structural changes with ultra-high field strengths.

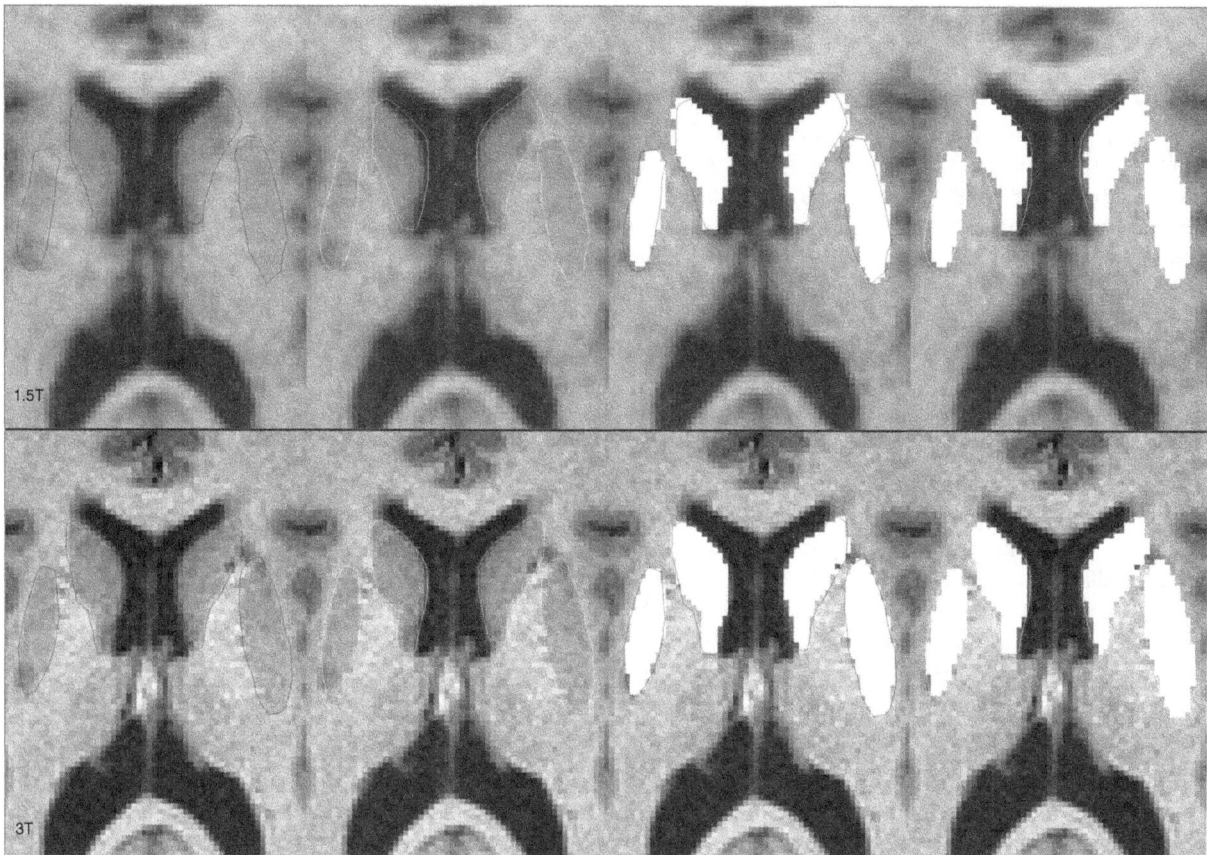

Fig. 4 Manual (expert) segmentation overlaid with automated segmentation output (white areas) of the caudate nucleus and putamen from 1.5T (upper row) and 3T (lower row) 3D T1-weighted MRI scans. Images are from a 51 year-old woman with multiple sclerosis and moderate physical disability. The total DGM volume was 28.4 ml at1.5T and 29.3 ml at 3T. For illustrative purposes, the ground truth contours are shown in both red and yellow colors. Automated segmentation was performed by the fully automated FSL-FIRST pipeline. The 3T automated output typically provided a larger and more accurate contour than 1.5T. At 1.5T, the interface between the caudate and the anterior and medial aspects of the ventricular CSF is underestimated vs. 3T. The interface between the putamen and the adjacent (lateral) white matter appears to be larger and more accurate at 3T

In the present study, we found atrophy of the DGM in patients with MS vs. NC in various nuclei. There are several mechanisms to consider in the pathogenesis of MS-related DGM atrophy. These include iron-deposition [25], oxidative stress [26], neurodegeneration [27], direct injury by the presence of DGM demyelinating lesions [28], and Wallerian degeneration due to damage of white matter tracts throughout the brain [29].

In a previous study, scan-rescan reliability for a variety of platforms at two field strengths was explored [30]. Their results showed that reliability of automatic brain morphometry obtained by FreeSurfer was generally higher with GE Signa Excite (1.5T) and Siemens Verio (3T) vs. Siemens Sonata (1.5T) and TrioTim (3T) acquisitions. The authors argued that, although TrioTim and Verio are both 3T MRI models from the same manufacture (Siemens), the results from the two machines differed significantly. Another group compared 3T Siemens scanners at seven sites to evaluate the difference between intra-scanner and inter-scanner reliability

of lesion and atrophy-related MS volumetrics in a human phantom study using a variety of processing pipelines [31]; the authors showed that, despite protocol harmonization and the use of high-resolution sequences, a large degree of variability in the data was caused by inter-scanner effects. In the present study, we showed high scan-rescan reliabilities for both 1.5T and 3T in the assessment of DGM volumetry. In the measurement of DGM raw volumes, there was perhaps slightly higher reliability at 3T. However, for DGM fractions, there was perhaps somewhat higher reliability at 1.5T. Raw volumes showed slightly higher reliability than the other two normalized methods. Also, the most sensitivity in detecting DGM atrophy was observed with raw DGM volumes. This probably reflects the inaccurate estimation of ICV and the brain contour, necessary for normalization, due to higher susceptibility artifacts at 3T.

Several limitations of our study are worthy of comment. First, aside from the field strength difference, the two acquisitions differed on the scanner vendor, type of head coil, and use of parallel imaging (only at 3T). The voxel sizes also slightly differed. One should also consider the potential effect of DMTs on brain volume; first because of their partial but significant therapeutic effects on limiting the rate of atrophy in MS [3, 5, 6, 32]. Because most of our patients were receiving DMT, the generazibility of our results to untreated patients is not established by this study. Furthermore, there is the potential for individuals to show pseudoatrophy in the few months after their initiation of therapy (for some but not all DMTs) [33]. However, in the present study, none of patients had newly started their DMT in the previous 3 months, thus indicating that pseudoatrophy did not have a major effect on our results. In addition, the sample size was small and no longitudinal data were available to compare the rate of atrophy between the two acquisitions. We did not test other fully automated segmentation pipelines such as FreeSurfer and others that are available to measure DGM atrophy [31, 34–36]. Finally, our patient population was dominated by subjects with relapsing forms of MS, with only four people in our study having progressive forms of the disease. Thus, the generalizability of our results to the full MS spectrum would require further study. Thus, taken together, these caveats suggest other factors that could have influenced the differences we observed between the two MRI scan platforms.

Conclusion

We conclude that MRI scan acquisition field strength should be considered in the design of longitudinal studies and multicenter clinical trials. Such differences may introduce bias in the obtained data and results. If such consistency cannot be maintained, statistically corrective modelling may be considered [37, 38].

Abbreviations

CI: Confidence interval; CIS: Clinically isolated demyelinating syndrome; CSF: Cerebrospinal fluid; DGM: Cerebral subcortical deep gray matter nuclei; ICC: Intraclass correlation coefficient; ICV: Intracranial volume; MS: Multiple sclerosis; NC: Normal controls; NIfTI: Neuroimaging informatics technology initiative; T25FW: Timed 25-ft walk

Acknowledgements
None.

Funding
There are no relevant external funding sources.

Authors' contributions

RB conceived the study and designed the protocol. RC performed the image analysis. ST provided technical assistance and study supervision. SH provided statistical analysis. RB and RC drafted the manuscript. ST and SH edited the manuscript for critical content. RB provided overall study supervision. All authors read and approved the final version of the manuscript.

Competing interests
The authors declare that they have no competing interests.

Author details
[1]Laboratory for Neuroimaging Research, Brigham and Women's Hospital, Harvard Medical School, 60 Fenwood Rd, Mailbox 9002L, Boston, MA 02115, USA. [2]Departments of Neurology, Brigham and Women's Hospital, Harvard Medical School, Boston, MA, USA. [3]Radiology, Brigham and Women's Hospital, Harvard Medical School, Boston, MA, USA. [4]Partners MS Center, Brigham and Women's Hospital, Harvard Medical School, Boston, MA, USA. [5]Department of Medicine, Brigham and Women's Hospital, Harvard Medical School, Boston, MA, USA.

References
1. Houtchens MK, Benedict RH, Killiany R, Sharma J, Jaisani Z, Singh B, et al. Thalamic atrophy and cognition in multiple sclerosis. Neurology. 2007;69:1213–23.
2. Bergsland N, Horakova D, Dwyer MG, Dolezal O, Seidl ZK, Vaneckova M, et al. Subcortical and cortical gray matter atrophy in a large sample of patients with clinically isolated syndrome and early relapsing-remitting multiple sclerosis. AJNR Am J Neuroradiol. 2012;33:1573–8.
3. Bakshi R, Dandamudi VSR, Neema M, De C, Bermel RA. Measurement of brain and spinal cord atrophy by magnetic resonance imaging as a tool to monitor multiple sclerosis. J Neuroimaging. 2005;15:30S–45S.
4. Nourbakhsh B, Azevedo C, Maghzi AH, Spain R, Pelletier D, Waubant E. Subcortical grey matter volumes predict subsequent walking function in early multiple sclerosis. J Neurol Sci. 2016;366:229–33.
5. Dupuy SL, Tauhid S, Hurwitz S, Chu R, Yousuf F, Bakshi R. The effect of dimethyl fumarate on cerebral gray matter atrophy in multiple sclerosis. Neurol Ther. 2016;5:215–29.
6. Kim G, Chu R, Yousuf F, Tauhid S, Stazzone L, Houtchens MK, et al. Sample size requirements for 1 year treatment effects using deep gray matter volume from 3T MRI in progressive forms of multiple sclerosis. Int J Neurosci. [Epub ahead of print]. doi:10.1080/00207454.2017.1283313.
7. Ontaneda D, Fox RJ, Chataway J. Clinical trials in progressive multiple sclerosis: lessons learned and future perspectives. Lancet Neurol. 2015;14:208–23.
8. Filippi M, Rocca MA, Arnold DL, Bakshi R, Barkhof F, De Stefano N, et al. EFNS guideline on the use of neuroimaging in the management of multiple sclerosis. Eur J Neurol. 2006;13:313–25.
9. Filippi M, Wolinsky JS, Comi G. CORAL Study Group. Effects of oral glatiramer acetate on clinical and MRI-monitored disease activity in patients with relapsing multiple sclerosis: a multicentre, double-blind, randomised, placebo-controlled study. Lancet Neurol. 2006;5:213–20.
10. Zivadinov R, Bakshi R. Role of MRI in multiple sclerosis I: inflammation and lesions. Front Biosci. 2004;9:665–83.
11. Li DK, Held U, Petkau J, Daumer M, Barkhof F, Fazekas F, et al. MRI T2 lesion burden in multiple sclerosis: a plateauing relationship with clinical disability. Neurology. 2006;66:1384–9.
12. Zurawski J, Lassmann H, Bakshi R. Use of magnetic resonance imaging to visualize leptomeningeal inflammation in patients with multiple sclerosis: A review. JAMA Neurol. 2017;74:100–9.
13. Sicotte NL, Voskuhl RR, Bouvier S, Klutch R, Cohen MS, Mazziotta JC. Comparison of multiple sclerosis lesions at 1.5 and 3.0 Tesla. Investig Radiol. 2003;38:423–7.
14. Stankiewicz JM, Glanz BI, Healy BC, Arora A, Neema M, Benedict RH, et al. Brain MRI lesion load at 1.5T and 3T versus clinical status in multiple sclerosis. J Neuroimaging. 2011;21:e50–6.
15. Chu R, Tauhid S, Glanz BI, Healy BC, Kim G, Oommen VV, et al. whole brain volume measured from 1.5T versus 3T MRI in healthy subjects and patients with multiple sclerosis. J Neuroimaging. 2016;26:62–7.
16. Polman CH, Reingold SC, Edan G, Filippi M, Hartung HP, Kappos L, et al. Diagnostic criteria for multiple sclerosis: 2005 revisions to the "McDonald Criteria". Ann Neurol. 2005;58:840–6.
17. Kurtzke JF. Rating neurologic impairment in multiple sclerosis: an expanded disability status scale (EDSS). Neurology. 1983;33:1444–52.
18. Fischer JS, Rudick RA, Cutter GR, Reingold SC. The multiple sclerosis functional composite measure (MSFC): an integrated approach to MS clinical outcome assessment. National MS Society Clinical Outcomes Assessment Task Force. Mult Scler. 1999;5:244–50.

19. Kalavathi P, Prasath VB. Methods on skull stripping of MRI head scan images–a review. J Digit Imaging. 2016;29:365–79.

20. Meng X, Rosenthal R, Rubin DB. Comparing correlated correlation coefficients. Psychol Bull. 1992;111:172–5.

21. Winer BJ, Dr B, Michels KM. Statistical Principles in Experimental Design. 2nd ed. New York: McGraw-Hill; 1971.

22. Jovicich J, Czanner S, Han X, Salat D, van der Kouwe A, Quinn B, et al. MRI-derived measurements of human subcortical, ventricular and intracranial brain volumes: Reliability effects of scan sessions, acquisition sequences, data analyses, scanner upgrade, scanner vendors and field strengths. NeuroImage. 2009;46:177–92.

23. Chow N, Hwang KS, Hurtz S, Green AE, Somme JH, Thompson PM, et al. Comparing 3T and 1.5T MRI for mapping hippocampal atrophy in the Alzheimer's Disease Neuroimaging Initiative. AJNR Am J Neuroradiol. 2015;36:653–60.

24. Kollia K, Maderwald S, Putzki N, Schlamann M, Theysohn JM, Kraff O, et al. First clinical study on ultra-high-field MR imaging in patients with multiple sclerosis: comparison of 1.5T and 7T. AJNR Am J Neuroradiol. 2009;30:699–702.

25. Neema M, Arora A, Healy BC, Guss ZD, Brass SD, Duan Y, et al. Deep gray matter involvement on brain MRI scans is associated with clinical progression in multiple sclerosis. J Neuroimaging. 2009;19:3–8.

26. Lassmann H, van Horssen J, Mahad D. Progressive multiple sclerosis: pathology and pathogenesis. Nat Rev Neurol. 2012;8:647–56.

27. Frischer JM, Bramow S, Dal-Bianco A, Lucchinetti CF, Rauschka H, Schmidbauer M, et al. The relation between inflammation and neurodegeneration in multiple sclerosis. Brain. 2009;132:1175–89.

28. Harrison DM, Oh J, Roy S, Wood ET, Whetstone A, Seigo MA, et al. Thalamic lesions in multiple sclerosis by 7T MRI: Clinical implications and relationship to cortical pathology. Mult Scler. 2015;21:1139–50.

29. Klawiter EC, Ceccarelli A, Arora A, Jackson JS, Bakshi S, Kim G, et al. Corpus callosum atrophy correlates with gray matter atrophy in patients with multiple sclerosis. J Neuroimaging. 2015;25:62–7.

30. Yang C-Y, Liu HM, Chen SK, Chen YF, Lee CW, Yeh LR. Reproducibility of brain morphometry from short-term repeat clinical MRI examinations: a retrospective study. PLoS One. 2016;11:e0146913.

31. Shinohara RT, Oh J, Nair G, Calabresi PA, Davatzikos C, Doshi J, et al. Volumetric analysis from a harmonized multisite brain MRI study of a single subject with multiple sclerosis. AJNR Am J Neuroradiol. [Epub ahead of print]. 10.3174/ajnr.A5254.

32. Tsivgoulis G, Katsanos AH, Grigoriadis N, Hadjigeorgiou GM, Heliopoulos I, Kilidireas C, et al. The effect of disease modifying therapies on brain atrophy in patients with relapsing-remitting multiple sclerosis: a systematic review and meta-analysis. PLoS One. 2015;10:e0116511.

33. Khoury SJ, Bakshi R. Cerebral pseudoatrophy or real atrophy after therapy in multiple sclerosis. Ann Neurol. 2010;68:778–9.

34. Ceccarelli A, Rocca MA, Pagani E, Colombo B, Martinelli V, Comi G, et al. Voxel-based morphometry study of grey matter loss in MS patients with different clinical phenotypes. NeuroImage. 2008;42:315–22.

35. Benedict RH, Ramasamy D, Munschauer F, Weinstock-Guttman B, Zivadinov R. Memory impairment in multiple sclerosis: correlation with deep grey matter and mesial temporal atrophy. J Neurol Neurosurg Psychiatry. 2009;80:201–6.

36. Popescu V, Schoonheim MM, Versteeg A, Chaturvedi N, Jonker M, Xavier de Menezes R, et al. Grey matter atrophy in multiple sclerosis: clinical interpretation depends on choice of analysis method. PLoS One. 2016;11:e0143942.

37. Jones BC, Nair G, Shea CD, Crainiceanu CM, Cortese IC, Reich DS. Quantification of multiple-sclerosis-related brain atrophy in two heterogeneous MRI datasets using mixed-effects modeling. Neuroimage Clin. 2013;3:171–9.

38. Chua AS, Egorova S, Anderson MC, Polgar-Turcsanyi M, Chitnis T, Weiner HL, et al. Handling changes in MRI acquisition parameters in modeling whole brain lesion volume and atrophy data in multiple sclerosis subjects: Comparison of linear mixed-effect models. Neuroimage: Clin. 2015;8:606–10.

8

The Swiss Multiple Sclerosis Registry (SMSR): study protocol of a participatory, nationwide registry to promote epidemiological and patient-centered MS research

Nina Steinemann[1], Jens Kuhle[2], Pasquale Calabrese[3], Jürg Kesselring[4], Giulio Disanto[5], Doron Merkler[6], Caroline Pot[7], Vladeta Ajdacic-Gross[1], Stephanie Rodgers[1], Milo Alan Puhan[1†], Viktor von Wyl[1*†] and the Swiss Multiple Sclerosis Registry

Abstract

Background: Multiple sclerosis (MS) is one of the most frequently observed neurological conditions in Switzerland, but data sources for country-wide epidemiological trend monitoring are lacking. Moreover, while clinical and laboratory MS research are generally well established, there is a gap in patient-centered MS research to inform care management, or treatment decisions and policy making not only in Switzerland but worldwide.

Methods: In light of these research gaps, the Swiss Multiple Sclerosis Society initiated and funded the Swiss Multiple Sclerosis Registry (SMSR) an open-ended, longitudinal and prospective, nationwide, patient-centered study.
The SMSR recruits adult persons with a suspected or confirmed MS diagnosis who reside or receive care in Switzerland. The SMSR has established a governance structure with clear rules and guidelines. It follows a citizen-science approach with direct involvement of persons with MS (PwMS), who contribute actively to registry development, operations, and research. Main scientific goals entail the study of MS epidemiology in Switzerland, health care access and provision, as well as life circumstances and wellbeing of persons with MS.
The innovative study design ("layer model") offers several participation options with different time commitments. Data collection is by means of regular surveys and medical record abstraction. Survey participation is offered in different modes (web, paper & pencil) and in the three main national languages (German, French, Italian). Participants also receive regular data feedbacks for personal use and self-monitoring, contextualized in the whole population of study participants. Data feedbacks are also used to solicit data corrections of key variables from participants.

Discussion: The SMSR combines the advantages of traditional and novel research methods in medical research and has recruited over 1600 PwMS in its first year. The future-oriented design and technology will enable a response not only to future technological innovations and research trends, but also to challenges in health care provision for MS.

Keywords: Multiple sclerosis, Health-related quality of life, Epidemiology, Switzerland, Patient-reported outcomes

* Correspondence: viktor.vonwyl@uzh.ch
†Milo Puhan and Viktor von Wyl contributed equally to this work.
[1]Epidemiology, Biostatistics and Prevention Institute, University of Zurich, Hirschengraben 84, CH-8001 Zurich, Switzerland
Full list of author information is available at the end of the article

Background

Multiple sclerosis (MS) is the most common cause of non-traumatic disability among young adults in industrialized countries [1]. With an estimated 110 MS cases per 100,000 inhabitants, [2] the MS prevalence in Switzerland surpasses the median estimate for Europe - the region with the highest MS prevalence worldwide (80 per 100,000 inhabitants) [3]. However, the Swiss estimate has not been updated in nearly 30 years, mostly because no easily accessible routine data are available, for example from clinical care or health insurances. Unlike countries with national health care systems, the highly fragmented Swiss health care landscape suffers from a lack of standardization in data collection, an inexistent legal basis for mandatory reporting of severe chronic illnesses, as well as limited information technology (IT) system interoperability between different care and health insurance providers. In light of these constraints, the establishment of a medical registry with active data collection from various sources is one of very few viable options for establishing a long-term monitoring of epidemiological trends, but also for promoting personalized medicine approaches in MS [4].

As illustrated by a systematic survey of European MS registries, the role of registries in MS research is not limited to monitoring purposes [5]. The international MS registry landscape is very diverse, and many of these studies have made important contributions to MS epidemiology, treatment, diagnosis, and care research. However, several other disease aspects are less well covered by some existing registries, such as cost of illness, quality management of healthcare, patient preferences, and patient reported outcomes [5]. These research limitations can weigh heavy in chronic illnesses such as MS, often characterized by a complex management, an unclear evidence base for treatment guidelines, and on the important role of patient preferences in treatment decisions.

These two issues, a lack of epidemiological data for Switzerland and the promotion of the patient-perspective in MS research, triggered the Swiss MS Society to establish a novel MS registry. The Swiss MS Registry (SMSR) not only contributes basic data on the epidemiology of MS in Switzerland, through its patient-centered design it can also fill an important niche in national and international research together with other studies [5, 6]. This manuscript describes the main philosophy behind the SMSR and elaborates on the study design, as well as the methods and contents of the data collection. Moreover, a companion paper illustrates how the SMSR merges traditional with novel, internet-driven research approaches to leverage the advantages of both while mitigating legal, ethical, and data security risks [7].

Methods/Design

Study objectives

The SMSR was established with three primary goals. First, the SMSR shall provide the basis for more accurate prevalence estimates and long-term monitoring of epidemiological trends of MS in Switzerland.

Second, the SMSR will establish a study base for patient-centered MS research in Switzerland, thereby focusing on assessments of the disease burden for persons with MS (PwMS) and their relatives and proxies. Along the same lines, the SMSR aims to contribute research to previously understudied topics concerning patients' life circumstances and experiences (e.g. MS and work), as well as on clinical and health care related aspects (e.g. access to specialized MS care).

Third, by creating a versatile database and a flexible study infrastructure, the SMSR offers a platform for nested investigations. From the outset, the SMSR aimed to be an interdisciplinary, open, collaborative project, designed to leverage other existing research efforts. In particular, by systematic analysis of the Swiss and the international MS research landscape [5], knowledge gaps were identified and subsequently taken into account during the study planning phase. Examples of such topics include health-related quality of life, alternative medicines, physiotherapy, or work and insurance, which have now become part of the SMSR core data collection. Furthermore, the SMSR data structures were designed for compatibility with ongoing national and international collaborations (EUReMS) [8]. Specifically, the SMSR has established a strategic partnership with the clinically-oriented Swiss MS Cohort (SMSC) study [9] and strives to complement the SMSC data collection by adding further data from the patients' perspectives on diagnosis, treatment, and general well-being. In both studies, informed consent documents include opt-in agreements to allow future data exchanges between the SMSR and the SMSC for data validation and research projects.

Study design

The SMSR is an open-ended, longitudinal and prospective, nationwide, patient-centered study (http://www.ClinicalTrials.gov identifier: NCT02980640). It follows a citizen-science approach with direct involvement of PwMS, who contribute to the SMSR development and research via representation in the Scientific Assembly.

Unlike other MS registries, the data are primarily collected directly from participants via structured questionnaires, that is, without intermediary health professionals. Consequently, surveys must be understandable by lay-persons and be provided in the three main Swiss official languages (German, French, Italian). Participation is offered via an online web system and as paper & pencil versions.

Design and the research strategy of the SMSR are based on three major tenets, which were flexibility regarding study contribution by PwMS (from one-time to longitudinal participation), provision of data feedbacks to participants and regular information on how data are being used, as well as the involvement of PwMS in study design and execution.

The SMSR includes four participation options for PwMS: (1) they can simply fill in a one-time survey, (2) additionally they can complete regular, semi-annual surveys on varying topics, (3) when signing the informed consent, they can decide to grant access to their medical records for abstraction by the SMSR, and (4) participants can allow the SMSR to exchange their data with the SMSC. Combinations of these options are possible. The decision for participation in either study module needs to be taken at time to informed consent signature (layer 1) on an opt-in basis but can be revised later, for example if a person wishes to withdraw her/his consent for medical record release.

These different participation forms are also reflected (and accommodated) in the SMSR study design, which entails different layers (Fig. 1) through which participants can gradually navigate. This layer concept was inspired by the amyotrophic lateral sclerosis registry in the USA [10]. The first, outermost layer 1 includes the deposition of contact information and informed consent signature. During these steps, prospective participants can also decide on which study modules they would like to contribute to.

The SMSR registration process is considered complete upon submission of a first, one-off questionnaire, which also demarks the second registry layer. The purpose of layer 2 is to collect basic demographic and medical data from as many PwMS as possible for epidemiological investigations (e.g. on MS prevalence in Switzerland).

In layer 3, the SMSR further offers regular participation by means of semi-annual surveys. The main objective of this third layer is a longitudinal data collection on disease burden, MS progression, physical and mental well-being, and changing life circumstances (Table 1). Layer 3 is open to all participants who have completed layer 2 and are willing to submit a confirmation of their diagnosis, signed by their treating physician.

The self-reported data from layers 1 to 3 are complemented by clinical data in layer 4, which stems from two sources. Participants may either elect to release their patient charts for medical record abstraction or they can allow data exchanges between the SMSR and the SMSC in case of dual participation in both studies. These clinical layer 4 data are of critical importance for validation of self-reported medical events such as symptoms, relapses, comorbidities, and treatments. The goal is to document up to 1000 participants, and the patient selection for layer 4 medical record abstraction is made by the SMSR study center based on age, gender, disease stage, and treatment setting in order to ensure representativeness.

Layers 3 and 4 also allow data collections for specific projects, which can either be included into regular follow-up surveys and data abstractions or be conducted as separate nested measurements outside the regular follow-up schedule (but possibly requiring its own ethical approval / informed consent). Combined, the layer design offers a very flexible structure, which not only accommodates specific research needs, but also offers participants a choice of different commitment levels.

Study population

The SMSR is open to all adults aged 18 years and older who were diagnosed with MS or a clinically isolated syndrome (CIS) and who live or are regularly receiving medical care in Switzerland. For contribution to layers 3 and 4, the MS/CIS diagnosis needs to be confirmed by a physician.

Study recruitment

The SMSR was initiated by and developed in close collaboration with the MS community in Switzerland, represented by the Swiss MS Society. The SMSR is

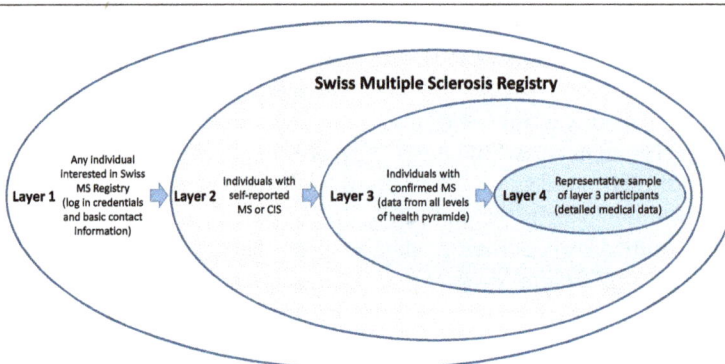

Fig. 1 Study design of the Swiss Multiple Sclerosis Registry (SMSR)

Table 1 Overview of assessments in the Swiss Multiple Sclerosis Registry

Topics	Layer 2 (one-off Survey)	Layer 3 Baseline (one-off Survey)	Layer 3 Follow-up 1 (every 6 months)	Layer 3 Follow-up 2 (every 12 months)	Layer 4 (Medical chart review every 12 months)
Sociodemographic variables					
Personal information	X	X		X	
Family and living situation	X	X		X	
Education, profession		X		X	
Working situation		X		X	
Occupational changes due to MS		X		X	
Societal context (e.g. disability insurance)		X		X	
Disease course					
First symptoms	X				X
Symptoms ever, current	X	X	X	X	X
Symptoms changes (prior and after diagnosis)					X
Disease stage, type of MS	X	X	X	X	X
EDSS-score		X	X	X	X
Mobility		X		X	
Relapses		X	X	X	X
Age of disease progression		X			
Diagnostic process					
Age at first symptoms	X				
Time of first medical doctor visit			X		
Personal experience of diagnostic process			X		
Treatment					
Disease modifying treatment ever/current	X	X	X	X	X
Non-drug therapies	X	X	X	X	X
Side effects / adverse events	X	X	X	X	X
Therapy stop / interruption	X	X	X	X	
Interventions against side effects		X	X	X	X
Alternative medicine	X	X	X	X	
Additional medicine / supplements	X	X	X	X	
Cannabis treatment		X	X	X	
Comorbidities					
Comorbidities		X	X	X	X
Medication for comorbidities		X	X	X	X
Risk factors and family history					
Weight		X		X	
Smoking behavior (and exposure)		X		X	
Alcohol consumption		X		X	
Nutrition	X			X	
Previous medical history		X			
Childhood illnesses		X			
Vaccination		X		X	
MS family history	X				X
Sun exposure		X			
Hormonal factors (only women)		X			

Table 1 Overview of assessments in the Swiss Multiple Sclerosis Registry *(Continued)*

Topics	Layer 2 (one-off Survey)	Layer 3 Baseline (one-off Survey)	Layer 3 Follow-up 1 (every 6 months)	Layer 3 Follow-up 2 (every 12 months)	Layer 4 (Medical chart review every 12 months)
Nutrition and Lifestyle					
Nutrition change since diagnosis	X			X	
Lifestyle change since diagnosis	X			X	
Physical Activity	X	X		X	
Care and medical aids					
Institutions visits	X	X		X	
Care types		X		X	
Contact with healthcare professionals	X	X		X	
Specialists consultation	X	X		X	
Confidence in specialists		X		X	
Medical aids		X		X	
Domestic assistance		X		X	
Housework		X		X	
Disclosure of MS		X		X	
Quality of Life					
Health related quality of life (EQ-5D-5 L;WHO 5-item well-being index)	X	X	X	X	
Mental health					
Psychological well-being	X	X	X	X	
Depression		X	X	X	
Burden of disease					
Individual burden (e.g. symptoms,...)	X	X	X	X	
Societal burden		X	X	X	
Economic burden				X	

executed by the University of Zurich and promoted as a project of the Swiss MS Society. The Society's extensive network and various media outlets (website, member magazine, social media activities, newsletters) allowed a quick and nationwide dissemination of information about the SMSR to potentially interested participants, as well as physicians.

Registry enrolment occurs by means of self-recruitment and peer referral. Clinics and private practices are involved in recruitment insofar as they provide postcards and leaflets about the SMSR and raise awareness of the Registry's existence among their patients. For SMSR enrolment, interested persons can either send in a postcard to the SMSR data center, upon which they will receive additional instructions for joining the SMSR. Alternatively, they can login directly to a website (www.ms-register.ch), create an account, and - after signing the informed consent- access the surveys.

Ethical aspects

The study has been approved for nationwide conduct as a multi-centric study by the Ethics Committee

Zurich (Study number PB-2016-00894). Informed consent is obtained from all participants, either electronically upon first access to the SMSR platform or as part of the registration process for participants who prefer paper & pencil versions. In line with the SMSR's strategy to offer various commitment levels, the informed consent offers three opt-in choices regarding study module participation.

The first module involves the diagnosis confirmation, which is prerequisite for participation in regular follow-up surveys (layer 3) and medical record abstraction (layer 4). That is, refusal of providing permission of the diagnosis confirmation by the treating physician implies that only participation in layer 2 is possible.

The second module is the medical record abstraction. Giving approval to this study option means providing the SMSR data center personnel access to medical records. Prior to first record access, participants are notified and given 3 weeks to notify the SMSR data center in case they wish to reconsider their decision.

Third, SMSR participants can agree to share their data with the SMSC study and vice versa. This study module only applies to persons enrolled in both studies. Overall, agreement to these three study modules is in excess of 90%. Withdrawal from any of these study modules or from SMSR participation is possible at any time and without provision of explanations, but very few persons have chosen to do so (< 20 participants).

Data acquisition

Data are collected directly from participants via structured questionnaires. The entry questionnaire, which constitutes layer 2, takes approximately 20 min to complete and collects data on a person's MS history, symptoms, treatments, diagnosis, risk factors, as well as changes in lifestyle behavior due to MS (Table 1). Approx. 75% of all layer 2 participants also contribute to the regular surveys in layer 3. These semi-annual questionnaires require 45 min and collect data on recent medical events, drug- and non-drug treatments, living and familial situation, work and evolving special topics (e.g. on patients' experiences of the diagnostic process). Participants are either informed via email when a new questionnaire is ready or, in case of participation on paper, the survey is mailed directly, along with a pre-stamped return envelope. The online system implements completeness and plausibility checks, as well as bifurcations if questions pertain only to a subgroup of respondents. It further allows users to pause the entry process and to store intermediary results. Upon completion and submission of the questionnaire, the answers are stored in the study database and can no longer be changed or updated by the participant. A help desk, located at the SMSR data center, is available via phone and email in case of questions.

For all layer 4 data collections, participants must have either agreed to release their medical records or to exchange data with the SMSC in case of dual enrolment. The SMSR data center manages all data collections and exchanges. Medical record abstraction is performed on site at clinics and private practices on an annual basis.

Technical aspects

The SMSR has established an online platform for survey delivery and data collection, which also includes a patient diary, as well as features for participants to analyze their own data. The data collection platform was developed in close collaboration with the S3IT (Science and IT) Division of the University of Zurich. The backend and the frontend applications are hosted on secure servers at the University. The backend consists of a Mongo Database and a set of Python scripts providing API functions for the frontend. The frontend is programmed in Java Script Angular by a dedicated Web Developer and also includes a Content Management System for simple creation and update of online study forms.

Security and data safety are of great concern. Safety measures include e-mail confirmation during account creation (double opt-in), password strength enforcement, 256-TLS secured SSL communication between clients and servers, as well as strict separation of identifiable and research data. For user administration and access authentication, a single sign-on system was developed (Mysql, PHP), which is hosted outside the University of Zurich by a certified Swiss Internet provider. All identifiable data are encrypted and IT security was assessed by an external, specialized company.

Measurements

One particular challenge for studying MS is its multifaceted manifestation. Therefore, in line with its patient-centered design, the SMSR data collection goes well beyond medical information also including data on socio-demographic factors, family history, (lifestyle) behaviors and exposures, risk factors, patient-reported outcomes and living and working conditions (Fig. 2). In addition, data on the general cultural, environmental and socio-economic conditions can be added based on where participants live. The breadth of data collection enables comprehensive study questions on disease burden, causes of disease, prognostic questions, therapeutic questions as well as research on health services for PwMS. The following paragraphs and Table 1 provide further details on the specific topics, as well as their assessment frequency.

Symptoms, relapses and progression

Data on symptoms and MS progression are collected by self-reporting in regular surveys. At baseline, participants are instructed to indicate all symptoms they have ever experienced, the first MS symptoms they ever noticed, as

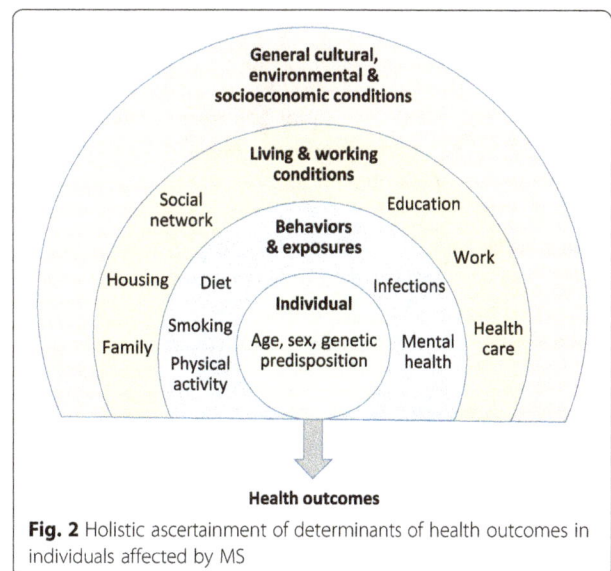

Fig. 2 Holistic ascertainment of determinants of health outcomes in individuals affected by MS

well as symptoms that have occurred during the past 6 months. The questionnaire further includes items on the number of relapses and corticosteroid treatments (including treatment settings or, where applicable, reasons for absence of treatment initiation). This information is updated on an annual basis in layer 3 and validated with clinical layer 4 data where available. Aspects of mobility are queried in layer 3 by use of the validated MS Questionnaire for Physiotherapists (MSQPT) [11].

Treatments, medication and adherence to disease-modifying treatment (DMT)

In the layer 2 survey, participants are asked to list all DMTs they have taken in the past 6 months, as well as all DMTs that were ever taken. The survey also collects basic data on alternative medications and non-pharmacological drug treatments. These data are updated semiannually in regular layer 3 questionnaires. Adherence to DMT is assessed at least annually in layer 3 on the basis of a short questionnaire that queries the number of missed doses over the past 4 weeks.

Health-related quality of life

The EuroQol- 5 Dimension (EQ5D) instrument is assessed on an annual basis [12, 13], for the first time in layer 2. The EQ5D is also integrated in the patient diary, which is accessible through the online data collection platform. The regular follow-up questionnaires also contain the Warwick-Edinburgh Scale [14] and the World Health Organization (WHO) 5-item well-being scale, which are also implemented annually [15]. In addition, a validated single-item questionnaire on (positive) health behavior is included [16].

Mental health, depression, and fatigue

In order to assess fatigue, which represents one of the most prominent symptoms of MS, the Modified Fatigue Impact Scale (MFIS-21) is applied [17, 18]. In addition, the well-established Multiple Sclerosis Impact Scale (MSIS-29) is assessed to address physical and psychological impact from the patient perspective in the last 2 weeks. [19]

Additional questions covering aspects of mental health and depression are assessed in specialized follow-up surveys by applying the standardized Beck Depression Inventory (BDI)-Fast Screen [20], and Mini SPIKE [21, 22].

Circumstances of life

The layer 3 questionnaire further includes a series of questions on education, living situation, work, disability insurance, social support ("Oslo 3 Social Support Scale" [23]) and benefit finding ("Benefit Finding in MS Scale" (BFiMSS)) [24]. These questions were developed in close collaboration with the Swiss MS Society, neuropsychologists, and PwMS. The work history and insurance status are updated annually.

Statistical analyses

The SMSR Data Center, located at the Epidemiology, Biostatistics and Prevention Institute of the University of Zurich, is responsible for data collection and quality assurance. Statistical analyses are performed continuously for monitoring purposes, for data feedbacks to study participants, and for specific scientific projects. One of the SMSR core aims is to establish a long-term, epidemiological monitoring of MS in Switzerland. As no single study is able to establish precise prevalence estimates for MS in Switzerland, the SMSR approaches this goal by combining information from different sources (e.g. the SMSC) to estimate the total size of the Swiss MS population. Thereby, the SMSR employs methods of sensitivity analysis [25], data triangulation [26], and individual-based mathematical modelling (e.g. [27]) in order to refine these estimates and assess the validity of results.

Study status

Since its launch on June 25, 2016, the SMSR has enrolled 1605 persons with MS who have signed the informed consent (status per September 27, 2017). Recruitment is ongoing, with 1–2 new enrolments daily. In total, 1343 persons have successfully completed the first layer 2 questionnaire. Moreover, 1005 persons also opted to participate in regular surveys and have successfully completed the first layer 3 questionnaire, which is the starting point for semi-annual follow-up surveys. Of those 1005 persons, 833 have already submitted a diagnosis confirmation. Overall, 80% of participants complete the questionnaires online, the remainder on paper.

Organization and funding

The SMSR was established at the initiative of the Swiss MS Society, which is also the financial sponsor of the study. The SMSR has a clearly defined governance structure and guidelines in place to ensure a cooperative, transparent operation. The main steering body of the SMSR is the Scientific Assembly, which oversees the research strategy, elects the SMSR president, and grants access to research data. It consists of elected representatives of major MS centers, the Swiss MS Society, the MS research community, neurorehabilitation clinics, and, last but not least, PwMS. Scientific Assembly members bring in diverse professional expertise such as neurology, nursing, physiotherapy, neuropsychology, IT, or neuroimmunology. The Scientific Assembly is structured into three thematic research committees, which oversee the operational aspects of the MS registry development and initiate research projects in their respective area of expertise. The first Research Committee is concerned with all patient and population-based research activities (including review of questionnaires and research instruments). A second Research Committee deals with all things related to IT, databases, and analysis of unstructured data. This IT Research Committee also initiates and develops technology-driven registry extensions. The third Research Committee oversees all clinical and laboratory research and has the lead in the development of the layer 4 data collection.

Anonymized SMSR data are - in principle – available to all qualified researchers for specific projects. Guidelines regulate procedures for data access, which consist of the submission of a research proposal to the Scientific Assembly. The proposal is then scored according to feasibility, scientific soundness, and alignment with overarching SMSR goals and examined by independent reviewers before being approved by the members of the Scientific Assembly. PwMS and the Swiss MS Society are also involved in this approval process.

Discussion

The SMSR is a longitudinal, patient-centered study, designed to fill important knowledge gaps on MS epidemiology and disease burden for patients in an environment where systematic compilation of routine data from providers and/or insurers is not feasible. The close collaboration with a patient-organization, PwMS, and MS researchers has created a unique approach and philosophy for data collection and research. In particular, the SMSR stands out for its participatory approach to registry development and research, a singular blend of patient-reported and clinical data, as well as a transparent governance.

Other web-based, patient-centered initiatives include, for example, the UK MS Register, which is a nationwide, web-based study for the UK [6], which also has participatory elements [28]. The UK Register gathers basic information on MS status and progression, socio-demographic factors, and a number of several patient-reported instruments and has recruited over 11,000 participants in 5 years [6, 29]. A second notable example is the Dutch MS Study, which also collects longitudinal data on quality of life and health status by means of validated, patient-reported instruments [30]. Although comparable in scope and methodology, we believe that the SMSR offers additional noteworthy features.

First, the SMSR pursues a participatory approach to study planning and research. PwMS and the Swiss MS Society are active contributors to the SMSR, which enhances motivation for participation and greatly improves the clarity and structure of the surveys, as well as communication of the findings.

Second, the layer model offers several participation options with different time commitments. The SMSR strives to obtain basic epidemiological data from as many PwMS as possible by means of a short one-off survey. Participants may also opt to contribute to semi-annual surveys, which are somewhat more time-demanding. Other additional study modules such as medical record abstraction come without any additional workload for patients and care providers, however.

Third, the SMSR offers regular data feedbacks for private use and self-monitoring. Feedbacks are contextualized in the whole population of study participants. That is, participants receive additional information on whether their specific survey response is rare or common among the other participants. Data feedbacks are also a very efficient means to solicit data corrections of key variables from participants.

Fourth, the SMSR has established a governance structure that involves PwMS via representation. The Scientific Assembly determines the scientific strategy and approves data requests for research. The inclusion of patient representatives and the Swiss MS Society in governing bodies guarantees influence of the MS patient community over project guidelines, research agenda and data usage.

Finally, by combining traditional and novel, web-based data collection methods the SMSR exploits the potential of societal and technological trends while mitigating legal and ethical risks. By offering different participation modes (web, paper & pencil) and in the three main national languages, the SMSR leverages benefits of modern technology for those who wish to participate online, without leaving less internet-savvy persons behind. Furthermore, unlike commercial initiatives, the SMSR operates under clear regulations and guidelines (Swiss Human Research Law), which guarantee the rights of participants.

Therefore, while the SMSR may not be the first participatory study in the field of MS research to take advantage of technical innovations, in particular by providing a web portal for data collection and visualization, it clearly takes patient participation to a new level, thereby distinguishing itself from other international MS registries.

Conclusion

The SMSR is an innovative, prospective study that combines advantages of traditional and novel research methods in medical research. Moreover, the SMSR is unique by taking the participatory approach further than any other study in the MS field and by covering a large variety of domains that are relevant to PwMS' experiences and life circumstances. What is more, the flexible IT infrastructure and clear governance rules support extensions to the core protocol and data collections, thus creating a future-oriented platform that is well suited to respond to future technological innovations and research trends, but also to challenges in health care provision in MS.

Abbreviations

BDI: Beck Depression Inventory; CIS: Clinically isolated syndrome; DMT: Disease-modifying treatment; EQ5D: EuroQol- 5 Dimension; IT: Information technology; MS: Multiple sclerosis; MSIS-29: Multiple Sclerosis Impact Scale; MSQPT: Multiple sclerosis questionnaire for physiotherapists; PwMS: Person with MS; SMSC: Swiss Multiple Sclerosis Cohort Study; SMSR: Swiss Multiple Sclerosis Registry; WHO: World Health Organization

Acknowledgements

Members of the Swiss Multiple Sclerosis Registry are:
Bernd Anderseck, Pasquale Calabrese, Andrew Chan, Giulio Disanto, Britta Engelhardt, Claudio Gobbi, Roger Häussler, Christian P. Kamm, Susanne Kägi, Jürg Kesselring (President), Jens Kuhle (Chair of Clinical and Laboratory Research Committee), Roland Kurmann, Christoph Lotter, Kurt Luyckx, Doron Merkler, Patricia Monin, Stephanie Müller, Krassen Nedeltchev, Caroline Pot, Milo A. Puhan, Irene Rapold, Anke Salmen, Sven Schippling, Claude Vaney (Chair of Patient- and Population Research Committee), Viktor von Wyl (Chair of IT and Data Committee).

Funding

The Swiss Multiple Sclerosis Registry is funded by a grant from the Swiss Multiple Sclerosis Society.

Authors' contributions

NS, MP & VvW wrote the first draft of the manuscript, GD, DM, CP, JKu, PC, JKe, SR & VA revised the manuscript critically. All authors read and approved the final manuscript.

Competing interests

The authors declare that they have no competing interests.

Author details

[1]Epidemiology, Biostatistics and Prevention Institute, University of Zurich, Hirschengraben 84, CH-8001 Zurich, Switzerland. [2]Neurological Policlinic, University Hospital Basel, Basel, Switzerland. [3]Department of Psychology, University of Basel, Basel, Switzerland. [4]Rehabilitation Clinic Valens, Valens, Switzerland. [5]Department of Neurology, Regional Hospital Lugano (EOC), Lugano, Switzerland. [6]Division of Clinical Pathology, Geneva University Hospital, Geneva, Switzerland. [7]Department of Clinical Neuroscience, Centre hospitalier universitaire vaudois, Lausanne, Switzerland.

References

1. Compston A, Coles A. Multiple sclerosis. Lancet. 2008;372:1502–17.
2. Beer S, Kesselring J. High prevalence of multiple sclerosis in Switzerland. Neuroepidemiology. 1994;13:14–8.
3. Organization WH: Atlas: multiple sclerosis resources in the world 2008. 2008.
4. Ziemssen T, Kern R, Thomas K. Multiple sclerosis: clinical profiling and data collection as prerequisite for personalized medicine approach. BMC Neurol. 2016;16:124.
5. Flachenecker P, Buckow K, Pugliatti M, Kes VB, Battaglia MA, Boyko A, Confavreux C, Ellenberger D, Eskic D, Ford D, et al. Multiple sclerosis registries in Europe - results of a systematic survey. Mult Scler. 2014;20: 1523–32.
6. Ford DV, Jones KH, Middleton RM, Lockhart-Jones H, Maramba ID, Noble GJ, Osborne LA, Lyons RA. The feasibility of collecting information from people with multiple sclerosis for the UK MS register via a web portal: characterising a cohort of people with MS. BMC Med Inform Decis Mak. 2012;12:73.
7. Puhan MA, Steinemann N, Kamm CP, Muller S, Kuhle J, Kurmann R, Calabrese P, Kesselring J, von Wyl V, Swiss Multiple Sclerosis Registry S. A digitally facilitated citizen-science driven approach accelerates participant recruitment and increases study population diversity. Swiss Med Wkly. 2018; 148:w14623.
8. Pugliatti M, Eskic D, Mikolcic T, Pitschnau-Michel D, Myhr KM, Sastre-Garriga J, Otero S, Wieczynska L, Torje C, Holloway E, et al. Assess, compare and enhance the status of persons with Multiple Sclerosis (MS) in Europe: a European register for MS. Acta Neurol Scand Suppl. 2012;126:24–30.
9. Disanto G, Benkert P, Lorscheider J, Mueller S, Vehoff J, Zecca C, Ramseier S, Achnichts L, Findling O, Nedeltchev K, et al. The Swiss Multiple Sclerosis Cohort-Study (SMSC): a prospective Swiss wide investigation of key phases in disease evolution and new treatment options. PLoS One. 2016;11: e0152347.
10. Horton DK, Mehta P, Antao VC. Quantifying a nonnotifiable disease in the United States: the National Amyotrophic Lateral Sclerosis Registry model. JAMA. 2014;312:1097–8.
11. van der Maas NA. Patient-reported questionnaires in MS rehabilitation: responsiveness and minimal important difference of the multiple sclerosis questionnaire for physiotherapists (MSQPT). BMC Neurol. 2017;17:50.
12. Brooks R. EuroQol: the current state of play. Health Policy. 1996;37:53–72.
13. EuroQol G. EuroQol--a new facility for the measurement of health-related quality of life. Health Policy. 1990;16:199–208.
14. Tennant R, Hiller L, Fishwick R, Platt S, Joseph S, Weich S, Parkinson J, Secker J, Stewart-Brown S. The Warwick-Edinburgh Mental Well-Being Scale (WEMWBS): development and UK validation. Health Qual Life Outcomes. 2007;5:63.
15. Topp CW, Ostergaard SD, Sondergaard S, Bech P. The WHO-5 well-being index: a systematic review of the literature. Psychother Psychosom. 2015;84: 167–76.
16. Wanner M, Probst-Hensch N, Kriemler S, Meier F, Bauman A, Martin BW. What physical activity surveillance needs: validity of a single-item questionnaire. Br J Sports Med. 2014;48:1570–6.
17. Fischer JS, LaRocca NG, Miller DM, Ritvo PG, Andrews H, Paty D. Recent developments in the assessment of quality of life in multiple sclerosis (MS). Mult Scler. 1999;5:251–9.
18. Guidelines MSCfCP: Fatigue and multiple sclerosis: evidence-based management strategies for fatigue in multiple sclerosis: clinical practice guidelines. The Council; 1998.
19. Hobart J, Lamping D, Fitzpatrick R, Riazi A, Thompson A. The Multiple Sclerosis Impact Scale (MSIS-29): a new patient-based outcome measure. Brain. 2001;124:962–73.
20. Beck A, Steer R, Brown G. Manual for the BDI–fast screen for medical patients. San Antonio: Psychological Corporation; 2000.
21. Ajdacic-Gross V, Muller M, Rodgers S, Warnke I, Hengartner MP, Landolt K, Hagenmuller F, Meier M, Tse LT, Aleksandrowicz A, et al. The ZInEP epidemiology survey: background, design and methods. Int J Methods Psychiatr Res. 2014;23:451–68.
22. Angst J, Gamma A, Neuenschwander M, Ajdacic-Gross V, Eich D, Rossler W, Merikangas KR. Prevalence of mental disorders in the Zurich cohort study: a twenty year prospective study. Epidemiol Psichiatr Soc. 2005;14:68–76.
23. Dalgard OS, Dowrick C, Lehtinen V, Vazquez-Barquero JL, Casey P, Wilkinson G, Ayuso-Mateos JL, Page H, Dunn G, Group O. Negative life events, social support and gender difference in depression: a multinational community survey with data from the ODIN study. Soc Psychiatry Psychiatr Epidemiol. 2006;41:444–51.
24. Pakenham KI, Cox S. The dimensional structure of benefit finding in multiple sclerosis and relations with positive and negative adjustment: a longitudinal study. Psychol Health. 2009;24:373–93.
25. Ding P, VanderWeele TJ. Sensitivity analysis without assumptions. Epidemiology. 2016;27:368–77.
26. Rutherford GW, McFarland W, Spindler H, White K, Patel SV, Aberle-Grasse J, Sabin K, Smith N, Tache S, Calleja-Garcia JM, Stoneburner RL. Public health triangulation: approach and application to synthesizing data to understand national and local HIV epidemics. BMC Public Health. 2010;10:447.

25. Ding P, VanderWeele TJ. Sensitivity analysis without assumptions. Epidemiology. 2016;27:368–77.
26. Rutherford GW, McFarland W, Spindler H, White K, Patel SV, Aberle-Grasse J, Sabin K, Smith N, Tache S, Calleja-Garcia JM, Stoneburner RL. Public health triangulation: approach and application to synthesizing data to understand national and local HIV epidemics. BMC Public Health. 2010;10:447.
27. Phillips AN, Pillay D, Miners AH, Bennett DE, Gilks CF, Lundgren JD. Outcomes from monitoring of patients on antiretroviral therapy in resource-limited settings with viral load, CD4 cell count, or clinical observation alone: a computer simulation model. Lancet. 2008;371:1443–51.
28. Osborne LA, Middleton RM, Jones KH, Ford DV, Noble JG. Desirability and expectations of the UK MS register: views of people with MS. Int J Med Inform. 2013;82:1104–10.
29. Jones KH, Jones PA, Middleton RM, Ford DV, Tuite-Dalton K, Lockhart-Jones H, Peng J, Lyons RA, John A, Noble JG. Physical disability, anxiety and depression in people with MS: an internet-based survey via the UK MS register. PLoS One. 2014;9:e104604.
30. Jongen PJ, Heerings M, Lemmens WA, Donders R, van der Zande A, van Noort E, Kool A. A prospective web-based patient-centred interactive study of long-term disabilities, disabilities perception and health-related quality of life in patients with multiple sclerosis in The Netherlands: the Dutch multiple sclerosis study protocol. BMC Neurol. 2015;15:128.

9

Comorbidity and metabolic syndrome in patients with multiple sclerosis from Asturias and Catalonia, Spain

Antoni Sicras-Mainar[1], Elena Ruíz-Beato[2], Ruth Navarro-Artieda[3] and Jorge Maurino[4*]

Abstract

Background: The impact of comorbidity on multiple sclerosis (MS) is a new area of interest. Limited data on the risk factors of metabolic syndrome (MetS) is currently available. The aim of this study was to estimate the presence of comorbid conditions and MetS in a sample of adult patients with MS.

Methods: A retrospective, cohort study was conducted using electronic medical records from 19 primary care centres in Catalonia and Asturias, Spain. The number of chronic diseases (diagnoses), the Charlson Comorbidity Index and the individual Case-mix Index were used to assess general comorbidity variables. MetS was defined using the National Cholesterol Education Program Adult Treatment Panel III. Patients were distributed into two groups according to the Expanded Disability Status Scale (EDSS) score: 0–3.5 and 4–10.

Results: A total of 222 patients were studied (mean age = 45.5 (SD 12.5) years, 64.4% were female and 62.2% presented a diagnosis of relapsing-remitting MS. Mean EDSS score was 3.2 (SD 2.0). Depression (32.4%), dyslipidaemia (31.1%), hypertension (23.0%) and obesity (22.5%) were the most common comorbidities. Overall MetS prevalence was 31.1% (95% CI: 25.0–37.2%). Patients with an EDSS ≥ 4.0 showed a significantly higher number of comorbidities (OR=2.2; 95% CI: 1.7–3.0; p<0.001).

Conclusion: MS patients had a high prevalence of MetS. Screening for comorbidity should be part of standard MS care. Further studies are necessary to confirm this association and the underlying mechanisms of MS and its comorbidities.

Keywords: Comorbidity, Metabolic syndrome, Multiple sclerosis, Electronic medical records

Background

Multiple Sclerosis (MS) is a chronic autoimmune disease that affects the central nervous system and has a high impact on the health-related quality of life of patients, their families and society [1, 2]. It is one of the most common causes of neurological disability in young adults and its prevalence is increasing throughout Europe [3]. Different epidemiological studies suggest that the prevalence of MS in Spain is also increasing [4, 5]. A recent article from the Malaga province in Spain found a prevalence of 125 cases/100,000 inhabitants (95% CI: 102–169) [6].

Comorbidity is common in patients who suffer chronic disease; including individuals suffering from MS [7]. The association of comorbidity with health-related quality of life and disability progression has resulted in comorbidity being an area of increasing importance in MS research [2, 8, 9]. Rates of mortality and comorbidities have been shown to be higher in MS patients compared to non-MS patients. A recent observational study of the United States Department of Defence administrative claims database showed that MS patients (vs. a non-MS cohort) had an increased risk of developing a broad spectrum of comorbidity such as sepsis, ischemic stroke, suicide ideation, ulcerative colitis, and cancer (lymphoproliferative disorders and melanoma) [10]. Furthermore, overall risk of postmenopausal breast cancer was 13% higher amongst MS patients according to the

* Correspondence: jorge.maurino@roche.com
[4]Medical Department, Roche Farma S.A., Madrid, Spain
Full list of author information is available at the end of the article

Swedish Cancer Registry (HR [95% CI] = 1.13 [1.02–1.26]) [11]. Recent evidence suggests that patients with MS and ≥1 comorbidities have a two-fold increased risk of non-MS-related hospitalisation compared to patients without comorbidity [12].

The metabolic syndrome (MetS) is a global public-health challenge and a complex disorder characterised by a cluster of interconnected factors which lead to an increased risk of cardiovascular disease (CVD) and diabetes mellitus type 2 [13]. Previous research has shown that for individuals with autoimmune diseases, such as rheumatoid arthritis and systemic lupus erythematosus, the prevalence of MetS is higher than national averages [14]. However, only limited and inconsistent data on MetS risk factors exists for patients with MS [15]. Therefore, the aim of this study was to analyse the presence of comorbidity in a population of patients with MS with especial emphasis on MetS and its individual components.

Methods

A retrospective, cohort study using electronic medical records from two regions of Spain (Catalonia and Asturias) was conducted. The study analysed patients from 19 primary care centres covering a population of 315,658 inhabitants in a predominantly industrial urban setting with a medium-low socioeconomic status. The study protocol was approved by the investigational review board of the Fundació Unió Catalana d'Hospitals (Barcelona, Spain).

The study included all outpatients who required care in 2015 and fulfilled the following criteria: age ≥ 18 years; a diagnosis of MS according to the International Classification of Primary Care (IPC-2, code N86) and the International Statistical Classification of Diseases (ICD-9, ninth revision, code 340); inclusion in the long-term prescriptions program (with a record of daily dose, time interval and duration of each treatment administered); and a guaranteed regular patient follow-up (presenting ≥2 healthcare records in the computer system) [16, 17]. McDonald 2010 criteria were not used in the study because our healthcare database collected diagnosis following only IPC-2 and ICD-9 classifications.

Variables and measurements instruments

The Expanded Disability Status Scale (EDSS) was used to assess disability [18]. For the purposes of this study, disability was defined as mild to moderate (EDSS score 0–3.5) or severe (4.0–10.0). The number of chronic diseases (diagnoses), the Charlson Comorbidity Index and the individual Case-mix Index (obtained from the Adjusted Clinical Groups [ACG] - a classification system based on the consumption of healthcare resources) were used to summarise general comorbidity variables for each patient [19, 20]. The ACG application provides resource utilization

bands (RUBs), so each patient was included in one of the five mutually exclusive categories depending on overall morbidity (1: healthy or very low morbidity, 2: low morbidity, 3: moderate morbidity, 4: high morbidity, and 5: very high morbidity).

The clinical, biochemical and anthropometric parameters analysed were: systolic and diastolic blood pressure (mm Hg), body mass index (BMI, kg/m^2), basal blood glucose (mg/dl), serum triglycerides (mg/dl), total cholesterol (mg/dl), high-density lipoprotein (HDL) cholesterol (mg/dl); low-density lipoprotein (LDL) cholesterol (mg/dl) and serum creatinine (mg/dl). The diagnosis of MetS was established when an individual had three or more components of the National Cholesterol Education Program Adult Treatment Panel III (NCEP-ATP III) diagnostic criteria: hypertriglyceridemia (fasting triglyceride concentration ≥ 150 mg/dl or treatment with triglyceride-lowering agents), dyslipidaemia (fasting HDL- cholesterol <40 mg/dl in males and <50 mg/dl in females), hypertension (systolic and diastolic blood pressure ≥ 130/85 mmHg or on antihypertensive medication), hyperglycaemia (fasting plasma glucose concentration of ≥110 mg/dl or on glucose-lowering drug treatment or a previous diagnosis of diabetes), and abdominal obesity (waist circumference > 102 cm in males and >88 cm in females) [21]. In this study, the waist circumference measurement was replaced by BMI; a BMI ≥ 28.8 kg/m^2 was considered to be equivalent to abdominal adiposity [22].

Statistical analysis

A descriptive analysis was performed for all variables of interest with mean values, standard deviation (SD) and percentages. The variables were analysed for the overall sample of valid patients and for stratified subgroups according to the EDSS scale score. The Chi-Square and Student's t-tests compared variables by EDSS division. In logistic regression, odds ratios (OR) were adjusted for age, gender, comorbidity (Charlson Comorbidity Index, RUBs) and EDSS score. The SPSSWIN version 19 was used for all analyses. A $p < 0.05$ was considered statistically significant.

Results

Amongst 299,875 subjects aged ≥18 years who required medical care, 225 patients presented a diagnosis of MS and 222 were analysed (Fig. 1).

Socio-demographic and clinical characteristics of the patients are shown in Table 1. The mean ± SD age was 45.5 ± 12.5 years and 64.4% were female; 62.2% of the patients presented a diagnosis of relapsing-remitting MS (RRMS). The mean ± SD EDSS score was 3.2 ± 2.0. Intramuscular interferon beta-1a (30.6%), subcutaneous interferon beta-1a (23.9%) and glatiramer acetate (18%) were the most common disease-modifying treatments

Table 1 Socio-demographic characteristics of the sample

	EDSS 0–3.5 n = 152	EDSS 4.0–10 n = 70	Total n = 222	p-value
Mean age, years (SD)	42.5 (11.5)	52.2 (12.2)	45.5 (12.5)	<0.001
Gender, female, %	68.4	65.7	64.4	0.292
Mean time since diagnosis, years (SD)	10.5 (7.6)	19.8 (10.2)	13.4 (9.5)	<0.001
MS type, %				
RRMS	74.3	35.7	62.2	<0.001
SPMS	13.8	50.0	25.2	<0.001
PPMS	7.2	14.3	9.5	0.094
CIS	4.6	0.0	3.2	0.001
Overall comorbidity, mean (SD)				
Number of comorbidities	4.5 (2.7)	6.0 (3.3)	5.0 (3.0)	0.001
Charlson Index	0.7 (0.6)	1.0 (0.7)	0.8 (0.6)	0.005
RUBs	2.9 (0.8)	3.2 (0.7)	3.0 (0.8)	0.003
Comorbid diagnoses, %				
Depression	34.2	28.6	32.4	0.404
Dyslipidaemia	25.7	42.9	31.1	0.010
Hypertension	17.8	34.3	23.0	0.007
Obesity	22.4	22.9	22.5	0.935
Active smoking	16.4	12.9	15.3	0.490
Neoplasm	9.2	15.7	11.3	0.154
COPD	6.6	14.3	9.0	0.062
Diabetes mellitus	6.6	10.0	7.7	0.373
Asthma	7.9	2.9	6.3	0.151
Ischemic stroke	4.6	8.6	5.9	0.242
Alcoholism	3.9	5.7	4.5	0.555
Ischemic cardiomyopathy	2.6	8.6	4.5	0.047

CIS Clinically Isolated Syndrome; *COPD* Chronic Obstructive Pulmonary Disease; *EDSS* Expanded Disability Status Scale; *MS* Multiple Sclerosis; *PPMS* Primary Progressive MS; *RRMS* Relapsing-Remitting MS; *RUBs* Resource Utilization Bands; *SD* Standard Deviation; *SPMS* Secondary Progressive MS

administered. A total of 48 patients (21.8%) were not receiving immunomodulatory treatment.

Depression (32.4%), dyslipidaemia (31.1%), hypertension (23.0%), and obesity (22.5%) were the most frequent comorbidities (Table 1). The impact of comorbidity was significantly greater in the severe disability group than in group of mild/moderate impairment group: mean number of comorbidities (severe vs. mild/moderate: 6.0 vs. 4.5; $p = 0.001$), Charlson index (1.0 vs. 0.7; $p = 0.005$), and RUBs (3.2 vs. 2.9; $p = 0.003$) (Table 1).

Table 2 shows the prevalence of the main cardiovascular risk factors and metabolic syndrome. The overall prevalence of MetS was 31.1% (95% CI: 25.0–37.2%). No statistically significant differences in the MetS prevalence and the number of its components between patients with an EDSS score < 4.0 vs. ≥ 4.0 were found. All biochemical and anthropometric parameters were similar between groups. The overall prevalence of cardiovascular risk factors was 14.4%

without statistically significant differences between patients with an EDSS score ≥ 4.0 (12.0%) and <4.0 (15.7), $p = 0.658$. Furthermore, patients with an EDSS ≥4.0 showed a significantly higher number of comorbidities (RUBs, OR = 2.2; 95% CI: 1.7–3.0; $p < 0.001$) and longer time to diagnosis (OR = 1.2; 95% CI: 1.1–1.3; $p = 0.023$).

Discussion

Comorbidity is associated with diagnostic delays, more severe disability at diagnosis, greater disability progression, cognitive impairment, increased healthcare use, and higher mortality [23]. A systematic review analysed 249 articles indicated that depression, anxiety, hypertension, hypercholesterolemia and chronic lung disease were five of the most prevalent comorbidities in MS patients, whereas thyroid disease and psoriasis were the most common autoimmune diseases [24].

Table 2 Prevalence of the main cardiovascular risk factors and metabolic syndrome

	EDSS 0–3.5 n = 152	EDSS 4.0–10 n = 70	Total n = 222	p-value
MetS prevalence, %	28.9	35.7	31.1	0.311
MetS components, %				
BMI >28.8 kg/m^2	30.9	30.0	30.6	0.890
BP >130/85 mmHg (or treatment)	30.8	40.0	33.7	0.199
Triglycerides >150 mg/dL (or treatment)	14.5	22.9	17.1	0.123
Fasting blood glucose >110 mg/dL	11.7	10.0	11.2	0.772
HDL-c < 40 (men) or <50 (women) mg/dL	36.8	42.9	38.7	0.393
Number of components, SD	1.4 (1,3)	1.7 (1,5)	1.5 (1,4)	0.265
Total				
1	28.9	24.3	27.5	0.532
2	11.2	10.0	10.8	0.822
3	23.0	22.9	23.0	0.758
4	5.3	10.0	6.8	0.163
5	0.7	2.9	1.4	0.234
Cardiovascular risk factors, mean (SD)				
Systolic BP, mmHg	127.3 (14.8)	127.9 (15.9)	127.6 (15.5)	0.870
Diastolic BP, mmHg	74.5 (10.1)	76.2 (9.9)	75.4 (10.0)	0.726
BMI, kg/m^2	25.9 (4.5)	26.1 (4.6)	26.0 (4.5)	0.949
Glucose, mg/dL	93.2 (17.6)	93 (19.1)	93.1 (18.1)	0.985
HbA1c, %	5.8	5.8	5.8	0.255
Triglycerides, mg/dL	105.7 (50.0)	115.1 (49.4)	108.7 (49.9)	0.545
Total cholesterol, mg/dL	198.4 (38.0)	202.2 (41.5)	199.6 (39.1)	0.691
LDL-C, mg/dL	119.5 (36.5)	124.1 (39.6)	121.0 (37.4)	0.458
HDL-C, mg/dL	59.2 (17.5)	60.3 (17.2)	59.5 (17.4)	0.366
Serum creatinine, mg/dL	1.1 (0.1)	1.1 (0.1)	1.1 (0.1)	0.888
High cardiovascular risk, %	12.0	15.7	14.4	0.658

BP Blood Pressure; *BMI* Body Mass Index; *EDSS* Expanded Disability Status Scale; *HbA1c* Glycated Haemoglobin; *HDL-C* high-density lipoprotein cholesterol; *LDL-C* low-density lipoprotein cholesterol; *MetS* Metabolic Syndrome; *SD* Standard Deviation

Our analysis of 222 MS patients from two different regions of Spain provides support for the presence of comorbidities and MetS in MS patients, as well as a trend for increasing comorbidity with increasing MS disability. Depression, dyslipidaemia, hypertension, and obesity were the most frequently observed comorbidities. Furthermore, a 31.1% prevalence of MetS was found.

The ENRICA study showed a MetS prevalence of 22.7% (95% CI: 21.7–23.7%) in a sample of 11,143 adult subjects in Spain [25]. Information about MetS in MS is still very scarce [15]. However the results of our study agree with previous research. Similarly, Pinhas-Hamiel et al. found a MetS prevalence of 30% with no gender difference in a sample of 130 MS patients with significant disability (EDSS score ≥ 3) [26].

In a systematic review analysing 34 studies, Wens et al. found an increased CVD risk in MS patients compared to healthy controls [15]. Lalmohamed et al. showed a 3.5-fold increased mortality rate in MS compared with the general population, which was mainly caused by increased deaths due to CVD (2.4-fold) [27]. However, it is not clear whether this increased risk of CVD is related to obesity or changes in body composition, dyslipidaemia, hypertension or type II diabetes [15]. Many symptoms of MS such as mobility disability and fatigue could increase the prevalence of sedentary behaviour and may have considerable implications for the development of cardiovascular comorbidities [28]. In this context, physical exercise may be a feasible intervention targeting the CVD risk.

Our study has several limitations inherent to research based on population databases, such as the presence of missing values or diagnostic codification differences [29]. In addition, socioeconomic levels, lifestyle factors and concomitant medications were not evaluated as factors associated with CVD risk.

Conclusions

In recent years there has been a big change in the management of MS. Treatment decisions are becoming more complex due to the introduction of several new disease-modifying treatments with a more diverse spectrum of risks and benefits [30]. Before starting a treatment, neurologists should carefully consider the state of the disease, its prognostic factors and comorbidities, response to previous treatments, and patient preferences [31, 32]. Comorbidity screening should be part of standard MS care [33]. The findings in this study may help to establish an expectation of comorbidities, identify high-risk patients, educate MS patients in preventive measures and facilitate decision-making in clinical practice [33, 34]. Further studies need to be undertaken in order to validate these finding, and to gain a better understanding of the underlying mechanisms of MS and its comorbidities.

Abbreviations
ACG: Adjusted clinical groups; BMI: Body mass index; BP: Blood pressure; CIS: Clinically isolated syndrome; COPD: Chronic obstructive pulmonary disease; CVD: Cardiovascular disease; EDSS: Expanded disability status scale; HbA1c: Glycated haemoglobin; HDL: High-density lipoprotein; HR: Hazard ratio; ICD-9: International statistical classification of diseases; IPC-2: International classification of primary care; LDL: Low-density lipoprotein; MetS: Metabolic syndrome; MS: Multiple sclerosis; NCEP-ATP III: National cholesterol education program adult treatment panel III; OR: Odd ratio; PPMS: Primary progressive multiple sclerosis; RRMS: Relapsing-remitting multiple sclerosis; RUBs: Resource utilization bands; SD: Standard deviation; SPMS: Secondary progressive multiple sclerosis

Acknowledgements
None.

Funding
The study was funded by Roche Farma SA, Spain.

Authors' contributions
ASM, ERB, RNA and JM developed the research question. ASM designed the study, wrote the protocol and performed the statistical analyses. All authors contributed to and have approved the final manuscript.

Competing interests
ERB and JM are employees of Roche Farma SA. None of the other authors report any conflict of interest.

Author details
[1]Fundación Rediss (Red de Investigación en servicios Sanitarios), Barcelona, Spain. [2]Health Economics and Outcomes Research Unit, Roche Farma S.A., Madrid, Spain. [3]Department of Medical Information, Hospital Universitari Germans Trias i Pujol, Badalona, Barcelona, Spain. [4]Medical Department, Roche Farma S.A., Madrid, Spain.

References

1. Ayuso GI. Multiple sclerosis: socioeconomic effects and impact on quality of life. Med Clin (Barc). 2014;143(Suppl 3):7–12.
2. Berrigan LI, Fisk JD, Patten SB, Tremlett H, Wolfson C, Warren S, Fiest KM, McKay KA, Marrie RA; CIHR Team in the Epidemiology and Impact of Comorbidity on Multiple Sclerosis (ECoMS). Health-related quality of life in multiple sclerosis: Direct and indirect effects of comorbidity. Neurology. 2016. [Epub ahead of print].
3. Howard J, Trevick S, Younger DS. Epidemiology of multiple sclerosis. Neurol Clin. 2016;34:919–39.
4. Otero-Romero S, Roura P, Solà J, Altimiras J, Sastre-Garriga J, Nos C, Vaqué J, Montalban X. Increase in the prevalence of multiple sclerosis over a 17-year period in Osona, Catalonia. Spain Mult Scler. 2013;19:245–8.
5. Candeliere-Merlicco A, Valero-Delgado F, Martínez-Vidal S, Lastres-Arias MDC, Aparicio-Castro E, Toledo-Romero F, Villaverde-González R. Prevalence of multiple sclerosis in Health District III, Murcia. Spain Mult Scler Relat Disord. 2016;9:31–5.
6. Fernández O, Fernández V, Guerrero M, León A, López-Madrona JC, Alonso A, Bustamante R, Tamayo JA, Romero F, Bravo M, Luque G, García L, Sanchís G, San Roman C, Romero M, Papais-Alvarenga M, de Ramon E. Multiple sclerosis prevalence in Malaga, southern Spain estimated by the capture-recapture method. Mult Scler. 2012;18:372–6.
7. Estruch BC. Comorbidity in multiple sclerosis and its therapeutic approach. Med Clín (Barc). 2014;143(Suppl 3):13–8.
8. Marrie RA, Rudick R, Horwitz R, Cutter G, Tyry T, Campagnolo D, Vollmer T. Vascular comorbidity is associated with more rapid disability progression in multiple sclerosis. Neurology. 2010;74:1041–7.
9. Culpepper WJ. The incidence and prevalence of comorbidity in multiple sclerosis. Mult Scler. 2015;21:261–2.
10. Capkun G, Dahlke F, Lahoz R, Nordstrom B, Tilson HH, Cutter G, Bischof D, Moore A, Simeone J, Fraeman K, Bancken F, Geissbühler Y, Wagner M, Cohan S. Mortality and comorbidities in patients with multiple sclerosis compared with a population without multiple sclerosis: an observational study using the US Department of defense administrative claims database. Mult Scler Relat Disord. 2015;4:546–54.
11. Hajiebrahimi M, Montgomery S, Burkill S, Bahmanyar S. Risk of premenopausal and postmenopausal breast cancer among multiple sclerosis patients. PLoS One. 2016;11:e0165027.
12. Marrie RA, Elliott L, Marriott J, Cossoy M, Tennakoon A, Yu N. Comorbidity increases the risk of hospitalizations in multiple sclerosis. Neurology. 2015; 84:350–8.
13. Kassi E, Pervanidou P, Kaltsas G, Chrousos G. Metabolic syndrome; definitions and controversies. BMC Med. 2011;9:48.
14. Versini M, Jeandel PY, Rosenthal E, Shoenfeld Y. Obesity in autoimmune diseases: not a passive bystander. Autoimmun Rev. 2014;13:981–1000.
15. Wens I, Dalgas U, Stenager E, Eijnde BO. Risk factors related to cardiovascular diseases and the metabolic syndrome in multiple sclerosis - a systematic review. Mult Scler. 2013;19:1556–64.
16. Lamberts H, Wood M, Hofmans-Okkes I. The international classification of primary Care in the European Community. With a multi-language layer. Second edition. Oxford: Oxford University Press; 1993.
17. World Health Organization. Ninth Revision, International Classification of Diseases (ICD-9). Geneva, 1999.
18. Kurtzke JF. Rating neurologic impairment in multiple sclerosis: an expanded disability status scale (EDSS). Neurology. 1983;33:1444–52.
19. Charlson ME, Pompei P, Ales KL, MacKenzie CR. A new method of classifying prognostic comorbidity in longitudinal studies: development and validation. J Chronic Dis. 1987;40:373–83.
20. Weiner JP, Starfield BH, Steinwachs DM, Mumford LM. Development and. application of a population-oriented measure of ambulatory care case-mix. Med Care. 1991;29:452–72.
21. National Cholesterol Education Program Expert Panel on Detection, Evaluation, and Treatment on High Blood Cholesterol in Adults (Adult Treatment Panel III). Third report of the National Cholesterol Education Program (NCEP) Expert Panel on Detection, Evaluation, and Treatment of High Blood Cholesterol in Adults (Adult Treatment Panel III) final report. Circulation. 2002;106:3143–421.
22. Sattar N, Gaw A, Scherbakova O, Ford I, O'Reilly DS, Haffner SM, Isles C, Macfarlane PW, Packard CJ, Cobbe SM, Shepherd J. Metabolic syndrome with and without C-reactive protein as a predictor of coronary heart disease and diabetes in the west of Scotland coronary prevention study. Circulation. 2003;108:414–9.

23. Marrie RA. Comorbidity in multiple sclerosis. Some answers, more questions. Int J MS. 2016;18:271–2.

24. Marrie RA, Cohen J, Stuve O, Trojano M, Sorensen PS, Reingold S, Cutter G, Reider N. A systematic review of the incidence and prevalence of comorbidity in multiple sclerosis: overview. Mult Scler. 2015;21:263–81.

25. Guallar-Castillón P, Pérez RF, López García E, León-Muñoz LM, Aguilera MT, Graciani A, Gutiérrez-Fisac JL, Banegas JR, Rodríguez-Artalejo F. Magnitude and management of metabolic syndrome in Spain in 2008-2010: the ENRICA study. Rev Esp Cardiol. 2014;67:367–73.

26. Pinhas-Hamiel O, Livne M, Harari G, Achiron A. Prevalence of overweight, obesity and metabolic syndrome components in multiple sclerosis patients with significant disability. Eur J Neurol. 2015;22:1275–9.

27. Lalmohamed A, Bazelier MT, Van Staa TP, Uitdehaag BM, Leufkens HG, De Boer A, De Vries F. Causes of death in patients with multiple sclerosis and matched referent subjects: a population-based cohort study. Eur J Neurol. 2012;19:1007–14.

28. Veldhuijzen van Zanten JJ, Pilutti LA, Duda JL, Motl RW. Sedentary behaviour in people with multiple sclerosis: Is it time to stand up against MS? Mult Scler. 2016;22:1250–6.

29. Motheral B, Brooks J, Clark MA, Crown WH, Davey P, Hutchins D, Martins BC, Stanq P. A checklist for retrospective database studies–report of the ISPOR task force on retrospective databases. Value Health. 2003;6:90–7.

30. Comi G, Radaelli M, Soelberg SP. Evolving concepts in the treatment of relapsing multiple sclerosis. Lancet. 2017;389:1347–56.

31. Brück W, Gold R, Lund BT, Oreja-Guevara C, Prat A, Spencer CM, Steinman L, Tintoré M, Vollmer TL, Weber MS, Weiner LP, Ziemssen T, Zamvil SS. Therapeutic decisions in multiple sclerosis: moving beyond efficacy. JAMA Neurology. 2013;70:1315–24.

32. Arroyo R, Sempere PA, Ruiz-Beato E, Carreño A, Roset M, Maurino J. Conjoint analysis to understand multiple sclerosis patients´ preferences for disease-modifying therapy attributes in Spain. BMJ Open. 2017;7:e014433.

33. Marrie RA. Comorbidity in multiple sclerosis: implications for patient care. Nat Rev Neurol. 2017. [Epub ahead of print].

34. Haghikia A, Gold R. Positive effect on multiple sclerosis with treatment of metabolic syndrome. JAMA Neurol. 2016;73:499–500.

10

Healthcare resource use and costs of multiple sclerosis patients in Germany before and during fampridine treatment

Tjalf Ziemssen[1], Christine Prosser[2], Jennifer Scarlet Haas[2*], Andrew Lee[3], Sebastian Braun[2], Pamela Landsman-Blumberg[4], Angela Kempel[5], Erika Gleißner[5], Sarita Patel[5] and Ming-Yi Huang[3]

Abstract

Background: Multiple sclerosis (MS) patients often suffer from gait impairment and fampridine is indicated to medically improve walking ability in this population. Patient characteristics, healthcare resource use, and costs of MS patients on fampridine treatment for 12 months in Germany were analyzed.

Methods: A retrospective claims database analysis was conducted including MS patients who initiated fampridine treatment (index date) between July 2011 and December 2013. Continuous insurance enrollment during 12 months pre- and post-index date was required, as was at least 1 additional fampridine prescription in the fourth quarter after the index date. Patient characteristics were evaluated and pre- vs post-index MS-related healthcare utilization and costs were compared.

Results: A total of 562 patients were included in this study. The mean (standard deviation [SD]) age was 50.5 (9.8) years and 63% were female. In the treatment period, almost every patient had at least 1 MS-related outpatient visit, 24% were hospitalized due to MS, and 79% utilized MS-specific physical therapy in addition to the fampridine treatment. Total MS-related healthcare costs were significantly higher in the fampridine treatment period than in the period prior to fampridine initiation (€17,392 vs €10,960, $P < 0.001$). While this difference was driven primarily by prescription costs, MS-related inpatient costs were lower during fampridine treatment (€1,333 vs €1,565, $P < 0.001$).

Conclusions: Physical therapy is mainly used concomitant to fampridine treatment. While healthcare costs were higher during fampridine treatment compared to the pre-treatment period, inpatient costs were lower. Further research is necessary to better understand the fampridine influence.

Keywords: Multiple sclerosis, Claims data, Germany, Fampridine

Background

Multiple sclerosis (MS) is a chronic and progressive autoimmune disease of the central nervous system. MS patients suffer from diverse symptoms, whereas gait disturbance is one of the major problems that occurs frequently [1–3]. An estimated 40 to 90% of patients with MS experience walking impairment [1, 4, 5]. Fampridine is the first and only available medical treatment for improving walking ability in patients with MS and it has been licensed since 07/2011 in Europe [6]. The fampridine tablets (10 mg) are given twice a day, and if no improvement is shown after 2 weeks, the treatment should be stopped [6].

Due to its relative novelty, no information on fampridine-treated patients under real-life conditions is available in Germany. This information can contribute to understanding the unmet needs of this patient group. Furthermore, limited data assessing the resource implications of treating MS mobility symptoms are available.

This study aims at identifying the treatment, patient characteristics, MS-related healthcare resource use, and costs of patients staying on fampridine therapy for 1 year after treatment initiation. Furthermore, a comparison of the MS-specific healthcare resource use and costs during

* Correspondence: jennifer.haas@xcenda.de
[2]Xcenda GmbH, Lange Laube 31, D-30159 Hannover, Germany
Full list of author information is available at the end of the article

fampridine treatment with the pre-treatment period without fampridine was also conducted.

Methods

This retrospective claims data analysis was conducted using data from the Health Risk Institute (HRI) research database.

Database

The HRI research database comprises claims data from 75 of the 120 statutory health insurances in Germany. The analysis sample includes the utilization and costs of services for approximately 4 million covered lives through 2014 on an anonymized, individual level. This sample represents 4.8% of the population in Germany and is already adjusted for age and gender for the German population. Furthermore, the HRI research database is considered to have good external validity to the German population in terms of morbidity, mortality, and drug use [7].

Patient selection

All adult patients initiating treatment with fampridine between July 2011 and December 2013 in the database were identified, and the first prescription fill of fampridine (Anatomical Therapeutic Chemical code N07XX07) in this period determined the index quarter. Patients were included if they were continuously enrolled 4 quarters before and 4 quarters after the index quarter. At least 1 MS diagnosis (International Classification of Diseases, 10th Revision, German Modification [ICD-10-GM] G35.XX) in the inpatient sector (main or secondary diagnosis) or in the outpatient sector (verified diagnosis) during the index quarter or the preceding quarters was required. Furthermore, at least 1 additional fampridine prescription fill in the fourth quarter after the index served as a proxy indicating continuous fampridine treatment within the post-index period.

The identified patients were then stratified by DMT use, age and by use of antispasmodics to identify differences related to specific patient characteristics.

The full study population was stratified according to their disease-modifying therapy (DMT) use during the study period, defined as "continuous DMT", "discontinuous DMT" and "no DMT". This stratification was performed to isolate the effect of fampridine from possible effects of DMT treatment. The included DMTs were intramuscular (IM) interferon (INF) beta-1a, subcutaneous (SC) INF beta-1a, INF beta-1b, glatiramer acetate, natalizumab, teriflunomide, dimethyl fumarate, and fingolimod. Continuous DMT users were required to have at least 1 prescription claim for a DMT in the fourth quarter before the index quarter, 1 in the index quarter itself, and 1 in the fourth quarter after the index quarter.

Switches between the DMTs were not permitted in this subgroup. The discontinuous DMT cohort was defined as having a prescription claim for at least 1 DMT in any of the 9 quarters (4 quarters pre-index, index quarter, and 4 quarters post-index) where DMT switches were allowed. The subgroup of patients with no DMT had no prescription claims for any DMT in any of the 9 study quarters.

The second stratification divided the study population by age, including the subgroups aged 18 to 49 years and ≥50 years of age.

For the third stratification, all fampridine patients were subdivided into users and non-users of antispasmodic treatment. Users were defined as having at least 1 prescription of an antispasmodic treatment (baclofen, botulinum toxin, dantrolene, tizanidine, tolperisone, tetrazepam, gabapentin, cannabinoids) anytime during the 24-month observation period. Non-users had no evidence of symptomatic treatment within the study period.

Outcomes

Patient characteristics, including demographics, co-medication use (including DMTs and other MS-related medications using Anatomical therapeutic chemical classification system [ATC] codes), and comorbidities measured with the Charlson Comorbidity Index (CCI), and the most frequent diagnoses (top 10) in the 4 quarters before the index fampridine prescription were assessed.

The outcomes consisted of MS-related healthcare resource use for the inpatient, outpatient, and pharmacotherapy sectors. For the inpatient stays, MS-specific hospital visits were those with the MS ICD-10-GM code G35.XX as the primary diagnosis. Outpatient diagnoses were coded by different physician specialties, including but not limited to: general practitioners, neurologists, emergency physicians, and internists. The diagnoses are only coded on a quarterly basis and not directly linked to an intervention in the German healthcare system; therefore, an approximation of MS-related outpatient visits was assessed by calculating the number of visits with an MS ICD-10-GM diagnosis code in the same quarter. The same method was applied for the physical therapy visits. Furthermore, corticosteroid prescription fills, MS-related sick leave days (with a MS ICD-10-GM diagnosis code), and prescriptions for mobility-related devices were also assessed (eg, wheelchair, cane, etc.).

The MS-related healthcare costs in Euros were calculated using the costs for the use of resources described above. Pharmacotherapy costs included the corticosteroid prescriptions, DMTs, fampridine, and other MS-related medications, including antidementia; antidepressants; antiepileptic; urinary antispasmodics; selected muscle relaxants such as baclofen, botulinum toxin, dantrolene, tizanidine, tolperisone, and tetrazepam; selected medications to manage fatigue such as amantadine and modafinil; selected drugs for sexual dysfunction such as sildenafil, tadalafil, and tibolone; selected drugs against tremor such as propranolol; as well as benzodiazepine, and cannabinoids, according to Deutsche Gesellschaft für Neurologie (German Neurological Society) [8], Hoer et al. [9], and Bonafede et al. [10] The costs were then adjusted for inflation for the year 2014 using the general rate of inflation for Germany [11].

Baseline patient characteristics were assessed in the pre-index period. Healthcare utilization and costs for the 1-year treatment period were analyzed using descriptive statistics. Baseline characteristics, healthcare resource use, and costs were also stratified by the subgroups previously noted. Mean change (pre – post) and SD were computed for continuous healthcare resource use and cost measures. One-sample t-tests or Wilcoxon signed-rank tests were used for the evaluation of change measures (pre – post), depending on the distributional properties of the measure under evaluation. A P-value <0.05 denoted statistical significance and the statistical software SAS version 9.2 (SAS Institute, Cary NC, USA) was used for all analyses.

Results

Patient characteristics

Out of 1318 identified patients treated with fampridine, 43% (N = 562) met all study criteria. Most of the patients were excluded because they did not have a fampridine prescription fill in the 4th quarter after the index quarter. The mean age was 50.5 years and 63% were female. The most frequently prescribed medications in the pre-index period were muscle relaxants with 40.4% (such as baclofen with 26.2%) and antidepressants (31.9%) (see Table 1). On average, fampridine was prescribed 11 times per patient in the 12-month post-index period (SD 3.4).

MS-related healthcare resource use and costs before and during fampridine treatment

Regarding the MS-related resource utilization, a high percentage of patients had at least 1 MS-related physical therapy and 1 MS-related outpatient visit during fampridine treatment. One-third of patients had a prescription claim for corticosteroids, and the average number of corticosteroid prescriptions was 0.78 (SD 1.38). Furthermore, 1 in 5 patients had at least 1 day of sick leave due to MS, with a total of 12.6 (SD 45.5) MS-related sick leave days on average.

Compared to the pre-index period, significant reductions were observed in inpatient stays and corticosteroid use during the fampridine treatment period. The mean number of sick leave days decreased by 2 days, although the difference was not statistically significant (14.7 days [SD 46.8] vs 12.6 days [SD 45.5] P = 0.195). The percentage of patients using physical therapy and with outpatient visits increased significantly between the time periods (see Fig. 1).

Data not shown for the pre- and post-index MS-related resource use has been added as supplementary material (Additional file 1).

The overall average number of MS-related outpatient visits was 19 per year (SD 10.4) during the treatment period, implying that 1.6 physician visits per month due to MS were usual for the fampridine-treated patients. The majority of patients had at least 1 MS-related visit at their general practitioner (GP) (7.5 visits on average, SD 7.4). Less than half of the patients visited a neurologist during the fampridine treatment period (4.1 visits on average, SD 5.9).

MS-related healthcare costs before and during fampridine treatment

After pharmacotherapy, the second highest costs were observed for the inpatient sector. Devices for mobility problems were the smallest cost component, with 0.05% of the total MS-related healthcare costs during the observation period.

Compared with the pre-index period, MS-related inpatient costs declined significantly during fampridine treatment (€1,565.42 vs €1,333.42; P < 0.001), whereas MS-related outpatient costs increased significantly during the same period (€518.09 vs €565.47; P < 0.0001) (see Table 2).

Stratified analyses

About one-quarter of the identified patients had continuous DMT treatment and most (46%) did not use any DMT during the whole study period. Just under one-half (48%) of patients were younger than 50 years of age and more than half (53%) used antispasmodics at least once (53%) (see Fig. 2).

DMT stratification

Overall, a greater proportion of patients (46%) had no evidence of DMT treatment during the full observation period, compared with discontinuous DMT use (29%), and continuous use (26%). These subgroups differed in age, comorbidities, MS-related inpatient stays and costs, and MS-related sick leave.

Concerning the inpatient stays, those with discontinuous DMT use had the highest proportion with MS-related hospitalizations (30%) in contrast to the no DMT (27%) and the continuous DMT (10%) subgroups. However, the decline in MS-related stays from the pre- to post-index period was the highest and only significant in the no DMT subgroup (35–27%, P = 0.007).

Table 1 Patient characteristics

Characteristic	N = 562
Age in years, mean (SD)	50.5 (9.8)
Median	50.5
Minimum, maximum	23.7, 79.2
Age group, n (%)	
18–34	30 (5.3%)
35–44	128 (22.8%)
45–54	229 (40.7%)
55–64	137 (24.4%)
65+	38 (6.8%)
Female, n (%)	352 (62.6%)
Index year, n (%)	
2011	185 (32.9%)
2012	265 (47.2%)
2013	112 (19.9%)
MS ICD-10-GM codes at index quarter, n (%)[a]	
G35.0: Initial manifestation of MS	92 (16.4%)
G35.1: Mainly relapsing/remitting MS	288 (51.2%)
G35.2: Primary progressive MS	121 (21.5%)
G35.3: Secondary progressive MS	175 (31.1%)
G35.9: MS, unspecified	450 (80.1%)
Exclusively unspecified diagnosis (G35.9)	85 (15.1%)
First prescribed DMT, n (%)[c]	
IM INF beta-1a	50 (8.9%)
SC INF beta-1a	48 (8.5%)
SC INF beta-1b	59 (10.5%)
Glatiramer acetate	85 (15.1%)
Natalizumab	41 (7.3%)
Teriflunomide	0 (0%)
Fingolimod	19 (3.4%)
Dimethyl fumarate	3 (0.5%)
None	257 (45.7%)
MS-related medications, n (%)[d]	
Corticosteroids	225 (40.0%)
Immunosuppressants	84 (14.9%)
Drugs for symptom relief, n (%)[d]	
Antidementia	6 (1.1%)

Table 1 Patient characteristics (Continued)

Antidepressants	179 (31.9%)
Antiepileptics	97 (17.3%)
Select muscle relaxants	227 (40.4%)
Urinary antispasmodics	122 (21.7%)
Medications to manage fatigue	37 (6.6%)
Medications for tremor	2 (0.4%)
CCI, mean (SD)[d]	1.08 (1.39)
Median	0
Minimum, maximum	0.00, 6.00
CCI, n (%)[d]	
0	210 (37.4%)
1	61 (10.9%)
2+	291 (51.8%)
Top 10 diagnoses using ICD-10-GM codes (n, %)[d]	
H52.2: Astigmatism	158 (28.1%)
I10.9: Essential (primary) hypertension not further specified	123 (21.9%)
F32.9: Depressive episode unspecified	122 (21.7%)
G82.4: Spastic tetraplegia	113 (20.1%)
H52.4: Presbyopia	107 (19.0%)
R26.8: Other and unspecified abnormalities of gait and mobility	107 (19.0%)
N31.9: Neuromuscular dysfunction of bladder unspecified	101 (18.0%)
N89.8: Other specified non-inflammatory disorders of vagina[b]	100 (28.4%)
N39.4: Other specified urinary incontinence	99 (17.6%)
G82.1: Spastic paraplegia	98 (17.4%)

Abbreviations: *CCI* Charlson Comorbidity Index, *DMT* disease-modifying therapy, *ICD-10-GM* International Classification of Diseases, 10th Revision, German Modification, *IM* intramuscular, *INF* interferon, *MS* multiple sclerosis, *SC* subcutaneous, *SD* standard deviation
[a]More than 1 diagnosis was possible during the index quarter; [b]calculated only for females
[c]measured in the whole period of 9 quarters (4 quarters pre-index, 1 quarter index, 4 quarters post-index)
[d]measured in the 4 quarters before the index fampridine prescription

In addition, the mean number of sick leave days and corticosteroid prescriptions declined significantly during the fampridine treatment period within the no DMT cohort (MS-related sick leave days: mean, 12.0–5.7 days, $P = 0.002$; corticosteroid prescriptions: 0.9–0.7, $P = 0.013$).

The inpatient costs declined significantly from the pre- to the post-index period in the no DMT subgroup

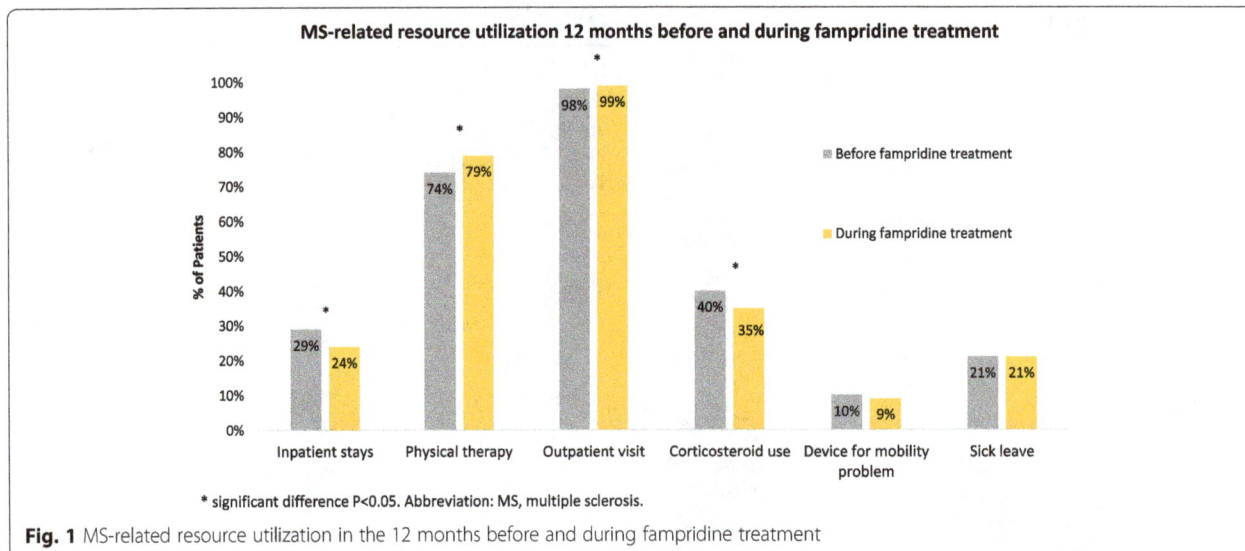

Fig. 1 MS-related resource utilization in the 12 months before and during fampridine treatment

(€2,004 vs €1,600, $P < 0.001$), whereas no significant differences could be observed within the other subgroups (€458 vs €457, $P = 0.872$ continuous DMT subgroup; €1,856 vs €1,691, $P = 0.174$ discontinuous DMT subgroup). Partly due to the lack of DMT costs, the no DMT subgroup had the lowest MS-related healthcare costs (€9,197), with €26,984 in the continuous DMT subgroup and €21,893 in the discontinuous DMT subgroup.

Stratification by age

Almost half of the patients were younger than 50 years (48%), and older patients had a higher CCI than younger patients (1.81 vs 1.06). Over half (57%) of the older and one-third (34%) of the younger age subgroups did not use DMTs. During fampridine treatment, 27% of the younger subgroup and 21% of the older subgroup had MS-related inpatient stays. These rates of MS-related hospitalization were significantly lower than in the pre-index period, with 33% in the younger age subgroup ($P < 0.05$) and 26% in the older age subgroup ($P < 0.05$) hospitalized.

Total MS-related healthcare costs in the treatment period for those aged ≥50 years were €14,920, and €20,804 for those aged 18 to 49 years. The second highest cost component next to pharmacotherapy was the inpatient sector among the younger aged subgroup and physical therapy in the older aged subgroup.

Stratification by antispasmodic treatment

Fifty-three percent ($n = 297$) of the fampridine patients had at least 1 prescription claim for antispasmodics during the study period. Twenty-seven percent of these had MS-related inpatient stays. Among the antispasmodic non-users, 20% were hospitalized due to MS in the post-

index period. In the pre-index period, the MS-related hospitalizations were significantly higher, with 33% ($P < 0.05$) and 26% ($P < 0.05$) compared to the post-index period for the users and non-users, respectively. The MS-related total costs were €18,100 in the antispasmodic non-user subgroup and €16,760 in the antispasmodic user subgroup (see Fig. 3).

Discussion

This study shows the differences in MS-related healthcare resource use and costs of patients in Germany initiating and continuing treatment with fampridine for at least 12 months compared to the 12 months prior to treatment initiation.

Patients starting fampridine treatment were, on average, 50 years old, which demonstrates that the disease had already progressed, as the average age for disease onset is 30 [12]. The mean age at the start of fampridine therapy, however, is slightly lower in Germany than in the United States (US), where the mean age is 55 years [13].

Before commencing fampridine treatment, many patients used medications such as muscle relaxants and antidepressants, which is similar to other findings [13]. The percentage of non-DMT users was slightly higher with 46% in this German population compared to 38% of MS patients in the US, as noted by M Jara, MF Sidovar and HR Henney [13] in 2014. Almost every patient had at least 1 outpatient visit, 24% were hospitalized due to MS in the treatment period, and 81% utilized physical therapy in addition to fampridine treatment. This study reveals that the combination of fampridine treatment and physical therapy is common in Germany, supporting the fact that fampridine is used complementary to rather than in place of physical therapy [14, 15] whereas

Table 2 MS-related healthcare costs before and during fampridine treatment

	Pre-index period (before fampridine treatment)	Observation period (during fampridine treatment)	P-value
	N = 562	N = 562	
Inpatient, mean (SD)	**€1,565.42** (€3,335.18)	**€1,333.42** (€3,882.73)	0.0005
Median	€0	€0	
Minimum, maximum	€0, €30,568.04	€0, €62,415.54	
Physical therapy, mean (SD)	**€810.89** (€887.80)	**€963.92** (€925.50)	<0.0001
Median	€613.28	€825.40	
Minimum, maximum	€0, €8,015.80	€0, €6,945.80	
Outpatient, mean (SD)	**€518.09** (€341.78)	**€565.47** (€338.85)	<0.0001
Median	€459.33	€508.52	
Minimum, maximum	€0, €2,794.88	€0, €2,851.23	
Pharmacotherapy			
DMTs, mean (SD)	**€7,684.42** (€8,908.24)	**€8,604.78** (€9,948.43)	<0.0001
Median	€0	€0	
Minimum, maximum	€0, €29,157.08	€0, €33,639.54	
Corticosteroids, mean (SD)	**€108.24** (€194.47)	**€88.88** (€181.15)	0.0054
Median	€0	€0	
Minimum, maximum	€0, €989.38	€0, €1,041.33	
Fampridine, mean (SD)	**€0** (€0)	**€5,519.32** (€1,565.83)	<0.0001
Median	€0	€5,908.53	
Minimum, maximum	€0, €0	€225.11, €10,033.99	
Other MS-related prescriptions, mean (SD)	**€267.10** (€525.92)	**€306.90** (€642.63)	0.1229
Median	€52.16	€55.53	
Minimum, maximum	€0, €4,782.96	€0, €7,358.06	
Devices for mobility problems, mean (SD)	**€6.09** (€26.95)	**€9.17** (€58.20)	0.7468
Median	€0	€0	
Minimum, maximum	€0, €344.01	€0, €1,146.39	
Total MS-related healthcare, mean (SD)	**€10,960.26** (€9,030.32)	**€17,391.86** (€10,325.65)	<0.0001
Median	€9,376.59	€14,447.76	
Minimum, maximum	€0, €44,126.80	€1,107.41, €67,001.71	

Bolded text indicates the main message – the mean values and the categories
Abbreviations: *DMT* disease-modifying therapy, *MS* multiple sclerosis, *SD* standard deviation

physical therapy was deemed the appropriate comparator in the fampridine German Arzneimittelmarkt-Neuordnungsgesetz AMNOG) (ie, evaluation of new pharmaceuticals in Germany) value dossier. However, as the requested comparison did not include sufficient data, no additional benefit was stated [14]. The significant reductions in corticosteroid use and inpatient stays after initiating fampridine might be due to improvement of mobility problems. Improvement could also be due to the increase in physical therapy. Furthermore, the increasing use of physical therapy might also suggest that patients became more active to deal with mobility issues after experiencing the benefit from fampridine. It is also possible that individuals motivated to initiate and adhere

to fampridine treatment might also be subsequently motivated to attend physical therapy sessions. In addition to physical therapy, other outpatient care played an important role in treating MS (approximately 19 visits per year per patient), as GPs were contacted at least twice and neurologists at least once per quarter. M Jara, MF Sidovar and HR Henney [13] reported that 79.1% of the first fampridine prescriptions were prescribed by neurologists in the US, which is higher than the estimated 45% of MS patients visiting a neurologist for their MS in our study.

The total MS-related healthcare costs were significantly higher in the fampridine treatment period compared to the period before fampridine treatment, mainly due to the increased pharmacotherapy costs.

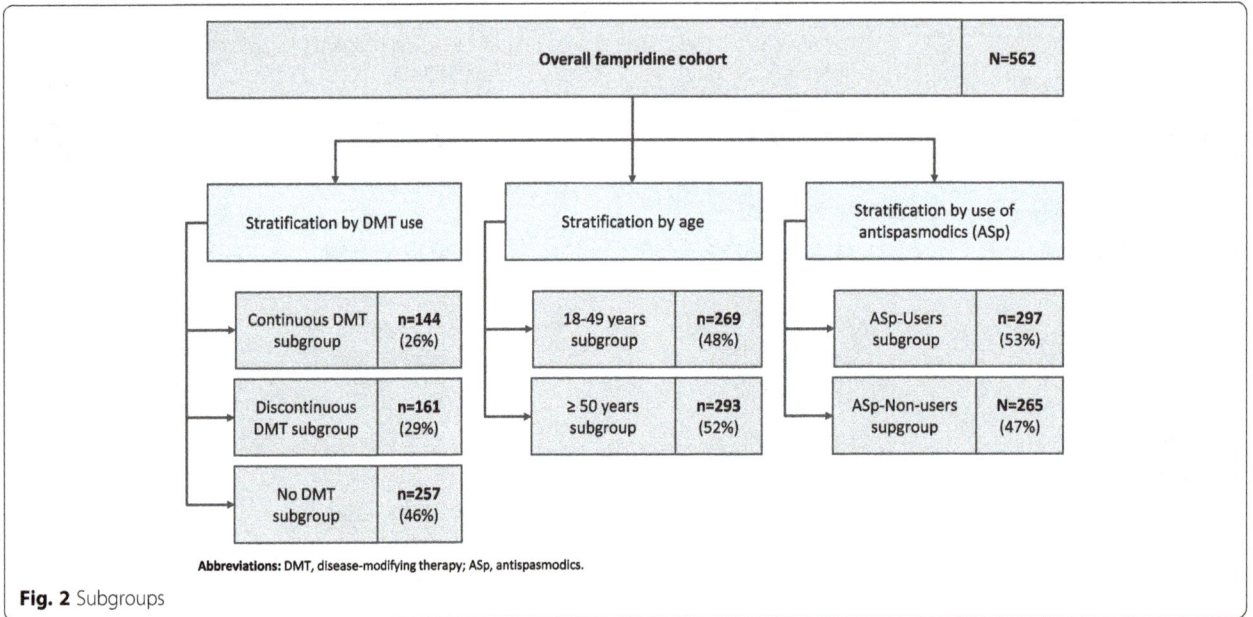

Fig. 2 Subgroups

Pharmacotherapy accounted for 82% of post-index MS-related costs, followed by the inpatient sector, with 8%. A high percentage of prescription costs relative to overall MS-related costs (65%) was also found by JD Prescott, S Factor, M Pill and GW Levi [16] in 2004. However, in contrast to the increasing pharmacotherapy costs, the MS-related inpatient costs declined during fampridine treatment compared to the pre-treatment period (€1,333 vs €1,565, *P* < 0.001). This means that while the main cost driver (pharmacotherapy) increased, the second highest cost component (inpatient costs) declined simultaneously.

The different patient subgroup analyses revealed findings that were consistent with the overall analysis. Prescription costs were the highest in all subgroups, followed by inpatient costs, except within the continuous DMT and ≥50-year-old subgroups, where physical therapy costs were higher than the inpatient costs. However, slight differences were observed, for example in the 3 subgroups measuring DMT treatment concerning characteristics such as age, comorbidity burden, and MS-related inpatient stays. The no DMT subgroup mostly had significant changes from pre- to post-fampridine initiation, including MS-related hospitalizations, corticosteroid use,

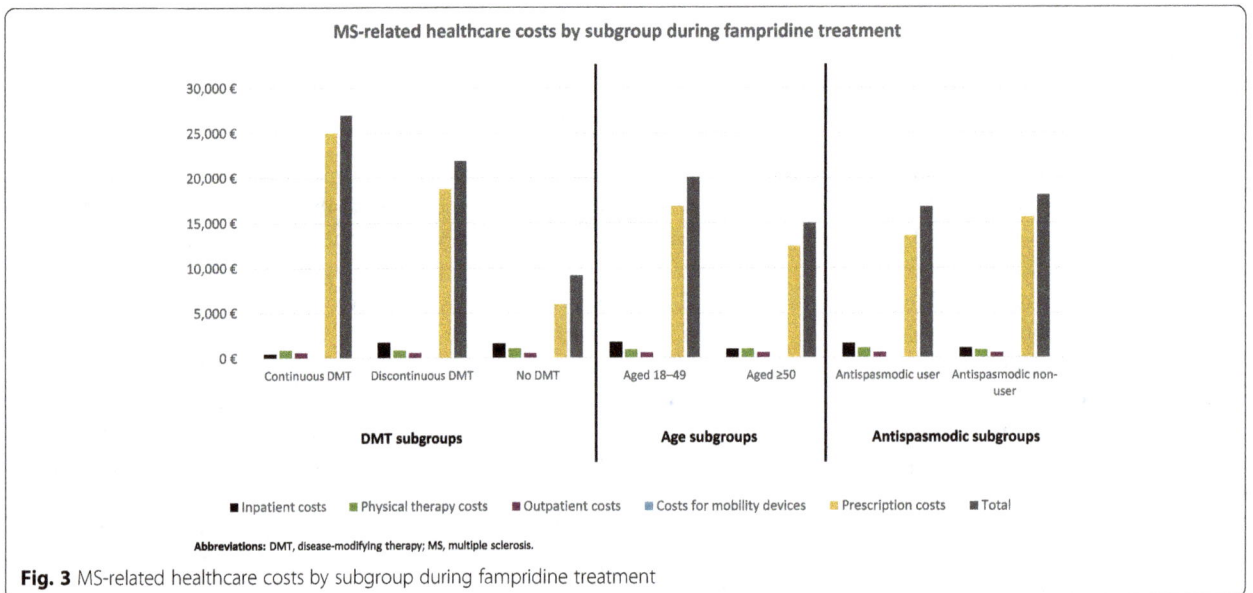

Fig. 3 MS-related healthcare costs by subgroup during fampridine treatment

and MS-related sick leave days. It was assumed that these patients were not relapsing-remitting MS patients; therefore, they had limited options for DMT treatment and may benefit the most from fampridine. Another explanation might be that without DMT treatment these patients were more willing to adhere to fampridine treatment and subsequently also physical therapy.

Several limitations of this study should be mentioned. First, there were no comparisons to fampridine discontinuers or non-users, and further research is warranted in these areas as the results cannot be generalized to those patient groups. Second, no information on clinical outcomes, such as Expanded Disability Status Scale scores, is available in claims data, so the severity of the disability could not be evaluated. Third, no adjustments, such as for the use of physical therapy, outpatient visits, or disease progression, were made and therefore the impact of these aspects on the outcomes could not be estimated. Fourth, claims data are not collected for research but instead for accounting purposes and therefore include only sectors that are reimbursed by the statutory health insurance. Therefore, indirect costs such as societal costs of MS-attributable informal care could not be assessed. Additionally, compliance with medication regimens could only be approximated based on prescription fills, as the actual intake is not observable in this data source. Last, the number of outpatient visits could only be approximated and may be underestimated, as flat charges for outpatient visits on a quarterly basis exist in Germany.

Conclusion

This study provides insights into the treatment of MS patients in Germany beginning treatment with fampridine and continuing treatment for at least 12 months. These patients visit the GP and neurologist regularly, and physical therapy is used in combination with fampridine treatment in almost every case. Besides the pharmacotherapy costs, the inpatient costs were the second most important cost driver in all but 2 patient subgroups. Inpatient stays, as well as the costs, declined during fampridine treatment compared to the pretreatment period. The overall costs, however, increased due to the pharmaceutical costs. This cost increase might be justified due to improved patient outcomes beyond the reduced healthcare utilization; however, patient reported outcomes are not available within the Statutory Health Insurance. To better understand fampridine influence in the real world, further research is necessary.

Abbreviations
AMNOG: Arzneimittelmarkt-Neuordnungsgesetz; ASp: Antispasmodics; ATC: Anatomical therapeutic chemical classification system; CCI: Charlson Comorbidity Index; DMT: Disease-modifying therapy; GP: General practitioner; HRI: Health Risk Institute; ICD-10-GM: International Classification of Diseases, 10th Revision, German Modification; IM: Intramuscular; INF: Interferon; MS: Multiple sclerosis; SC: Subcutaneous; SD: Standard deviation; US: United States

Acknowledgements
Not applicable

Funding
This study was sponsored by Biogen.

Authors' contributions
TZ, MYH, CP, JSH, SB, PLB were involved in the design of the study, interpretation of the data and drafting the manuscript. Furthermore TZ, MYH, CP, JSH, SB, PLB, AL, AK, EG, and SP interpreted the data, critically revised the manuscript, gave final approval of the version to be published and agree to be held accountable for all aspects of the work.

Author's information (optional)
Not applicable

Competing interests
AL, EG, SP and MYH are employees of and hold stock/stock options in Biogen. AK is a contract employee of Biogen.
TZ has received reimbursements for participation in scientific advisory boards from Bayer Healthcare, Biogen Idec, Novartis Pharma AG, Merck Serono, Teva, Genzyme, and Synthon. He has also received speaker honorarium from Bayer Healthcare, Biogen Idec, Genzyme, Merck Sharp & Dohme, GlaxoSmithKline, Novartis Pharma AG, Teva, Sanofi Aventis, and Almirall. He has also received research support from Bayer Healthcare, Biogen Idec, Genzyme, Novartis Pharma AG, Teva, and Sanofi Aventis.
CP, JSH, SB, and PLB are employees of Xcenda, which has a research consultancy agreement with Biogen.
The data analysis was performed in cooperation between Xcenda and Elsevier Health Analytics.
This study was sponsored by Biogen.

Ethics approval and consent to participate
The current analysis was conducted using the InGef (formerly known as Health Risk Institute after re-branding) research database, which contains anonymized, patient-level inpatient, outpatient, sick leave, and pharmacy claims data from around 75 health insurance companies, representing a large proportion of the approximately 120 health insurances that comprise the SHI in Germany and providing good external validity. For 2009–2014, the InGef research database contained individual, de-identified claims data for about 4 million people, with a patient sample that is representative of the German population for age and gender. The database is fully compliant with all data protection regulations in Germany and has been certified as such. Since the InGef research database includes verified accounting data of the participating insurance companies, these claims data are regularly audited by the insurance companies for reimbursement purposes and are prepared in accordance with German Social Law (paragraphs 287 SGB V and 75 SGB X). This study utilized an existing dataset in line with all data protection regulations, and patients were not identified for the purpose of this study.
This study is a retrospective database analysis based on fully anonymized claims data, and claims data are recorded for accounting purposes and not for clinical research. No electronic medical records or other clinical parameters were used. As a result, no ethical approval or consent from an ethics committee or review board was required for this study.

Author details
[1]Universitätsklinium Dresden, Fetscherstraße 74, 01307 Dresden, Germany. [2]Xcenda GmbH, Lange Laube 31, D-30159 Hannover, Germany. [3]Biogen, Cambridge, MA, USA. [4]Xcenda LLC, Palm Harbor, FL, USA. [5]Biogen GmbH, Carl-Zeiss-Ring 6, 85737 Ismaning, Germany.

References

1. Paltamaa J, Sarasoja T, Leskinen E, Wikstrom J, Malkia E. Measures of physical functioning predict self-reported performance in self-care, mobility, and domestic life in ambulatory persons with multiple sclerosis. Arch Phys Med Rehabil. 2007;88(12):1649–57.

2. Panitch H, Applebee A. Treatment of walking impairment in multiple sclerosis: an unmet need for a disease-specific disability. Expert Opin Pharmacother. 2011;12(10):1511–21.

3. Zwibel HL. Contribution of impaired mobility and general symptoms to the burden of multiple sclerosis. Adv Ther. 2009;26(12):1043–57.

4. Van Asch P. Impact of mobility impairment in multiple sclerosis 2-patients' perspectives. Eur Neurol Rev. 2011;6(2):115–20.

5. Larocca NG. Impact of walking impairment in multiple sclerosis: perspectives of patients and care partners. Patient. 2011;4(3):189–201.

6. EPAR summary for the public - Fampyra (fampridine) - EMA/430040/2011, EMEA/H/C/002097 [http://www.ema.europa.eu/docs/en_GB/document_library/EPAR_-_Summary_for_the_public/human/002097/WC500109958.pdf]. Accessed 1 July 2016.

7. Andersohn F, Walker J. Characteristics and external validity of the German Health Risk Institute (HRI) Database. Pharmacoepidemiol Drug Saf. 2016; 25(1):106–9.

8. Deutsche Gesellschaft für Neurologie (German Neurological Society). Diagnose und therapie der multiplen sklerose. 2014. Leitlinie S2e. AWMF-Registernummer: 030/050 2014.

9. Hoer A, Schiffhorst G, Zimmermann A, Fischaleck J, Gehrmann L, Ahrens H, Carl G, Sigel KO, Osowski U, Klein M, et al. Multiple sclerosis in Germany: data analysis of administrative prevalence and healthcare delivery in the statutory health system. BMC Health Serv Res. 2014;14:381.

10. Bonafede MM, Johnson BH, Wenten M, Watson C. Treatment patterns in disease-modifying therapy for patients with multiple sclerosis in the United States. Clin Ther. 2013;35(10):1501–12.

11. Consumer Price Index and Inflation Rate. [https://www.destatis.de/EN/FactsFigures/NationalEconomyEnvironment/Prices/ConsumerPriceIndices/ConsumerPriceIndices.html].

12. Flachenecker P, Stuke K, Elias W, Freidel M, Haas J, Pitschnau-Michel D, Schimrigk S, Zettl UK, Rieckmann P. Multiple sclerosis registry in Germany: results of the extension phase 2005/2006. Dtsch Arztebl Int. 2008;105(7):113–9.

13. Jara M, Sidovar MF, Henney HR. Prescriber utilization of dalfampridine extended release tablets in multiple sclerosis: a retrospective pharmacy and medical claims analysis. Ther Clin Risk Manag. 2015;11:1–7.

14. Zusammenfassende Dokumentation über die Änderung der Arzneimittel-Richtlinie (AM-RL): Anlage XII - Beschlüsse über die Nutzenbewertung von Arzneimitteln mit neuen Wirkstoffen nach § 35a SGB V - Fampridin, Stand: 28. November 2012 [https://www.g-ba.de/informationen/nutzenbewertung/14/#tab/beschluesse].

15. Anlage III - Vorlage zur Abgabe einer schriftlichen Stellungnahme zur Nutzenbewertung nach § 35a SGB V Stellungnahme Arzneimittelkommission Fampridine Vergleichstherapie, 23.05.2012 [http://www.akdae.de/Stellungnahmen/AMNOG/A-Z/Fampridin/Fampridin.pdf]. Accessed 1 July 2016.

16. Prescott JD, Factor S, Pill M, Levi GW. Descriptive analysis of the direct medical costs of multiple sclerosis in 2004 using administrative claims in a large nationwide database. J Manag Care Pharm. 2007;13(1):44–52.

11

Seasonal adherence to, and effectiveness of, subcutaneous interferon β-1a administered by RebiSmart® in patients with relapsing multiple sclerosis: results of the 1-year, observational GEPAT-SMART study

Spyros N. Deftereos[1][*] (iD), Evangelos Koutlas[2], Efrosini Koutsouraki[3], Athanassios Kyritsis[4], Panagiotis Papathanassopoulos[5], Nikolaos Fakas[6], Vaia Tsimourtou[7], Nikolaos Vlaikidis[3], Antonios Tavernarakis[8], Konstantinos Voumvourakis[9], Michalis Arvanitis[10], Dimitrios Sakellariou[1] and Filippo DeLorenzo[1]

Abstract

Background: Little is known about whether tolerability and adherence to treatment can be influenced by weather and temperature conditions. The objective of this study was to assess monthly and seasonal adherence to and safety of sc IFN-β1a (Rebif®, Merck) in relapsing-remitting multiple sclerosis (RRMS) patients using the RebiSmart® electronic autoinjector.

Methods: A multicentre, prospective observational study in Greece in adult RRMS patients with EDSS < 6, under Rebif®/RebiSmart® treatment for ≤6 weeks before enrollment. The primary endpoint was monthly, seasonal and annual adherence over 12 months (defined in text). Secondary endpoints included number of relapses, disability, adverse events.

Results: Sixty four patients enrolled and 47 completed all study visits (Per Protocol Set - PPS). Mean annual adherence was 97.93% ± 5.704 with no significant monthly or seasonal variations. Mean relapses in the pre- and post- treatment 12-months were 1.1 ± 0.47 and 0.2 ± 0.54 ($p < 0.0001$, PPS). 10 patients (22%) showed 3-month disability progression, 19 (40%) stabilization and 18 (38%) improvement. EDSS was not correlated to pre- ($r = 0.024$, $p = 0.87$) or post-treatment relapses ($r = 0.022$, $p = 0.88$).

Conclusion: High adherence with no significant seasonal or weather variation was observed over 12 months. While the efficacy on relapses was consistent with published studies, we could not identify a relationship between relapses and disability.

Keywords: Multiple sclerosis, Interferons, Rebif, Rebismart, Treatment adherence and compliance, Clinical efficacy

* Correspondence: spyros.deftereos@external.merckgroup.gr
[1]Merck Hellas, 41-45 Kifisias av, 15123 Athens, Greece
Full list of author information is available at the end of the article

Background

Adherence to treatment in Multiple Sclerosis (MS) is an important determinant of long-term outcomes, as suggested by the World Health Organization [1] and evidenced by several published studies [2–4]. However, the need for long-term treatment and the frequently debilitating nature of the disease make treatment adherence particularly challenging. This may impact disease progression, as on the one hand up 72% of patients do not adhere to disease-modifying MS treatments according to published studies [2, 5, 6], while on the other poor adherence has been associated with a higher rate of relapse [6].

The interferons (beta-1a and beta-1b) are among the first Disease Modifying Drugs (DMDs) that were approved for MS. These platform therapies are frequently associated with flu-like syndrome and injection-site reactions, which are among the reasons of non-adherence according to some studies [7]. Taking into account that the flu-like syndrome comprises a constellation of symptoms some of which may be more difficult to tolerate when the weather is hot, such as fever, chills and headache, we asked whether seasonal variation of weather conditions affects adherence to interferon treatment. As higher temperatures are typically observed in the Mediterranean countries, especially during the summer period, any effects of seasonal variation on adherence would be expected to be more pronounced in these countries. We, therefore, studied the seasonal variation of the adherence to sc IFN-β1a tiw (Rebif®), administered through the RebiSmart® autoinjector device, for a 12-month period, in patients with Relapsing-Remitting Multiple Sclerosis (RRMS) in Greece. Rebif® safety, including the occurrence of flu-like, was also studied.

Methods

The GEPAT-SMART study (Greece Epidemiological Project on Adherence and Temperature Using RebiS-MART®) was a multicentre, prospective, observational study carried out at 9 sites in Greece (Greek registry of non-interventional clinical trials id: 200136, date of registration: February 18th, 2013 [8]). The recruitment period lasted from February 2013 to February 2014. The last patient follow-up ended on April 2015. The study was carried out in accordance with the Declaration of Helsinki and applicable national regulatory requirements and was approved by local ethics committees at each study site [ethics committee of the Papageorgiou Hospital of Thessaloniki (reference number 161/20.9.2012), ethics committee of the AHEPA Hospital (reference number 32/5.12.2012), ethics committee of the University Hospital of Ioannina (reference number 754/12.11.2012), ethics committee of the University Hospital of Patras (reference number 83/7.2.2013), ethics committee of the 401 Army Hospital of Athens (reference number 15/2012), ethics committee of the University

Hospital of Larissa (reference number 19/13.11.2012), ethics committee of the Papanikolaou Hospital of Thessaloniki (reference number 11/3.10.2012), ethics committee of the Evangelismos Hospital (reference number 345/13.12.12), ethics committee of the Attiko Hospital (reference number 10/5.10.2012)]. Patients were enrolled after written informed consent had been obtained.

Participants

Inclusion criteria were 1) RRMS diagnosis (revised McDonald criteria (2010)), 2) Rebif® multi-dose injected by RebiSmart® prescribed according to the approved Summary of Product Characteristics (SmPC) within six (6) weeks prior to their enrolment into the study, 3) capable to handle RebiSmart®, 4) willing and capable to comply will all study requirements and procedures, 5) 18 to 65 years old and 6) Expanded Disability Scale Score (EDSS) < 6 at enrollment.

Exclusion criteria were 1) presence of any contraindication mentioned in the locally approved SmPC, 2) severe relapse within 30 days before study treatment commencement, 3) visual or physical impairment precluding them from self-injecting with RebiSmart®, 4) MS therapy within 6 months prior to study, 5) current or past (within the last 2 years prior to study enrolment) history of alcohol or drug abuse, 6) participation in another clinical trial during the last 30 days prior to study treatment commencement. Female subjects who were pregnant or breast-feeding were also excluded. Female patients with childbearing potential had to utilize a highly effective method of contraception for the duration of the study.

Administration of the study drug

All patients were provided with a RebiSmart® device (Merck, Darmstadt, Germany) for self-administration of serum-free Rebif® 44 μg or 22 μg sc three times weekly (tiw) for 12 months or until early discontinuation (ED). RebiSmart® is a CE-certified medical device. The dose of Rebif® was titrated over the first 4 weeks in accordance with the drug labeling information; the final dose was at the discretion of the treating physician and based on the recommendations in the drug labeling information.

Patient assessments

Following a pre-study evaluation visit, patients attended the study site at Study Day 1 (baseline), Month 6, and Month 12. At the baseline visit, all patients provided written informed consent and information on demographics, medical history, concomitant diseases, and MS history, including the number and characteristics of relapses in the past 12 months, was collected. At each post-baseline visit, the investigators recovered adherence data from the autoinjector. Reasons for missed injections were recorded in a patient diary. Relapse assessment, EDSS score, MS-related concomitant medication, vital signs, on-going therapy with Rebif® (including dose), and adverse events (AEs) were also recorded.

Study endpoints

The primary endpoint was the monthly, seasonal and annual adherence rate over the 12-month study treatment. Adherence rate was defined as 100 × number of injections actually administered divided by the expected number of injections over the defined time period (month, season, year), as captured by RebiSmart®. Secondary endpoints were: 1) reasons for missed injections, 2) proportion of patients free of relapses at month 12, 3) mean number of relapses at 12 months, 4) proportion of patients without progression of 3-month confirmed disability, at 12 months. Disability progression was defined as worsening by at least 0.5 EDSS points from baseline, 5) proportion of patients who discontinued prematurely the study treatment and the reasons for discontinuation. All (Serious) Adverse Events [(S)AEs] and Adverse Drug Reactions [(S)ADRs] were also recorded, 6) Patient evaluation of RebiSmart® based on a Convenience Questionnaire.

The following criteria were to be met for establishing an MS relapse: 1) Neurological abnormality, either newly appearing or re-appearing, at least 30 days after the onset of a preceding clinical event, with > = 24 h duration, 2) absence of fever (temperature > 37.5C) or known infection and 3) objective neurological impairment, correlating with the patient's reported symptoms, defined as either increase in at least one of the functional systems of the EDSS domain or increase of the total EDSS score. Severity of relapses was described as mild, moderate, or severe according to the Activities of Daily Living criteria [9]. AEs were classified according to MedDRA v14.0 [10].

Sample size

The calculation of the sample size was based on the primary endpoint of the study. Due to the lack of literature data regarding the seasonal and monthly adherence, the adherence over the 12-month treatment period was used. According to available data the expected adherence during the study period was expected to be approximately 70% and the standard deviation 15% [11]. Therefore, 70 patients would be required to estimate the mean adherence rate with accuracy of less than ± 4%.

Statistical analyses

This manuscript was development according to the STROBE (STrengthening the Reporting of OBservational studies in Epidemiology) guideline for reporting observational studies [12]. Descriptive statistics were calculated for all study variables. Summary statistics for categorical variables were presented as the number and percent of subjects in each category.

Seasonal and monthly variance of the adherence level was analyzed by One Way Analysis of Variance (ANOVA). Pre- and post-treatment relapse rate was compared by the Wilcoxon signed-rank test. Pearson's r was used to study correlation between variables. The level of significance was set to 5% (two-sided). Descriptive statistics were used for AEs and SAEs. Adverse events where handled according to the study protocol.

Statistical analyses sets were performed in the following sets:

- Full analysis set (FAS): all recruited subjects who fulfilled the inclusion/exclusion criteria.
- Per-protocol set (PPS): all FAS subjects who completed all study visits.
- Safety set: all study patients who actually received at least one dose of treatment for MS following informed consent.

No replacement policy existed in this study for drop-out patients and missing data.

Results
Patient demographics

Sixty four of the 66 patients that started documentation received at least one dose of Rebif® and were included in the Safety Set and FAS, while the remaining two did not fulfill the inclusion/exclusion criteria and were not enrolled. Of these, 58 patients (87.9%) completed the month-6 visit, and 47 (71.2%) completed the month-12 visit. Patient disposition is shown in Fig. 1 and demographics are shown in Table 1. Baseline MS characteristics are shown in Table 2.

Primary endpoint: 12-month and seasonal adherence

Mean adherence to Rebif®, administered through RebiSmart®, was 97.93% (±5.704) in FAS and 98.32% (±2.628) in PPS respectively (Table 3). No significant variations in monthly and seasonal adherence were noted (one-way ANOVA). Adherence did not vary significantly among different subgroups of the various demographic factors (Table 4).

Thirty-one patients missed at least one dose of the study treatment. The main reasons for non-adherence were forgotten dose and other (12 subjects each, 18.8%), followed by presence of viral infection (flu, 15.6%) and absence from home (10.9%, Table 5).

Secondary endpoints
Efficacy

Among the 47 patients that completed all study visits (PPS), 6 (12.8%) relapsed with a mean number of

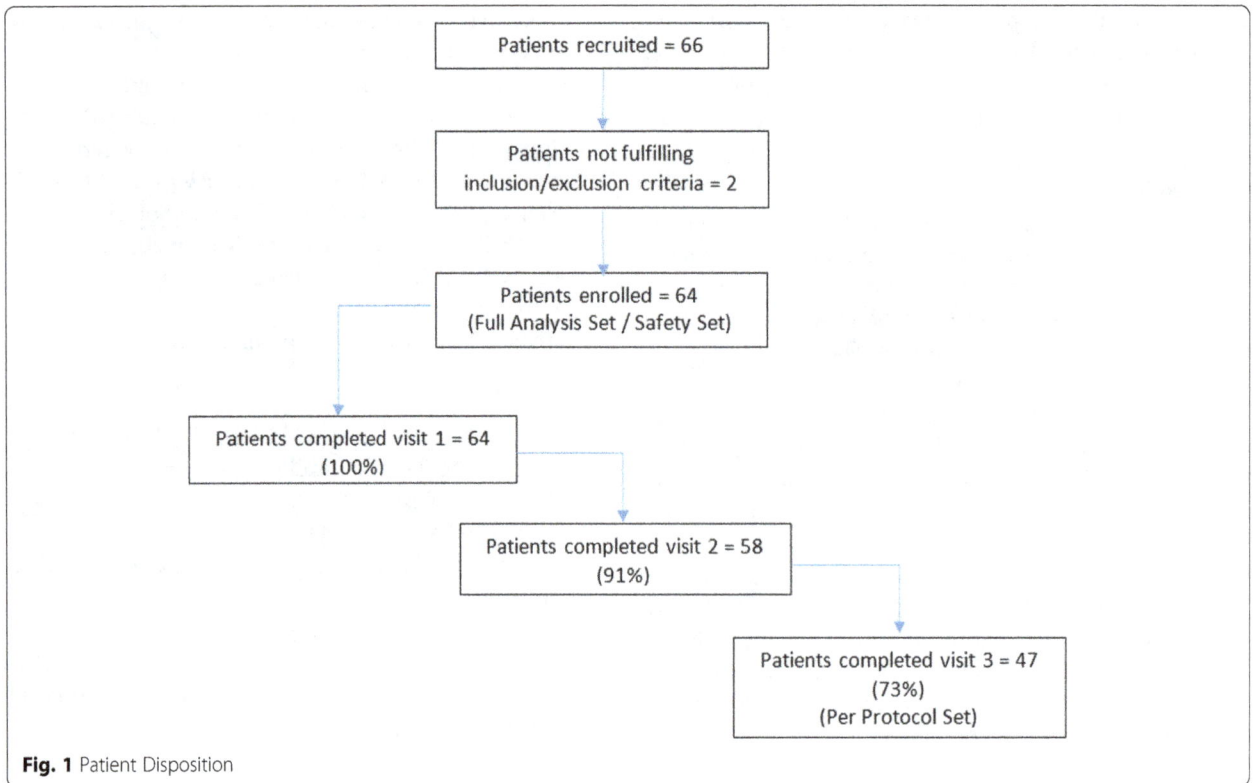

Fig. 1 Patient Disposition

relapses 1.3 ± 0.8 and 41 (87.2%) did not relapse. In the FAS 10 patients relapsed (15.6%) with a mean number of relapses 1.3 ± 0.6 and 54 (84.4%) did not relapse. Annual mean number of relapses in the PPS was 0.2 ± 0.54. This value was significantly lower compared to the mean number of relapses in the 12-month pre-Rebif® period (1.1 ± 0.47, $p < 10^{-15}$, Wilcoxon rank-sum test) (Fig. 2).

3-month confirmed disability progression at the end of the study period was observed in 10 patients (21%), while in 19 (40%) patients EDSS remained stable and improved in 18 (39%). Median EDSS progression was 1 point (range 0.5–2.5) in the former group, while median improvement was 0.5 points (range 0.5–2) in the latter group. Overall, in the PPS mean EDSS change was not significantly different from zero with a mean of 0.17 ± 1.13 points (median 0). EDSS was related neither to the 12-month pre-treatment number of relapses ($r = 0.024$, $p = 0.87$), nor to the 12-month post-treatment number of relapses ($r = 0.022$, $p = 0.88$) (Fig. 3). Furthermore, mean 12-month relapses pre- and post-treatment were not significantly different among those in whom EDSS improved, remained stable or deteriorated (one-way ANOVA, $p = 0.94$ and 0.24 respectively, Fig. 4).

Safety

Of the 64 patients in the FAS, 58 (90%) assessed RebiSmart®. Median score was 5 (highest) for all questionnaire items, while mean values are shown in Fig. 5. ED was

documented for 19 patients (29% of the Safety Population). The most common reason was 'patient's decision to quit treatment' (8/64, 12.5%), followed by 'adverse event' (4/64, 6.2%). Among the four cases where the drug was discontinued due to AEs, pregnancy was the reason in one, while in the other three cases the reasons were fatigue, malaise, anorexia, pyrexia and infections.

Treatment with Rebif® using RebiSmart® was well tolerated. No new safety signals were detected through this study. Sixty two reports of flu-like syndrome and of related symptoms (headache, malaise, myalgia) were obtained. Figure 6 shows the monthly distribution of these reports. While the distribution is not even throughout the year ($p < 0.001$, χ^2 test), peaks are observed in the spring, summer and autumn; this speaks against an effect of hot weather on the frequency and gravity of flu-like syndrome. Furthermore, monthly reports of flu-like syndrome did not correlate with monthly adherence ($r = 0.14$, $p = 0.66$).

RebiSmart® was evaluated by study participants as easy to use and convenient, giving an average score of 4.5 or above in most items of the convenience questionnaire (Fig. 5). The lower score (average 3.5 ± 1.79) was given to the item "it has easy connection needle".

Discussion

To our knowledge, this is the first prospective study to assess yearly, seasonal and monthly adherence to, and efficacy, safety, and tolerability of Rebif® for RRMS

Table 1 Patient demographic characteristics (Full Analysis Set)

		n (%)
Gender	Males	14 (21.9)
	Females	50 (78.1)
Age (yrs)	n, mean ± sd	64, 36.2 ± 11.22
	min-max	18.3–68.8
Weight (kg)	n, mean ± sd	64, 69.9 ± 15.2
	min-max	47–127
Height (cm)	n, mean ± sd	64, 166.7± 9.24
	min-max	116–186
BMI (kg/m^2)	n, mean ± sd	64, 25.16± 5.16
	min-max	18.40–46.2
Race	Caucasian	64 (100)
Place of Residence	Urban	46 (71.9)
	Semi urban	6 (9.4)
	Rural	12 (18.8)
Region	Attica	17 (26.6)
	Peloponnese	10 (15.6)
	Epirus	2 (3.1)
	Central Greece	2 (3.1)
	Central Macedonia	17 (26.6)
	Western Macedonia	7 (10.9)
	Eastern Macedonia / Thrace	1 (1.6)
	Crete	6 (9.4)
	Thessaly	2 (3.1)
	Ionian Islands	7 (10.9)
	North Aegean islands	0 (0.0)
	South Aegean Islands	0 (0.0)
Marital Status	Not married	29 (45.3)
	Married	32 (50)
	Widow/er	2 (3.1)
	Divorced	0 (0.0)
	Separated	1 (1.6)
Educational Status	0 yrs	0 (0.0)
	Elementary (1–6 yrs)	4 (6.3)
	High School/Lyceum (7–12 yrs)	32 (50.0)
	University (> 12 yrs)	28 (43.8)
Working status	Private Sector Employee	18 (28.1)
	Public Sector Employee	12 (18.8)
	Retired	2 (3.1)
	Free lancer	8 (12.5)
	Student	6 (9.4)
	Unemployed	18 (28.1)

Table 2 Summary of MS History (Full Analysis Set)

	n	mean ± sd	median	min-max
Years since MS diagnosis	64	2.1 ± 4.00	0.2	0.04–14.3
Mean number of relapses within the last 24 months prior to Rebif® Rebismart™ initiation	62	1.5 ± 0.76	1.0	0–4
Mean number of relapses in which corticosteroids were usedwere used were used	62	0.9 ± 0.71	1.0	0–3
Mean number of relapses within the last 12 months prior to Rebif® Rebismart™ initiation	63	1.1 ± 0.47	1.0	0–2
Mean number of relapses in which corticosteroids were used	62	0.9 ± 0.57	1.0	0–2

means of patient-administered questionnaire [7]. Here, adherence data was objectively captured by the autoinjector electronically and therefore not subject to patient reporting errors [2, 13].

In our study cumulative 12-month adherence to Rebif® was very high (97.93 ± 5.704, FAS), confirming the

Table 3 12-month, seasonal and monthly adherence

	n	mean ± sd	median	min-max
12 month adherence to Rebif® - Rebismart® (Per Protocol Set)	46	98.32 ± 2.628	99.09	90.30–100
Study adherence to Rebif® - Rebismart® (Full Analysis Set)	62	97.93 ± 5.704	100	90.30–100
Seasonal adherence				
Jan-Mar	61	98.02 ± 6.879	100	57.97–100
Apr-Jun	57	98.36 ± 5.678	100	60.94–100
Jul-Sep	55	98.58 ± 3.276	100	81.63–100
Oct-Dec	56	97.91 ± 6.837	100	52.0–100
Monthly adherence				
Jan	60	97.54 ± 10.409	100	33.33–100
Feb	60	97.56 ± 8.513	100	54.55–100
March	59	98.34 ± 7.192	100	54.17–100
April	57	98.60 ± 6.826	100	50.00–100
May	57	98.67 ± 6.795	100	52.00–100
June	53	98.21 ± 5.560	100	65.00–100
July	52	98.45 ± 5.777	100	60.87–100
August	49	98.873 ± 2.935	100	86.67–100
September	52	98.46 ± 4.073	100	81.25–100
October	53	99.01 ± 2.963	100	86.67–100
November	52	97.933 ± 6.282	100	68.42–100
December	59	98.14 ± 6.721	100	52.00–100

Annual adherence: 100 × (total no of injections in 12 months) / expected no of infections in the respective months
Seasonal adherence: 100 × (total no of injections in a 3 month-period) / expected no of infections during the same period
Monthly adherence: 100 × (total no of injections in specific month) / expected no of infections

administered with an electronic autoinjector. In a previous study seasonal adherence to the interferons and glatiramer acetate had been studied retrospectively, by

Table 4 Comparison of adherence in different subgroups, according to demographic factors

		12 months Compliance to			
		n	mean ± sd	min-max	p-value
Gender,	Males	13	98.55 ± 2.501	90.67–100	0.712
	Females	33	98.23 ± 2.708	90.30–100	
Age (yrs)	< 65	45	98.28 ± 2.645	90.30–100	NA
	≥ 65	1	100.00	100–100	
Race	Caucasian	46	98.32 ± 2.623	90.30–100	NA
	African	(–)			
	Asian	(–)			
	Other	(–)			
Place of Residence	Urban	33	98.42 ± 2.600	90.30–100	0.322
	Semi urban	4	99.66 ± 0.676	98.65–100	
	Rural	9	97.35 ± 3.105	90.67–100	
Region	Attica	10	98.05 ± 3.099	90.30–100	NA
	Peloponnese	6	97.89 ± 3.485	90.91--100	
	Epirus	2	98.81 ± 0.025	98.80–98-83	
	Central Greece	2	100 ± 0	100–100	
	Central Macedonia	14	98.68 ± 1.721	93.85–100	
	Western Macedonia	5	97.73 ± 4.041	90.67–100	
	Eastern Macedonia	(–)			
	Thrace	(–)			
	Crete	(–)			
	Thessaly	5	97.42 ± 3.108	92.09–100	
	Ionian Islands	2	100 ± 0	100–100	
	Northern/Southern Aeg. islands	(–)			
Marital Status	Unmarried	22	98.36 ± 2.914	90.30–100	0.988
	Married	22	98.26 ± 2.465	90.67–100	
	Widow/er	2	98.48 ± 2.143	96.97–100	
	Divorced	(–)			
	Separated	(–)			
Educational Status	0 yrs	(–)			
	Elementary (1–6 yrs)	4	96.64 ± 3.150	92.09–98.80	0.243
	High School/Lyceum (7–12 yrs)	22	98.08 ± 2.823	90.67–100	
	University (> 12 yrs)	20	98.92 ± 2.222	90.30–100	
Working status	Private sector employee	14	98.35 ± 2.619	90.30–100	0.993
	Public sector employee	9	98.73 ± 3.061	90.67–100	
	Retired	2	98.63 ± 0	98.63–98.63	
	Free lancer	5	98.12 ± 0.896	96.89–98.83	
	Student	4	98.46 ± 3.073	93.85–100	
	Unemployed	12	97.96 ± 3.185	90.91–100	

findings of a previous 12-month and of two 12-week user trials with the same autoinjector [2, 11, 14], (97.0 ± 7.3% cumulative 12-month adherence [2], 90.3% of patients with > 90% adherence [14], and 88.2% of patients having administered ≥80% of scheduled injections, with 67% administering all scheduled injections [11] respectively). The use of an intramuscular IFN b-1a autoinjector in another study resulted in monthly compliance rates of 87.5–96.2%, supporting the notion that an autoinjector may contribute to high compliance [15].

Table 5 Reasons for non-adherence (Full Analysis Set)

	n (%)	Period of no injections	Events	Subject's Location	Events
Subjects that missed at least one injection	31 (48.4)				
Reasons for missing the injections					
1. They forgot the injection	12 (18.8)	Week days	22	Home Area	25
		Bank Holidays	3	Out of Residence	2
		Holidays	2		
		Total Events	27		
2. They were not willing to inject for cosmetic reasons	0				
3. Absence from home	7 (10.9)	Week days	13	Home Area	11
		Bank Holidays	2	Out of Residence	6
		Holidays	3		
		Total Events	17		
4. Other reasons	12 (18.8)	Week days	55	Home Area	54
		Bank Holidays	2	Out of Residence	3
		Holidays	0		
		Total Events	57		
5. Pain reaction at injection site	0				
6. Flu-like illness	10 (15.6)	Week days	55	Home Area	53
		Bank Holidays	0	Out of Residence	2
		Holidays	0		
		Total Events	55		

Interestingly, the COMPLIANCE study investigators [7], which took place in Spain, where weather conditions are similar to Greece's, reported findings seemingly opposite to ours, namely that seasons had a considerable impact on adherence. The authors comment in the discussion that they found a correlation between summer months and non-adherence, however they acknowledge that this association was not statistically significant. Furthermore, 81% of their patients reported that seasons did not affect their adherence. Hence, the data in the COMPLIANCE study support our finding that seasons do not affect adherence.

Thirty one patients (48%) missed at least one injection during the study period. The main reasons for non-adherence (Table 5) are in agreement with previous reports [2, 5, 16]. RebiSmart® was evaluated by study

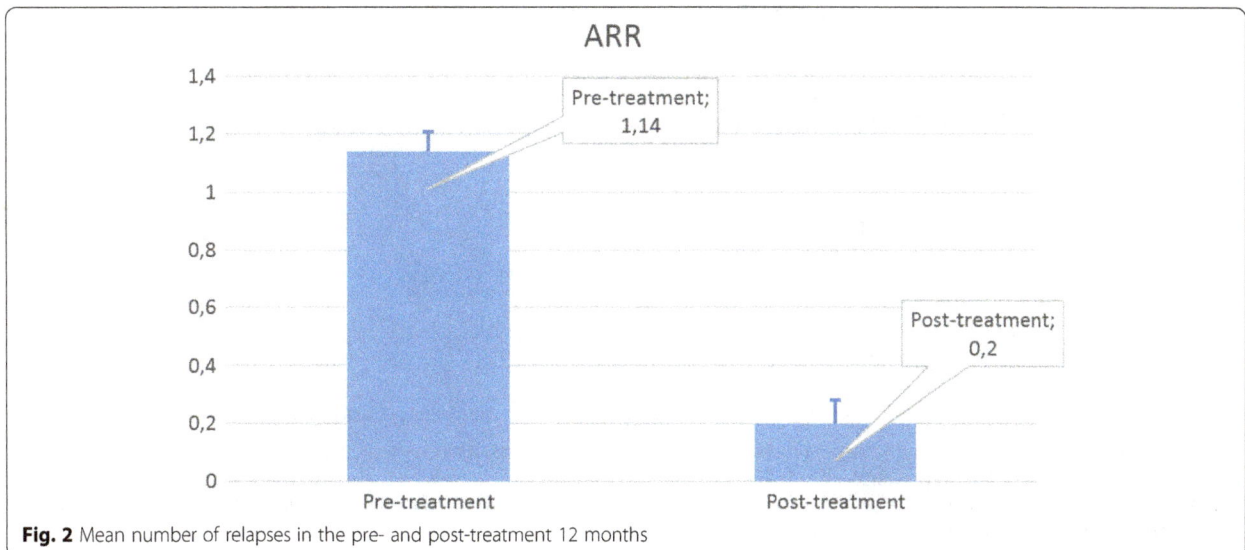

Fig. 2 Mean number of relapses in the pre- and post-treatment 12 months

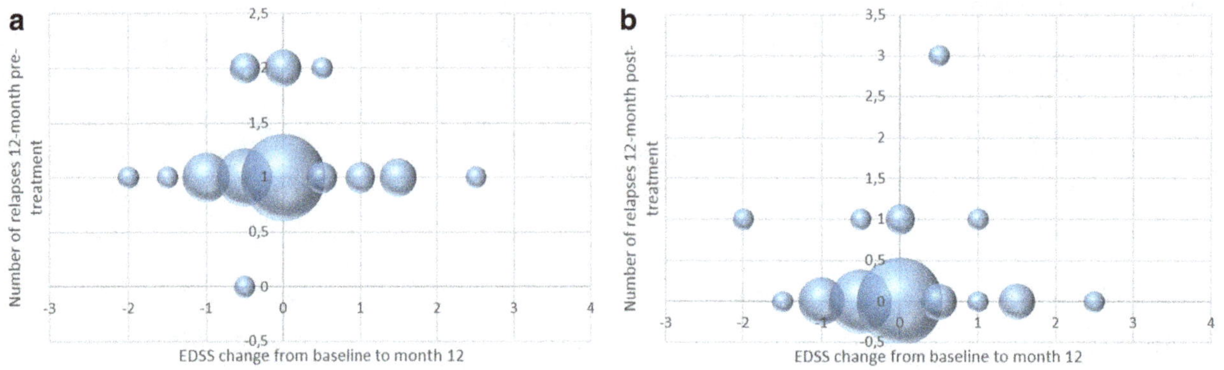

Fig. 3 Change of EDSS between baseline and visit 3, at 12 months vs number of 12-month pre-treatment relapses (*n* = 47) (**a**) and 12-month post-treatment relapses (*n* = 47) (**b**). The size of the bubbles represents the number of observations at each point on the graph

participants as easy to use and convenient (Fig. 5). The lower score was given to the item "it has easy connection needle" and this might be an aspect of the device that can be improved.

Treatment with Rebif® was efficacious; 87% of the per-protocol population were relapse free at month 12, which compares favorably with the rates of 66.8% at 48 weeks and 53.3% at 96 weeks with the same serum-free Rebif® formulation administered manually or with a mechanical autoinjector [16, 17]. Mean number of relapses was significantly lower at month 12 compared to the pre-treatment year. These numbers are consistent with those recently reported for RebiSmart® [2], yet lower compared to the ARR obtained for Rebif® in a series of recent clinical trials where the latter was used a comparator (Rebif® vs Alemtuzumab in CARE-MS-I and CARE-MS-II

where ARR for Rebif® was 0.39 ± 0.907 and 0.52 ± 1.01 respectively [18, 19] and Rebif® vs Ocrelizumab in OPERA-I and OPERA-II where ARR for Rebif® was 0.29 ± 0.72 and 0.29 ± 0.73 respectively [20]. The mean number of relapses in the 12 months pre-treatment was also higher in these studies: 1.33 ± 0.64 and 1.34 ± 0.73 in OPERA-I and II [20], 1.8 ± 0.8 and 1.5 ± 0.75 in CARE_MS I and II respectively [18, 19]. These differences in the study populations, as well as in the design of the trials, might account for the lower post-treatment relapse rate that we have observed. On the other hand, in the SMART trial, which recruited a similar patient population in terms of pre-treatment relapses, the one-year pre- and post- treatment ARR was comparable [2].

3-month confirmed disability progression at the end of the study period was observed in 10 patients (21%), while

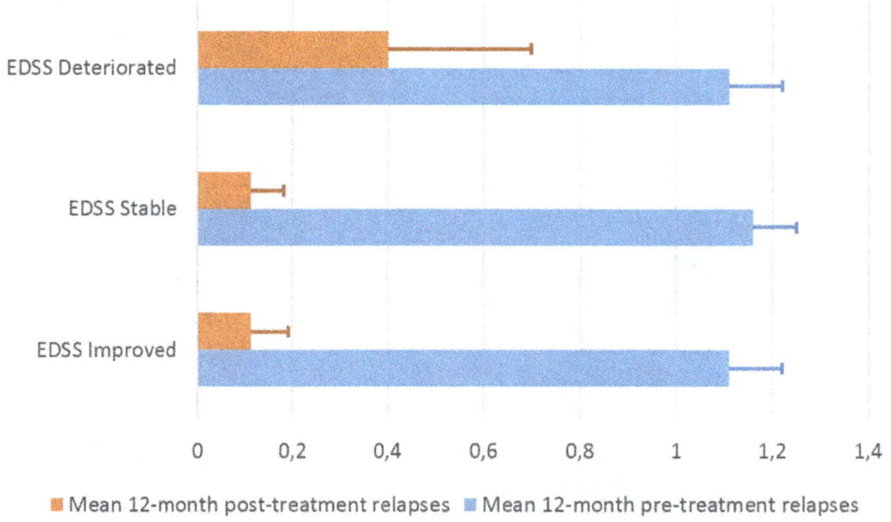

Fig. 4 The mean number of relapses in the 12-month pre-treatment period did not differ significantly among patients in whom EDSS at the end of the trial was improved, stable or had worsened (one way anova, *p* = 0.94). Similarly, there were no statistically significant differences among these groups in the mean number of relapses in the 12-month post-treatment period (one way anova, *p* = 0.24). This result is in support of a dissociation between disability progression and relapses

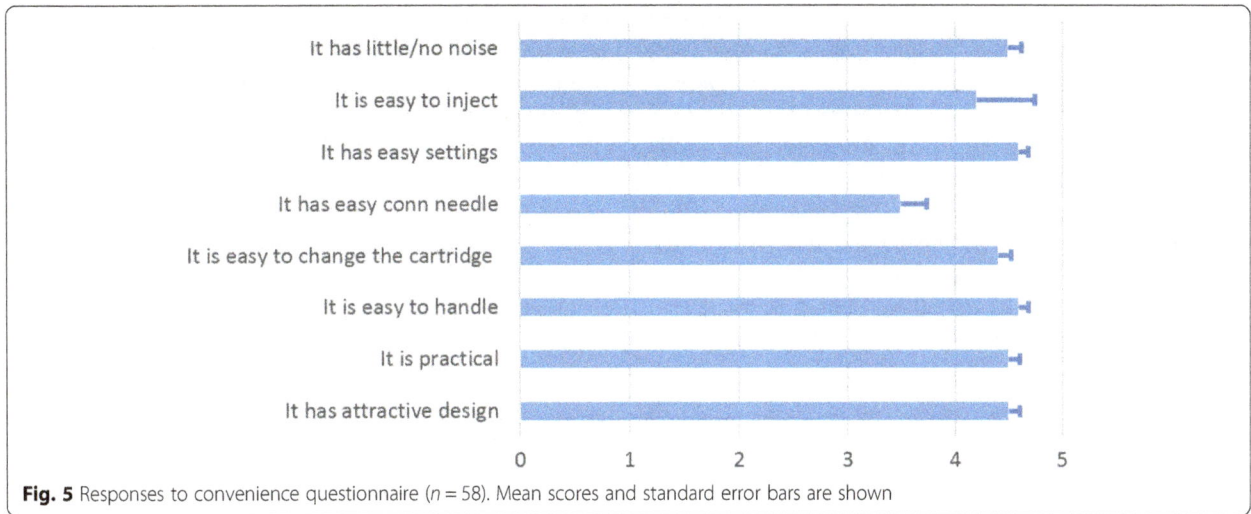

Fig. 5 Responses to convenience questionnaire (*n* = 58). Mean scores and standard error bars are shown

in 19 (40%) patients EDSS remained stable and in 18 (39%) it improved. Overall, in the PPS mean EDSS change of 0.17 ± 1.13 was not significant. It is notable that the change in EDSS from baseline was not related to the 12-month either pre- or post-treatment relapses (Fig. 3), while the mean number of relapses in the 12-month pre- and post- treatment period did not differ significantly among patients in whom EDSS had progressed, remained stable or improved at the end of the study (Fig. 4). Albeit there was a trend towards a higher mean number of relapses in the 12-month post-treatment period in those with EDSS progression, this difference did not reach statistical significance. It should be noted that these correlation analyses are post-hoc and should be treated with caution, as they are statistically under-powered.

Despite the relatively short observation period, these findings add to the on-going debate on the relation between relapses and disability in MS. Relapses and disability progression are two important clinical characteristics of MS. Relapses are the clinical expression of inflammatory insults localized at different parts of the central nervous system, whereas disability progression is the phenotypic expression of ongoing demyelination, axonal loss and gliosis [21]. In an earlier study of 1844 patients who had MS for 11 ± 10 years, it was found that once a certain clinical threshold is reached (namely, 4 on the EDSS), the progression of disability is not further affected by relapses. This, according to the authors, suggests that there is a dissociation between the pathophysiological mechanisms underpinning relapses and disability progression [21]. A more recent observational study of 162 MS patients treated with interferon beta for at least 2 years, found that compared to patients with no relapses in the first 2 years, those with 1 or ≥ 2 relapses were more likely

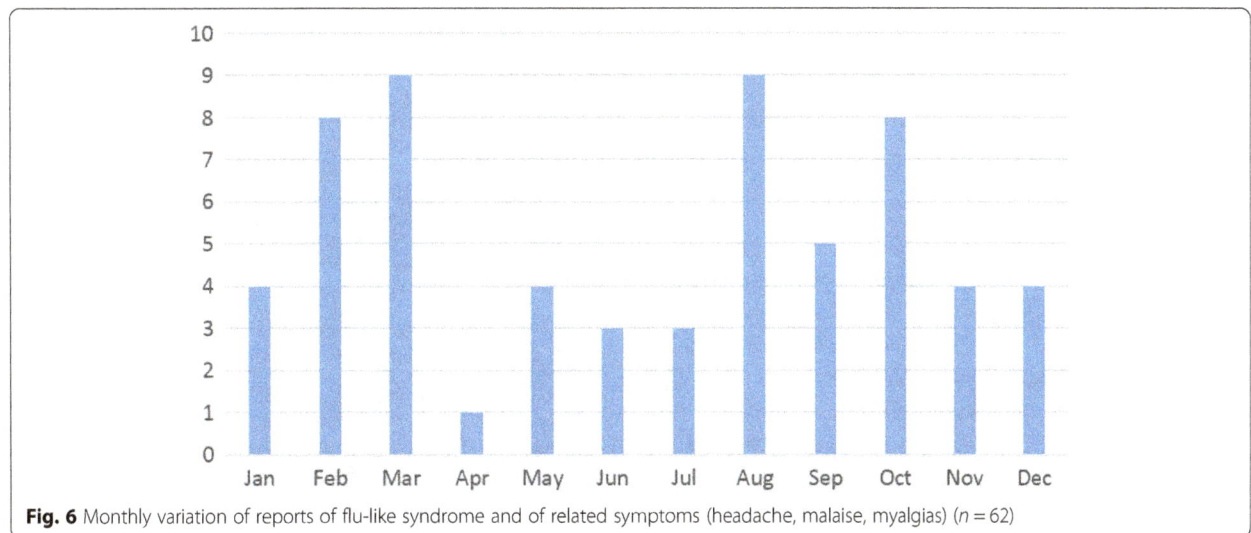

Fig. 6 Monthly variation of reports of flu-like syndrome and of related symptoms (headache, malaise, myalgias) (*n* = 62)

to exhibit early sustained disability progression (Hazard Ratio for 1 relapse: 3.4, $p = 0.05$; Hazard Ratio for ≥ 2 relapses: 4.3, $p < 0.001$). However, there was no statistically significant difference between patients that had 1 or ≥ 2 relapses [22]. Finally, a real world evidence study comparing alemtuzumab, interferon beta, fingolimod, or natalizumab in terms of relapses and disability progression showed that despite the fact that alemtuzumab was associated with a lower ARR than Rebif® (0.19 [95% CI 0.14–0.23] vs 0.53 [0.46–0.61], $p < 0.0001$), it was associated with similar probabilities of both disability accumulation (hazard ratio 0.66 [95% CI 0.36–1.22], $p = 0.37$) and disability improvement as Rebif® (0.98 [0.65–1.49], $p = 0.93$) at 5 years [23]. Our results favor those studies that support a dissociation between relapses and disability progression, calling for more research on the pathophysiological mechanisms underpinning this phenomenon and on the appropriate treatment strategies.

A limitation of our study is its relatively small size. However, it is the only study that we are aware of, in which seasonal adherence to interferon treatment for MS is evaluated by means of an autoinjector, rather than by patient-administered questionnaires. This increases the objectivity of the measurements. Furthermore, the sample size for this study was calculated based on the primary endpoint, namely 12-month adherence, due to the lack of published data regarding the seasonal and monthly adherence. As, according to our findings, 12-month, seasonal and monthly adherence are similar and have higher mean values and lower standard deviations than what was assumed during sample size calculations, the recruited number of patients was adequate to also estimate seasonal and monthly adherence.

The very high adherence rate that we have observed could have been confounded by factors such as higher educational level, occupation or willingness to participate in a clinical study. While the latter is a common factor in all studies, our sample was balanced in terms of educational level (high school – university), social status (married or not) and occupation (public/private sector). Furthermore, we did not observe any discrepancies in the adherence rates, which was high in all these subgroups.

While the observational design of the study and its 12-month duration are suitable for evaluating adherence (primary endpoint), they are less relevant to the efficacy measurements (relapse rate and disability progression), which were however secondary endpoints and should be interpreted with caution. Nevertheless, the results that we have obtained on relapse rate are consistent with those published in the literature, while our finding that pre- and post-treatment relapses are not related to disability progression or improvement at 12-months adds to the on-going discussion on the matter.

Conclusions
In conclusion, treatment with Rebif® using RebiSmart® was well tolerated and adherence exceeded 97% in a real world setting. There was no association of adherence with specific time periods of the year or geographical areas of Greece, which implies that weather conditions are not among its important determinants. Our data shows that Rebif® is effective in decreasing annual relapse rates, however there no correlation between ARR and disability progression.

Abbreviations
ADR: Adverse Drug Reaction; AE: Adverse Event; ANOVA: Analysis of Variance; DMD: Disease Modifying Drug; ED: Early Discontinuation; EDSS: Expanded Disability Scale Score; FAS: Full Analysis Set; MS: Multiple Sclerosis; PPS: Per Protocol Set; RRMS: Relapsing Remitting Multiple Sclerosis; SADR: Serious Adverse Drug Reaction; SAE: Serious Adverse Event; scIFN-β1a: Subcutaneous Interferon β1a; SmPC: Summary of Product Characteristics; STROBE: STrengthening the Reporting of OBservational studies in Epidemiology

Acknowledgements
None.

Funding
This study was funded by Merck Hellas S.A., who participated in the design of the study, in the analysis and interpretation of the data and in the writing of this manuscript.

Authors' contributions
SND analyzed and interpreted the patient data and was the main contributor in writing the manuscript. EvK, EfK, AK, PP, NF, VT, NV, AT and KV evaluated patients and were major contributors in writing the manuscript. MA, DS and FDL analyzed and interpreted the patient data and were major contributors in writing the manuscript. All authors read and approved the final manuscript.

Competing interests
Spyros N Defteros, Dimitrios Sakellariou and Filippo DeLorenzo are employees of Merck Hellas S.A. Michalis Arvanitis was an employee of Merck Hellas S.A when the study was conducted.

Author details
[1]Merck Hellas, 41-45 Kifisias av, 15123 Athens, Greece. [2]Neurology Department, Papageorgiou Hospital, Thessaloniki, Greece. [3]Neurology Department, Aristotle University of Thessaloniki, Thessaloniki, Greece. [4]University of Ioannina Neurology Department, Ioannina, Greece. [5]Neurology Department, University of Patras, Patras, Greece. [6]Neurology Department, 401 Army Hospital of Athens, Athens, Greece. [7]Neurology Department, University of Thessaly, Larissa, Greece. [8]Neurology Department, Evangelismos Hospital, Athens, Greece. [9]B Neurology Department, University of Athens, Athens, Greece. [10]Private Practice, Athens, Greece.

References
1. Sabate EE. Adherence to long-term therapies: evidence for action. General: World Health Organization; 2003. http://apps.who.int/iris/bitstream/10665/42682/1/9241545992.pdf. Accessed 25 Sept 2017.
2. Bayas A, Ouallet JC, Kallmann B, et al. Adherence to, and effectiveness of, subcutaneous interferon β-1a administered by RebiSmart® in patients with relapsing multiple sclerosis: results of the 1-year, observational SMART study. Expert Opin Drug Deliv. 2015;12:1239–50.

3. Kappos L, Kuhle J, Multanen J, et al. Factors influencing long-term outcomes in relapsing-remitting multiple sclerosis: PRISMS-15. J Neurol Neurosurg Psychiatry. 2015;86:1202–7.

4. Kappos L, Edan G, Freedman MS, et al. The 11-year long-term follow-up study from the randomized BENEFIT CIS trial. Neurology. 2016;87:978–87.

5. Treadaway K, Cutter G, Salter A, et al. Factors that influence adherence with disease-modifying therapy in MS. J Neurol. 2009;256:568–76.

6. Menzin J, Caon C, Nichols C, et al. Narrative review of the literature on adherence to disease-modifying therapies among patients with multiple sclerosis. J Manag Care Pharm. 2013;19(1 Suppl A):S24–40.

7. Saiz A, Mora S, Blanco J. Therapeutic compliance of first line disease-modifying therapies in patients with multiple sclerosis. COMPLIANCE Study. Neurologia. 2015;30:214–22.

8. Hellenic Association of Pharmaceutical Companies. Registry of non-interventional studies. https://www.dilon.sfee.gr/studiesp_d.php?meleti_id=200136. Accessed 25 Sept 2017.

9. Costello K, Kennedy P, Scanzillo J. Recognizing nonadherence in patients with multiple sclerosis and maintaining treatment adherence in the long term. Medscape J Med. 2008;10:225.

10. Medical Dictionary for Regulatory Activities. https://www.meddra.org/. Accessed 25 Sept 2017.

11. Lugaresi A, Florio C, Brescia-Morra V, et al. Patient adherence to and tolerability of self-administered interferon β-1a using an electronic autoinjection device: a multicentre, open-label, phase IV study. BMC Neurol. 2012;12:7.

12. von Elm E, Altman DG, Egger M, et al. The Strengthening the reporting of observational studies in epidemiology (STROBE) statement: guidelines for reporting observational studies. PLoS Med. 2007;4:e296.

13. Blaschke TF, Osterberg L, Vrijens B, et al. Adherence to medications: insights arising from studies on the unreliable link between prescribed and actual drug dosing histories. Annu Rev Pharmacol Toxicol. 2012;52:275–301.

14. Singer B, Wray S, Miller T, et al. Patient-rated ease of use and functional reliability of an electronic autoinjector for self-injection of subcutaneous interferon beta-1a for relapsing multiple sclerosis. Mult Scler Relat Disord. 2012;1:87–94.

15. Hupperts R, Becker V, Friedrich J, et al. Multiple sclerosis patients treated with intramuscular IFN-β-1a autoinjector in a real-world setting: prospective evaluation of treatment persistence, adherence, quality of life and satisfaction. Expert Opin Drug Deliv. 2015;12:15–25.

16. Devonshire V, Lapierre Y, Macdonell R, et al. The global adherence project (GAP): a multicenter observational study on adherence to disease-modifying therapies in patients with relapsing-remitting multiple sclerosis. Eur J Neurol. 2011;18:69–77.

17. Giovannoni G, Barbarash O, Casset-Semanaz F, et al. Immunogenicity and tolerability of an investigational formulation of interferon-beta1a: 24- and 48-week interim analyses of a 2-year, single-arm, historically controlled, phase IIIb study in adults with multiple sclerosis. Clin Ther. 2007;29:1128–45.

18. Cohen JA, Coles AJ, Arnold DL, et al. Alemtuzumab versus interferon beta 1a as first-line treatment for patients with relapsing-remitting multiple sclerosis: a randomised controlled phase 3 trial. Lancet. 2012;380:1819–28.

19. Coles AJ, Twyman CL, Arnold DL, et al. Alemtuzumab for patients with relapsing multiple sclerosis after disease-modifying therapy: a randomised controlled phase 3 trial. Lancet. 2012;380:1829–39.

20. Hauser SL, Bar-Or A, Comi G, et al. Ocrelizumab versus interferon Beta-1a in relapsing multiple sclerosis. N Engl J Med. 2017;376:221–34.

21. Confavreux C, Vukusic S, Moreau T, et al. Relapses and progression of disability in multiple sclerosis. N Engl J Med. 2000;343:1430–8.

22. Bosca I, Coret F, Valero C, et al. Effect of relapses over early progression of disability in multiple sclerosis patients treated with beta-interferon. Mult Scler. 2008;14:636–9.

23. Kalincik T, Brown JWL, Robertson N, et al. Treatment effectiveness of alemtuzumab compared with natalizumab, fingolimod, and interferon beta in relapsing-remitting multiple sclerosis: a cohort study. Lancet Neurol. 2017;16:271–81.

12

Outcome of MS relapses in the era of disease-modifying therapy

Muriel Stoppe[1,2†], Maria Busch[1†], Luise Krizek[1] and Florian Then Bergh[1,2*]

Abstract

Background: In multiple sclerosis (MS), neurological disability results from incomplete remission of relapses and from relapse-independent progression. Intravenous high dose methylprednisolone (IVMP) is the established standard treatment to accelerate clinical relapse remission, although some patients do not respond. Most studies of relapse treatment have been performed when few patients received disease-modifying treatment and may no longer apply today.

Methods: We prospectively assessed, over one year, the course of patients who presented with a clinically isolated syndrome (CIS) or MS relapse, documenting demographic, clinical, treatment and outcome data. A standardized follow-up examination was performed 10–14 days after end of relapse treatment.

Results: We documented 119 relapses in 108 patients (31 CIS, 77 MS). 114 relapses were treated with IVMP resulting in full remission (29.2%), partial remission (38.7%), no change (18.2%) or worsening (4.4%). In 27 relapses (22.7%), escalating relapse treatment was indicated, and performed in 24, using double-dose IVMP ($n = 18$), plasmapheresis ($n = 2$) or immunoadsorption ($n = 4$).

Conclusions: Standardised follow-up visits and outcome documentation in treated relapses led to escalating relapse treatment in every fifth relapse. We recommend incorporating scheduled follow-up visits into routine relapse management. Our data facilitate the design of prospective trials addressing methods and timelines of relapse treatment.

Keywords: Multiple Sclerosis, Relapse, Relapse treatment, Relapse management, Relapse outcome, Methylprednisolone, Immunoadsorption, Plasmapheresis, Prospective study

Background

Multiple sclerosis (MS) is the most common non-traumatic disease that causes permanent neurological deficits in young adults. It is a progressive, autoimmune disorder of the central nervous system (CNS), characterized by inflammatory lesions and demyelination which result in injury of myelin sheaths, oligodendrocytes, and of axons as well as entire neurons [1, 2]. Neurological disability results from accumulating residual deficits of acute MS relapses throughout the individual's disease course, and from insidious progression at later stages. Although MS relapses can spontaneously recover, several studies proved superior clinical outcome with high dose intravenous methylprednisolone (IVMP) treatment [3–6]. However, duration and degree of recovery of acute MS attack vary not only inter-individually but also intraindividually over the course of the disease. Some relapses do not fully remit despite treatment. The data quantifying clinical outcome of MS relapses are based on randomised trials which were performed before availability and common use of disease-modifying therapy (DMT) [7–11], and may no longer reflect clinical reality. Moreover, escalating relapse treatment has become more common. Besides the application of a second course of high dose IVMP, extra-corporeal procedures such as plasma exchange (PLEX) and immunoadsorption (IA) are increasingly used in steroid-resistant MS relapses [12–17]. Nevertheless, due to the lack of comparative studies, there is no standard approach for indication and employment of

* Correspondence: ThenBerF@medizin.uni-leipzig.de
†Equal contributors
[1]Department of Neurology, University of Leipzig, Liebigstraße 20, 04103 Leipzig, Germany
[2]Translational Centre for Regenerative Medicine, University of Leipzig, Liebigstraße 20, 04103 Leipzig, Germany

escalating relapse treatment in ongoing relapse. Evaluating how well severity and duration of the exacerbation are improved represents the most valuable and clinically meaningful assessment in determining the efficacy of relapse treatment. Thus, data investigating the clinical outcome in acute MS relapses in the era of wide-spread use of DMT needs to be collected and analysed systematically.

Methods

We prospectively assessed, over one year, data of patients who presented to the Department of Neurology at the University of Leipzig with either a relapse of established MS or clinically isolated syndrome (CIS) of CNS demyelination, including both outpatients and inpatients. Based on prior approval by the University of Leipzig's Ethics Committee, patients are requested, upon admission to our hospital, to consent to statistical analyses of anonymous diagnostic and treatment information for scientific and quality assurance purposes. We included only anonymous data from patients who consented to this request. To facilitate systematic analysis, we developed a documentation sheet to collect demographic data, MS history (onset, disease-modifying therapy (DMT), latest neurological evaluation before current relapse), characteristics of the current relapse (symptoms, Kurtzke's Expanded Disability Status Scale (EDSS) and Functional Systems Scale (FS), visual acuity (VA), primarily affected FS, date of relapse onset) and treatment of current relapse (drug, dose, application route, duration). A standardized follow-up examination was performed and documented in the Neuroimmunology outpatient clinic after primary relapse treatment in order to evaluate the clinical outcome and to decide whether an escalation of treatment was necessary; if escalation treatment was performed, an equivalent follow-up visit was performed after each treatment cycle. History was taken and examination performed by physicians experienced in evaluation of MS patients, including former neurostatus training and certification (www.neurostatus-systems.net). Recovery was defined based on both subjective symptoms and objective findings on neurological examination related to the current relapse (scored by Kurtzke Functional System and EDSS ratings). "Complete recovery" denotes complete resolution of symptoms and a neurological examination as documented pre-relapse (or, in first episodes, a normal neurological examination, EDSS 0). Accordingly, "partial response" refers to improvement in symptoms or/and FS score not returning to pre-relapse score, "no response" to unchanged symptoms and neurological findings, and "worsening" to an increase in the FS score relevant to the current relapse (which was always paralleled by an increase in symptoms). Descriptive statistics was calculated as indicated in the text and tables. Data are presented as mean ± standard deviation (SD) unless indicated otherwise. To analyse potential differences in the outcome of relapse treatment in different patient groups, we used Fisher's exact test (SPSS 11, SPSS Inc.).

Results

Overall, we documented 119 acute relapses in 108 patients (Table 1, Fig. 1). The average age of the 73 women (67.6%) and 35 men (32.4%) was 34.7 ± 9.7 years. Of these 108 patients, 31 presented with CIS, 72 with relapsing-remitting MS (RRMS) and 5 patients with a relapse during secondary-progressive MS (SPMS).

In the 77 patients with established MS, the disease was diagnosed 5.7 ± 15.4 years before current relapse; 41 patients (53.2%) had received a DMT for 2.10 ± 2.45 years: Interferon beta in 15 patients (36.6%), glatiramer acetate in 9 patients (22.0%), fingolimod in 6 patients (14.4%), natalizumab in 4 patients (9.8%), a B-cell depleting antibody in 2 patients within clinical trial (4.9%), teriflunomide, interferon beta plus teriflunomide within a clinical trial, dimethyl fumarate, mitoxantrone or monthly methylprednisolone in one patient each (2.4%). For the 88

Table 1 Demographic characteristics

Sex, n (%)	
Female	73 (67.6)
Male	35 (32.4)
Age at relapse onset (years)	34.7 ± 9.7
Clinical course, n (%)	
CIS	31 (28.7)
RRMS	72 (66.7)
SPMS	5 (4.6)
DMT in RRMS/SPMS, n (%)	
DMT	41/77 (53.2)
No DMT	36/77 (46.8)
DMT distribution, n (%)	
Interferon beta	15 (36.6)
Glatiramer acetate	9 (22.0)
Fingolimod	6 (14.6)
Natalizumab	4 (9.8)
B-cell depleting antibody[a]	2 (4.9)
Dimethyl fumarate	1 (2.4)
Teriflunomide	1 (2.4)
Mitoxantrone	1 (2.4)
Interferon + Teriflunomid[a]	1 (2.4)
Methylprednisolone[b]	1 (2.4)
DMT duration (years)	2.1 ± 2.5
Relapses, n	119

CIS clinically isolated syndrome, DMT disease-modifying therapy, RRMS relapse-remitting multiple sclerosis, SMPS secondary-progressive multiple sclerosis.
[a] = within clinical trial. [b] = monthly methylprednisolone as individual approach

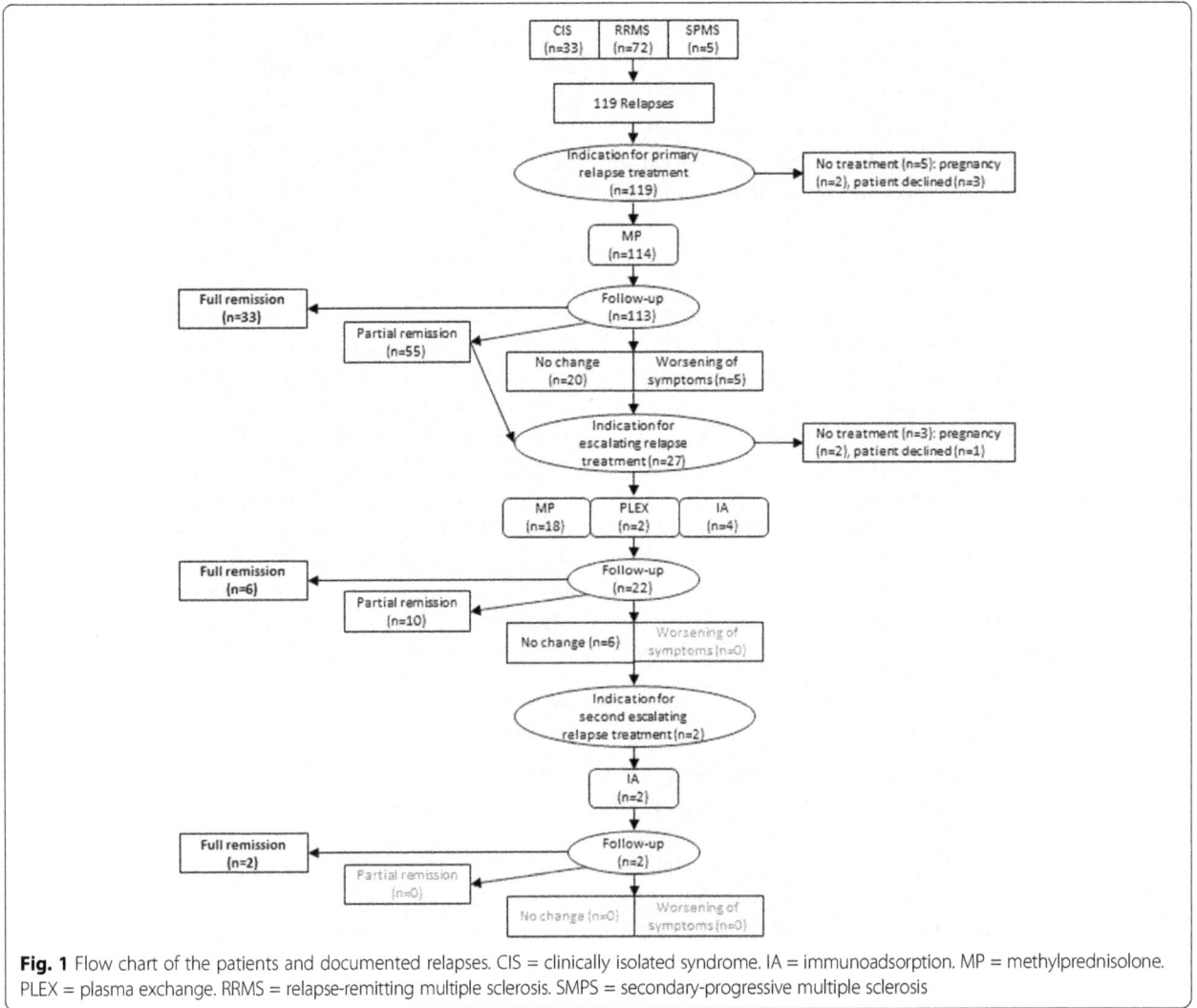

Fig. 1 Flow chart of the patients and documented relapses. CIS = clinically isolated syndrome. IA = immunoadsorption. MP = methylprednisolone. PLEX = plasma exchange. RRMS = relapse-remitting multiple sclerosis. SMPS = secondary-progressive multiple sclerosis

relapses observed in established MS, the mean EDSS before relapse was 2.2 ± 2.0, while prior EDSS was unknown in 6 cases.

The 31 patients presenting with CIS did not receive DMT. EDSS before symptom onset was, of course, unavailable and was defined as zero.

One hundred fourteen of the 119 documented relapses (95.8%) were treated, all with high dose IVMP with an average of 3531.6 mg ± 1164.3 mg over 3.6 ± 1.0 days (985 ± 151 mg/d). Treatment was initiated 13.8 ± 19.4 days after the onset of relapse symptoms. For all treated relapses (CIS, RRMS, and SPMS, n = 114), the mean onset EDSS was 3.1 ± 1.6 and improved to 2.6 ± 1.8 after primary relapse treatment. In MS relapses (n = 88), the mean EDSS at relapse onset was 3.5 ± 1.6 and improved to 3.0 ± 1.8 after primary relapse treatment. In CIS (n = 31), the mean EDSS at relapse onset was 2.2 ± 1.0 and improved to 1.4 ± 1.1 after primary relapse treatment. Mainly affected FS in all relapses (n = 119) were sensory (n = 51, 42.9%), motor (n = 35, 29.4%) and visual system (n = 29,

24.4%), followed by brainstem, cerebellum, ambulation, bladder function and cognition. In 38 relapses (31.9%), more than one FS was affected (Table 2). In 47 relapses (39.5%), symptoms occurred in a previously affected FS. For the remaining 72 relapses (60.5%), the affected FS

Table 2 Affected functional systems in all documented relapses (n = 119)

Affected FS in all relapses, n (%)	
Sensory	51 (42.0)
Motor	35 (29.4)
Visual	29 (24.4)
Brainstem	20 (16.8)
Cerebellum	15 (12.6)
Ambulation	14 (11.8)
Bowel and bladder	7 (5.9)
Cerebral	1 (0.8)
Relapses with more than one affected FS, n (%)	38 (31.9)

FS functional system

was zero before symptom onset (CIS: $n = 31$, 100%; RRMS: $n = 40$, 43.1%; SPMS: $n = 1$, 1.3%).

For CIS only ($n = 31$), mainly affected FS were visual ($n = 15$, 48.8%), sensory ($n = 7$, 22.6%), brainstem ($n = 6$, 19.4%) and motor system ($n = 5$, 16.1%), followed by cerebellum and cognition. Bladder function and ambulation were not affected in CIS. In 4 CIS relapses (12.9%), more than one FS was affected (Table 3).

In 23 relapses (19.3%), the symptoms were reflected by an increase in the FS score, while the overall EDSS remained unchanged. In 16 relapses (13.4%), there was neither a change in FS nor in EDSS score (as compared to the latest available examination).

Follow-up examination was scheduled 10 to 14 days after the end of primary relapse treatment to evaluate clinical outcome and the indication for escalating relapse treatment. Of all 114 treated relapses, the follow-up visit was done in all but one, at a median of 14 days (interquartile range 7–38 days) after end of primary relapse treatment. In 88 relapses (77.9%), follow-up occurred within 42 days allowing for the initiation of escalation steps. In the remaining 25 relapses, patients declined an extra visit, and follow-up took place during regular appointment within a 3-to-6-months interval.

Follow-up of relapses treated with primary relapse treatment (Fig. 2) revealed full remission ($n = 33$, 29.2%), partial remission ($n = 55$, 48.7%), no change ($n = 20$, 17.7%) or worsening of symptoms ($n = 5$, 4.4%).

In 27 of all 119 relapses (22.7%) and 113 follow-up visits (23.9%), escalating relapse treatment was indicated. In these relapses, primarily affected functional systems were visual ($n = 11$, 40.7%), motor ($n = 7$, 25.9%) or sensory ($n = 4$, 14.8%). Escalating relapse treatment was performed by a second course of IVMP ($n = 18$, 66.7%) treated with 3866.5 mg ± 2832.1 mg for 3.9 ± 1.1 days (1528 ± 539 mg/d), plasma exchange (5 sessions, $n = 2$, 7.4%) or immunoadsorption (5 sessions, $n = 4$, 14.8%). In the remaining three relapses (11.1%), further escalation

was indicated but not performed due to pregnancy ($n = 2$, 7.4%) or decline by the patient ($n = 1$, 3.7%). Treatment with escalating relapse treatment ($n = 24$, but loss of follow-up in 2 patients) yielded full remission ($n = 6$, 27,3%), partial remission ($n = 10$, 45.4%) or no change ($n = 6$, 27,3%).

In two relapses, the indication for a second escalation step was confirmed. In both relapses, primary and escalating relapse treatment was performed with IVMP but with no change of relapse symptoms (loss of visual acuity or ataxia). Second escalation relapse treatment was performed as immunoadsorption (5 cycles) in both relapses and resulted in full recovery.

In the relapses manifesting as optic neuritis (ON, $n = 29$), the mean visual acuity (VA) of the affected eye before relapse was 0.97 ± 0.10. Except for one patient (VA 0.9), all ON were treated with primary relapse treatment (i.e. first-time IVMP) with VA amelioration from 0.40 ± 0.25 in acute relapse ($n = 28$) to 0.62 ± 0.33 ($n = 27$, one loss of follow-up). In 11 ON, indication for escalating relapse treatment was confirmed. Due to pregnancy in one ON, only 10 ON were treated with escalating relapse treatment and VA improved from 0.33 ± 0.16 at ON onset and 0.47 ± 0.31 after primary treatment to 0.58 ± 0.30. One of these ON was treated with a second escalating relapse treatment and VA recovered from 0.33 at ON onset and 0.33 after primary treatment to 0.70; this constituted full recovery to the latest pre-ON VA (Table 4).

Forty five relapses (37.8% of all relapses, 51.1% of relapses in established MS) occurred under ongoing DMT with full remission in 18 relapses (40.0%), partial remission in 19 relapses (42.2%), no change in 7 relapses (15.6%) and worsening in 1 relapse (2.2%) after primary relapse treatment. In MS relapses without DMT, outcome after primary relapse treatment was full remission in 9 (20.9%), partial remission in 22 (51.2%), no change in 10 (23.3%) and worsening and loss of follow-up in 1 relapse (2.3%) each. This suggestive trend did not reach statistical significance for outcome of MS relapses under ongoing DMT vs. relapse outcome without DMT (Fisher's exact test, $p = 0.169$). Outcome of CIS attacks (all without DMT) was full remission in 10 (32.3%), partial remission in 15 (48.4%), no change in 3 (9.7%) and worsening in 3 attacks (9.7%) after primary treatment. Adding all 74 relapses (62.2%) in patients who were either therapy-naïve or had stopped former DMT, outcome was full remission in 19 (25.7%), partial remission in 37 (50.0%), no change in 13 (17.6%), worsening in 4 (5.4%) and 1 relapse with unknown outcome (1.4%) after primary relapse treatment. Of the 27 relapses where indication for escalating treatment was raised, 10 occurred under ongoing DMT and 17 in therapy–naïve patients (7 CIS and 10 MS).

Table 3 Affected functional systems in clinically isolated syndrome ($n = 31$)

Affected FS in CIS, n (%)	
Visual	15 (48.4)
Sensory	7 (22.6)
Brainstem	6 (19.4)
Motor	5 (16.1)
Cerebellum	3 (9.7)
Cognition	1 (3.2)
Ambulation	0 (0)
Bowel and bladder	0 (0)
Relapses with more than one affected FS, n (%)	4 (12.9)

CIS clinically isolated syndrome FS functional system

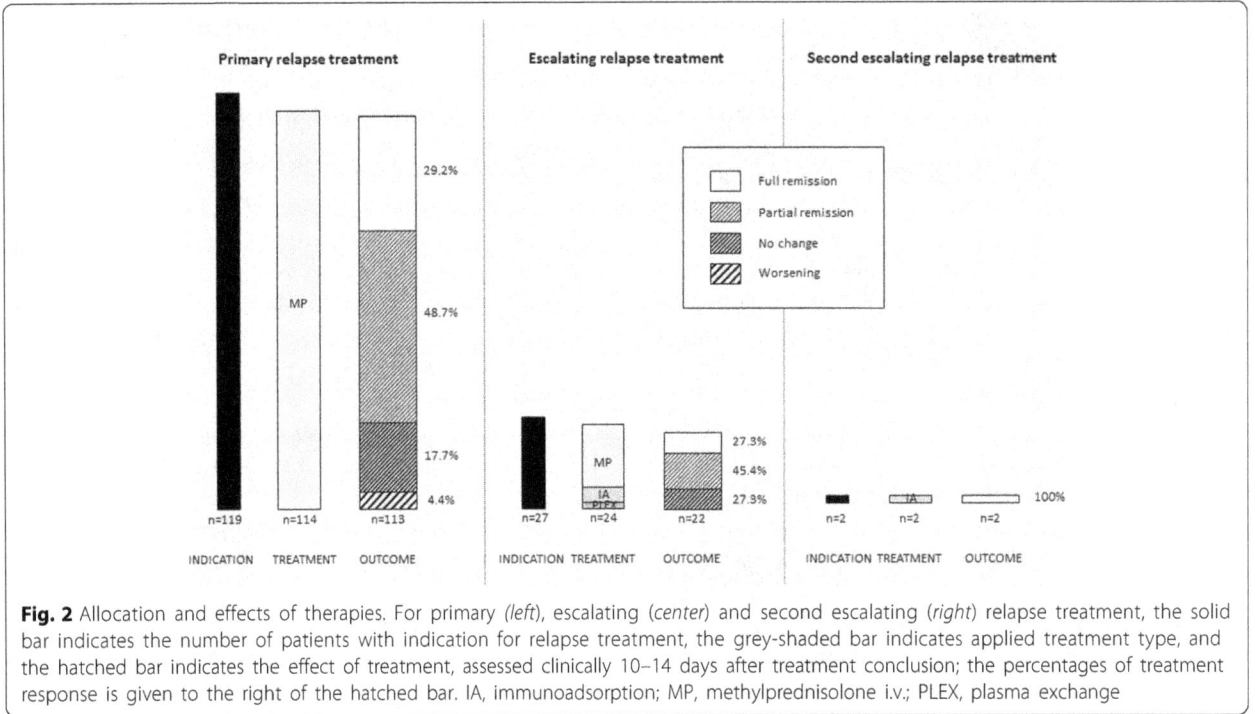

Fig. 2 Allocation and effects of therapies. For primary *(left)*, escalating *(center)* and second escalating *(right)* relapse treatment, the solid bar indicates the number of patients with indication for relapse treatment, the grey-shaded bar indicates applied treatment type, and the hatched bar indicates the effect of treatment, assessed clinically 10–14 days after treatment conclusion; the percentages of treatment response is given to the right of the hatched bar. IA, immunoadsorption; MP, methylprednisolone i.v.; PLEX, plasma exchange

Either full remission or improvement by at least one full EDSS point occurred at the first follow-up visit in 48.4% of all patients with EDSS-relevant relapses (65.5% of CIS patients and 40.6% of patients with established MS, respectively). When differentiating outcome according to DMT, the same criteria for treatment response were met by 50.0% of patients with established MS on DMT and 32.0% of those without DMT (Fisher's exact test, $p = 0.119$).

To address the question of optimal timing of the follow-up visit, we analysed outcome and treatment decision in the patients seen early (within 14 days) or later (15–42 days) after primary relapse treatment, based on the median time to follow-up. This revealed full remission in 24 and 28%, partial remission in 46 and 43%, no response in 19 and 23%, and worsening in 8.7 and 2.3%, respectively. Escalation treatment was indicated in 24 and 21%, respectively.

Discussion

High-dose intravenous methylprednisolone (IVMP) is the established treatment for relapses in MS to accelerate the remission of relapse symptoms [18]. However, there are different regimes concerning dosage and form of administration of methylprednisolone (MP), and variable recommendations as to the interval within which therapy should be initiated. Oral MP appears to be equally efficacious as IVMP at equivalent doses [7, 8, 19, 20], whereas higher doses of IVMP have been proven to be more efficient than lower doses, concerning both clinical outcome and reduction of contrast-enhancing lesions on MRI [21]. Experimental data also support higher doses [22]. Regardless of the variants of MP treatment, only a fraction of treated patients fully recover from their symptoms. According to current guidelines, this clinical problem is dealt with by administration of a second course of IVMP at a higher dose, and eventually plasma exchange or immunoadsorption [18, 23, 24].

In our sample, 37.8% of the observed relapses (51.1% of all RRMS/SPMS-patients) occurred under DMT, while the remaining relapses were either initial presentations (CIS)

Table 4 Visual acuity in all ON that received primary treatment ($n = 28$)

	Number	Visual acuity
Before ON onset	28	0.97 ± 0.11
At ON onset	28	0.40 ± 0.25
After primary relapse treatment		
All	27[a]	0.62 ± 0.33
Indication for escalating relapse treatment	11	0.47 ± 0.31
Escalating relapse treatment performed	10	0.47 ± 0.30
After escalating relapse treatment		
All	10	0.58 ± 0.33
Indication for second escalating relapse treatment	1	0.33
Escalating relapse treatment performed	1	0.33
After second escalating relapse treatment	1	0.70

ON optic neuritis [a] = one loss of follow-up

or occurred in MS patients off DMT. This limits the conclusions we can draw regarding relapses during ongoing DMT, one of our primary goals. Interestingly, however, success of primary relapse therapy, defined as full remission of relapse symptoms was more often observed in patients with ongoing DMT (40.0%) than in those without DMT (26.0%). Together with the lower number of relapses on DMT, this supports a firm therapy attitude as demanded in current guidelines [18, 24].

Previous studies show remarkably variable response rates (improvement of at least 1 EDSS point) between 50 and 80% after 28 days [7, 8, 19, 20]. All four studies were designed to compare oral with intravenous methylprednisolone in patients with acute relapse but only including patients with clinically definite MS [7, 8] or fulfilling the 2005 McDonald criteria [19, 20], whereas we included all relapses in CIS, RRMS and SPMS. Alam et al. [7] report 20 patients receiving 500 mg IVMP for 5 days of whom 80% improved, from a mean Kurtzke disability score of 4.85 at baseline to 3.5 at day 28. Barnes et al. [8] report 36 patients receiving 1000 mg IVMP for 3 days, with 18 patients (50%) improving after 4 weeks on the pyramidal FS (not mentioning the absolute value of improvement) and over all patients, an improvement of a mean of 0.5 points in the EDSS. The more recent work of Ramo-Tello et al. [19] and Le Page et al. [20] report an improvement of at least one EDSS point after 28 days in 65% of 23 patients and 80% of 90 patients, respectively. However, full recovery was reached only in 40% [20]. Despite the different follow-up schedule, our response rates after 10–14 days (48.4% full remission or EDSS improvement) are consistent with the additionally reported 39% after 7 days of Ramo-Tello et al. [19] but differ from Barnes et al. who report no improvement of EDSS after 1 week. However, Barnes et al. do not describe their cohort in terms of DMT but have excluded patients on immunosuppressants. Since the study was published in 1997, we suppose DMT rates to be low. Ramo-Tello et al. state a DMT rate of 56.4%, comparable to our cohort.

Relating to DMT, our data suggest a trend to better steroid-responsiveness in MS under DMT than without DMT. However, comparing more recent data from cohorts with 55–56.4% of patients under DMT [19, 20] and our current data on the one hand, to results of older studies [7, 8], response rates are still comparable. As to average EDSS scores at relapse onset, our data are comparable with the recent studies [19, 20], whereas the EDSS in the older cohorts is clearly higher [7, 8]. As observed in a standardized follow-up examination, we indicated escalating relapse treatment in 22.7% of all relapses (23.9% of all follow-up visits) due to insufficient improvement after primary relapse treatment. Scheduled follow-up visit and detailed outcome documentation

including EDSS after primary relapse treatment appears to lead to a fairly high rate of escalations. Unfortunately, data for relapse outcome without the explicit intention of follow-up are unavailable (and for systematic reasons may remain impossible to acquire). Also, our cohort is presumably not entirely comparable with relapses that present to neurological practitioners: we may have observed more severe relapses, given that we collected our sample from an outpatient clinic linked to a university hospital. This possible bias may limit the generalizability of our conclusion while, however, focussing the observation on the subgroup of MS patients who require the most efficient relapse treatment. In either case, integrating a follow-up visit 10 to 14 days after the end of relapse treatment into the routine of medical MS management, rather than relying on patients to return if unsatisfied, will – in our opinion - raise patients' expectations towards improvement of relapse symptoms, and encourage them to ask for escalating relapse treatment. At the same time, this will apply to treating neurologists' expectations as well, and scheduled follow-up should improve treatment quality. This is exemplified by (admittedly rare) relapses with irrelevant improvement after primary and escalating relapse treatment, in which full recovery emerged after second escalating relapse treatment. The need for scheduled follow-up visits is also supported by our observation that primary treatment achieves full recovery in less than one-third of relapses. With respect to optimal timing of the follow-up visit, longer follow-up (2–6 weeks) yielded a slightly higher proportion of "full recovery" while "worsening" was stated more often when follow-up was shorter (up to 2 weeks). Interestingly, however, the indication for escalating relapse treatment was confirmed in a remarkably similar proportion. Thus, patients recovering, but also those requiring escalation treatment can be identified early after primary relapse treatment. Taking into consideration that any relapse treatment is probably most successful within 6 weeks after symptom onset, and given that some patients require second escalation treatment, this argues for a follow-up visit at around two weeks after primary treatment, to allow for an equivalent period to evaluate the effect of escalated therapy. On the other hand, integrating relapse-specific documentation and follow-up visits into medical routine challenges clinic capacity, requires networking between in-patient and out-patient departments to organize escalating relapse treatment and schedule follow-up visits, flexible clinic schedules, and compliant patients.

Evaluation of the relative effectiveness of therapies in relapse treatment requires valid outcome measures that reflect the initial aggravation and subsequent improvement of the patients' symptoms in relapses [25]. We observed that in 23 relapses (19.3% of all relapses), clinical aggravation was reflected in at least one FS but not the integrated EDSS, and in 16 relapses (13.5% of all relapses) both values remained unchanged. This confirms that the indication for treatment of an acute MS-relapse should not be based solely on changes in FS or EDSS but always integrate the impact upon the individual patient's daily activities. At the same time, this shortcoming should not discourage neurologists from documenting relapse severity using quantitative scales. This is certainly best achieved in optic neuritis, and decline of visual acuity accounted for one quarter of MS relapses and almost half of CIS cases in our series. Importantly, visual acuity should be investigated regardless of reported relapse symptoms, since it revealed an additional affected FS in almost one-third of this cohort, increasing the sensitivity of the follow-up investigation. The mechanisms of action of IVMP include a wide range of effects on the immune system; DMTs may impact these effects in different ways [26, 27].

In the recent past, different possibilities of treatment for acute MS-relapses were explored, proposing plasmapheresis and immunoadsorption as alternatives to oral or intravenous MP either for steroid unresponsive MS relapses [13, 15] or when primary application of IVMP is not suitable (e.g. during pregnancy, MP intolerance, MP allergy) [18, 28, 29]. So far, these treatments are based on retrospective case series, and controlled trials to establish their risk-benefit ratio are not available. In order to design such prospective clinical trials to investigate the relative effectiveness of the different relapse therapies, our data provide a basis for estimating effects and derive required sample sizes.

Conclusion

Intravenous methylprednisolone continues to improve relapse outcome. While its effect appears superior in patients with concomitant disease-modifying treatment, this effect may be confounded by a trend toward less severe relapses in the era of DMT. Nevertheless, we recommend scheduled follow-up visit and detailed outcome documentation after primary relapse treatment in order to identify the fairly high number of patients whose outcome can be further improved by employing escalating relapse treatment.

Abbreviations
CIS: Clinically isolated syndrome; CNS: Central nervous system; DMT: Disease-modifying therapy; EDSS: Expanded disability status scale; FS: Functional systems scale; IA: Immunoadsorption; IVMP: Intravenous high dose methylprednisolone; MRI: Magnetic resonance imaging; MS: Multiple sclerosis; ON: Optic neuritis; PLEX: Plasma exchange; RRMS: Relapsing-remitting multiple sclerosis; SD: Standard deviation; SPMS: Secondary-progressive multiple sclerosis; VA: Visual acuity

Acknowledgements
Not applicable.

Funding
The Translational Centre for Regenerative Medicine was funded by the Federal Ministry of Education and Research (BMBF, PtJ-Bio, 0315883). The funding body took no role in the study design or in the collection, analysis and interpretation of data, nor in the decision to publish or writing this manuscript.

Authors' contributions
MS made substantial contributions to conception and design, acquisition of data, analysis and interpretation of data. She is accountable for all aspects of the work and ensures that questions related to the accuracy or integrity of any part of the work are appropriately investigated and resolved. She was substantially involved in drafting and revising the manuscript. MB made substantial contributions to conception and design, analysis and interpretation of data. She was substantially involved in drafting and revising the manuscript. LK made substantial contributions to acquisition of data. She was involved in revising the manuscript. FTB made substantial contributions to conception and design, analysis and interpretation of data. He was substantially involved in revising the manuscript critically for important intellectual content. He is accountable for all aspects of the work and ensures that questions related to the accuracy or integrity of any part of the work are appropriately investigated and resolved. All authors have given final approval of the version to be published.

Authors' information
MS holds a position as a resident physician (neurologist) at the Department of Neurology, University of Leipzig. She has several years of clinical experience in neuroimmunological disorders, from both inpatient and outpatient perspective. Her research has focused on multiple sclerosis, where she has initiated her own clinical projects employing electrophysiological and other surrogate markers. She has served as an investigator in the German Competence Network Multiple Sclerosis (KKNMS) prospective cohort study, in an investigator-initiated trial funded by the German Federal Ministry of Education and Research (BMBF) and in several multicenter clinical trials in multiple sclerosis, neuromyelitis optica and myasthenia gravis (phases I-III).
FTB is a professor of Neurology at the Department of Neurology, University of Leipzig. He is an associated partner of the German Competence Network Multiple Sclerosis (KKNMS), serving on the biosamples board. He has initiated several clinical studies in multiple sclerosis, partly funded by the German Federal Ministry of Education and Research (BMBF), the Deutsche Forschungsgemeinschaft (DFG) or by industry. He has been co-investigator, principal investigator or (national and international) lead investigator of several phase I to III trials in multiple sclerosis, neuromyelitis optica and myasthenia gravis. He has received funding from the Deutsche Forschungsgemeinschaft (DFG) for laboratory research in the field of neural stem cells.

Competing interests
The authors declare that they have no competing interests.

References
1. Weinshenker BG, Bass B, Rice GP, et al. The natural history of multiple sclerosis: a geographically based study. 2. Predictive value of the early clinical course. Brain. 1989;112(Pt 6):1419–28.
2. Ferguson B, Matyszak MK, Esiri MM, Perry VH. Axonal damage in acute multiple sclerosis lesions. Brain. 1997;120(Pt 3):393–9.
3. Milligan NM, Newcombe R, Compston DA. A double-blind controlled trial of high dose methylprednisolone in patients with multiple sclerosis: 1 clinical effects. J Neurol Neurosurg Psychiatry. 1987;50:511–6.
4. Grauer O, Offenhäusser M, Schmidt J, Toyka KV, Gold R. Glukokortikosteroid-Therapie bei Optikusneuritis und Multipler Sklerose. Evidenz aus klinischen Studien und praktische Empfehlungen. Nervenarzt. 2001;72:577–89.
5. Burton JM, O'Connor PW, Hohol M, Beyene J. Oral versus intravenous steroids for treatment of relapses in multiple sclerosis. Cochrane Database Syst Rev. 2009:CD006921.
6. Burton JM, O'Connor PW, Hohol M, Beyene J. Oral versus intravenous steroids for treatment of relapses in multiple sclerosis. Cochrane Database Syst Rev. 2012;12:CD006921.

7. Alam SM, Kyriakides T, Lawden M, Newman PK. Methylprednisolone in multiple sclerosis: a comparison of oral with intravenous therapy at equivalent high dose. J Neurol Neurosurg Psychiatry. 1993;56:1219–20.

8. Barnes D, Hughes RA, Morris RW, et al. Randomised trial of oral and intravenous methylprednisolone in acute relapses of multiple sclerosis. Lancet. 1997;349:902–6.

9. Durelli L, Cocito D, Riccio A, et al. High-dose intravenous methylprednisolone in the treatment of multiple sclerosis: clinical-immunologic correlations. Neurology. 1986;36:238–43.

10. Filippini G, Brusaferri F, Sibley WA, et al. Corticosteroids or ACTH for acute exacerbations in multiple sclerosis. Cochrane Database Syst Rev. 2000;(4): CD001331.

11. Sellebjerg F, Frederiksen JL, Nielsen PM, Olesen J. Double-blind, randomized, placebo-controlled study of oral, high-dose methylprednisolone in attacks of MS. Neurology. 1998;51:529–34.

12. Koziolek MJ, Tampe D, Bähr M, et al. Immunoadsorption therapy in patients with multiple sclerosis with steroid-refractory optical neuritis. J Neuroinflammation. 2012;9:80.

13. Trebst C, Bronzlik P, Kielstein JT, Schmidt BMW, Stangel M. Immunoadsorption therapy for steroid-unresponsive relapses in patients with multiple sclerosis. Blood Purif. 2012;33:1–6.

14. Heigl F, Hettich R, Arendt R, Durner J, Koehler J, Mauch E. Immunoadsorption in steroid-refractory multiple sclerosis: clinical experience in 60 patients. Atheroscler Suppl. 2013;14:167–73.

15. Trebst C, Reising A, Kielstein JT, Hafer C, Stangel M. Plasma exchange therapy in steroid-unresponsive relapses in patients with multiple sclerosis. Blood Purif. 2009;28:108–15.

16. Ehler J, Koball S, Sauer M, et al. Response to therapeutic plasma exchange as a rescue treatment in clinically isolated syndromes and acute worsening of multiple sclerosis: a retrospective analysis of 90 patients. PLoS One. 2015;10:e0134583.

17. Meca-Lallana JE, Hernández-Clares R, León-Hernández A, Genovés Aleixandre A, Cacho Pérez M, Martín-Fernández JJ. Plasma exchange for steroid-refractory relapses in multiple sclerosis: an observational, MRI pilot study. Clin Ther. 2013;35:474–85.

18. Gold R. Leitlinie Diagnostik und Therapie der Multiplen Sklerose. 5., vollst. überarb. Aufl. Stuttgart: Thieme; 2012.

19. Ramo-Tello C, Grau-López L, Tintoré M, et al. A randomized clinical trial of oral versus intravenous methylprednisolone for relapse of MS. Mult Scler. 2014;20:717–25.

20. Le Page E, Veillard D, Laplaud DA, et al. Oral versus intravenous high-dose methylprednisolone for treatment of relapses in patients with multiple sclerosis (COPOUSEP): a randomised, controlled, double-blind, non-inferiority trial. Lancet. 2015;386:974–81.

21. Oliveri RL, Valentino P, Russo C, et al. Randomized trial comparing two different high doses of methylprednisolone in MS: a clinical and MRI study. Neurology. 1998;50:1833–6.

22. Schmidt J, Gold R, Schönrock L, Zettl UK, Hartung HP, Toyka KV. T-cell apoptosis in situ in experimental autoimmune encephalomyelitis following methylprednisolone pulse therapy. Brain. 2000;123(Pt 7):1431–41.

23. Sellebjerg F, Barnes D, Filippini G, et al. EFNS guideline on treatment of multiple sclerosis relapses: report of an EFNS task force on treatment of multiple sclerosis relapses. Eur J Neurol. 2005;12:939–46.

24. Goodin DS, Frohman EM, Garmany GP, et al. Disease modifying therapies in multiple sclerosis: report of the therapeutics and technology assessment Subcommittee of the American Academy of neurology and the MS Council for clinical practice guidelines. Neurology. 2002;58:169–78.

25. Goodin DS. Disease-modifying therapy in multiple sclerosis: update and clinical implications. Neurology. 2008;71:S8–13.

26. La Mantia L, Eoli M, Milanese C, et al. Double trial of dexamethasone versus methylprednisolone in multiple sclerosis acute relapses. Eur Neurol. 1994;34:199–203.

27. Kupersmith MJ, Kaufman D, Paty DW, et al. MEgadose corticosteroids in multiple sclerosis. Neurology. 1994;44:1–4.

28. Park-Wyllie L, Mazzotta P, Pastuszak A, et al. Birth defects after maternal exposure to corticosteroids: prospective cohort study and meta-analysis of epidemiological studies. Teratology. 2000;62:385–92.

29. Hoffmann F, Kraft A, Heigl F, et al. Tryptophan-Immunadsorption bei Multipler Sklerose und Neuromyelitis optica: Therapieoption bei akuten Schüben in der Schwangerschaft und Stillphase. Nervenarzt. 2015;86:179–86.

13

Mindfulness-based stress reduction for people with multiple sclerosis

Robert Simpson[*], Frances S. Mair and Stewart W. Mercer

Abstract

Background: Multiple sclerosis (MS) is a stressful condition. Mental health comorbidity is common. Stress can increase the risk of depression, reduce quality of life (QOL), and possibly exacerbate disease activity in MS. Mindfulness-Based Stress Reduction (MBSR) may help, but has been little studied in MS, particularly among more disabled individuals.

Methods: The objective of this study was to test the feasibility and likely effectiveness of a standard MBSR course for people with MS. Participant eligibility included: age > 18, any type of MS, an Expanded Disability Status Scale (EDSS) $\leq$ 7.0. Participants received either MBSR or wait-list control. Outcome measures were collected at baseline, post-intervention, and three-months later. Primary outcomes were perceived stress and QOL. Secondary outcomes were common MS symptoms, mindfulness, and self-compassion.

Results: Fifty participants were recruited and randomised (25 per group). Trial retention and outcome measure completion rates were 90% at post-intervention, and 88% at 3 months. Sixty percent of participants completed the course. Immediately post-MBSR, perceived stress improved with a large effect size (ES 0.93; $p < 0.01$), compared to very small beneficial effects on QOL (ES 0.17; $p = 0.48$). Depression (ES 1.35; $p < 0.05$), positive affect (ES 0.87; $p = 0.13$), anxiety (ES 0.85; $p = 0.05$), and self-compassion (ES 0.80; $p < 0.01$) also improved with large effect sizes. At three-months post-MBSR (study endpoint) improvements in perceived stress were diminished to a small effect size (ES 0.26; $p = 0.39$), were negligible for QOL (ES 0.08; $p = 0.71$), but were large for mindfulness (ES 1.13; $p < 0.001$), positive affect (ES 0.90; $p = 0.54$), self-compassion (ES 0.83; $p < 0.05$), anxiety (ES 0.82; $p = 0.15$), and prospective memory (ES 0.81; $p < 0.05$).

Conclusions: Recruitment, retention, and data collection demonstrate that a RCT of MBSR is feasible for people with MS. Trends towards improved outcomes suggest that a larger definitive RCT may be warranted. However, optimisation changes may be required to render more stable the beneficial treatment effects on stress and depression.

Background

Multiple sclerosis (MS) is a stressful condition, with unpredictable relapses and disease progression [1], problematic comorbidity [2], complex drug regimens [3], and manifold social and role difficulties [1]. Stress may contribute to disease activity in MS [4, 5], is burdensome, can negate health-promoting behaviors [6], may contribute to the development of anxiety and depression and impair quality of life (QOL) in MS [7, 8]. Anxiety and depression are common in MS [2]. Evidence to support the use of pharmacological treatments for mental health comorbidities in MS is limited, with problematic side effects noted [9]. Amongst psychological interventions, cognitive behavioural therapy (CBT) approaches are often used, but evidence is limited and reviews consistently highlight a need for further high quality research to identify other effective and acceptable interventions [10]. CBT has the strongest evidence for treating depression [10] and stress [11] in MS, but effective treatments for anxiety are lacking [10].

* Correspondence: Robert.Simpson@glasgow.ac.uk
General Practice and Primary Care, Institute of Health and Wellbeing, University of Glasgow, House 1, 1 Horselethill Road, Glasgow, Scotland G12 9LX, UK

Mindfulness-based interventions (MBIs) are increasingly used to manage mental health problems and stress in long-term conditions (LTCs), with meta-analytic studies reporting comparable efficacy to both CBT and antidepressants [12]. MBIs are multicomponent complex interventions that teach a variety of meditation skills to facilitate the development of 'mindfulness' [13]. The term mindfulness is often defined as; *'paying attention in a particular way: on purpose, in the present moment, and non-judgmentally'* [14]. How MBIs work is not fully understood, but improved executive skills and enhanced emotion regulation are thought key mechanisms [15, 16]. Mindfulness-Based Stress Reduction (MBSR) was the original model for MBIs, first used for people with chronic pain [17]. MBIs have since been applied to a wide range of other LTCs, with existing evidence supporting their use in anxiety [18], recurrent depression [18], and somatisation [19].

In people with MS, a recent systematic review found limited evidence that MBIs may improve anxiety, depression, pain, fatigue, balance, and QOL [20]. Since then, further evidence suggests potential cost-effectiveness [21]. However, how best MBIs should be delivered to diverse MS populations remains unclear. Differing demographic factors such as age, sex, socio-economic status (SES), ethnicity, comorbidity, and greater levels of disability could conceivably impact on effectiveness. Prior studies have largely focused on distinct disease phenotypes [21, 22], or less disabled individuals [23–27], meaning that previous findings suggesting benefit from MBSR [24] may not apply to the wider spectrum of people with MS. Only one prior study has reported detailed feasibility findings for the use of MBIs in people with MS, where data is limited to people with progressive disease [21]. Very little is thus known about the feasibility, acceptability, accessibility, and implementability of standard MBSR for people with MS.

The aim of the study described in this paper was to determine the feasibility of conducting a definitive phase-3 randomised controlled trial (RCT) of standard MBSR and to obtain initial estimates of likely effectiveness.

Methods

Trial design and participants
This was a phase-2 exploratory RCT to assess the feasibility (engagement and retention), and likely effectiveness of MBSR in people with MS. It was conducted in Glasgow, Scotland, United Kingdom (UK). Acceptability, accessibility, and implementability were also assessed via nested qualitative semi-structured interviews (recently submitted for publication) and will be reported elsewhere.

The study employed a wait-list control design, meaning that all study participants eventually received MBSR. We aimed to recruit 50 adults with MS within 3 months. Between June and August 2014, participants were recruited from National Health Service (NHS) sites in Greater Glasgow. Participants were recruited directly by clinical staff on NHS sites providing MS services; by alerting all GPs in this health board area by email; advertising via NHS/third-sector bodies (MS Revive); through internet adverts (MS Society UK), and the University of Glasgow Twitter/Facebook social media outlets. Full inclusion and exclusion criteria are provided below (Table 1).

A priori stopping criteria were for trial discontinuation in the occurrence of any adverse event(s) strongly suggesting harm from the intervention.

Recruited participants had baseline measures and informed consent collected face-to-face, prior to randomisation. All measures were self-completed; firstly with a researcher present, then on subsequent iterations by the participant alone. Follow-up measures were collected by post, at intervention completion (2 months), and then again 3 months later (at 5 months). Those who did not return postal measures within 14 days were telephoned to confirm ongoing participation. After waiting 2 weeks for response, the average number of reminder calls required was 4.4. Participants received a £5 gift voucher as a gesture of appreciation for completing each questionnaire.

Randomisation and blinding
An independent, blinded statistician from the Robertson Centre for Biostatistics (RCB) at the University of Glasgow undertook randomisation and sequence generation, once all baseline measures had been collected. Block sizes of two were generated, to prevent over-allocation to either group. Blinded staff at the University of Glasgow with no prior knowledge of participants handled treatment allocation. Questionnaire data was identifiable

Table 1 Study eligibility criteria

Inclusion	1) Over 18 years of age; 2) Neurologist confirmed diagnosis of MS (Poser or McDonald criteria depending on year of diagnosis); 3) Able to understand spoken and written English; 4) A score of less than or equal to 7.0 on the Expanded Disability Status Scale (EDSS) [49]
Exclusion	1) Life-threatening physical or mental health comorbidities (i.e. suicidal ideation, active psychosis, or terminal/life threatening inter-current medical illness), or such conditions expected to significantly limit participation and adherence (eg dementia, pregnancy, on going substance abuse); 2) Those currently receiving another form of psychological intervention (non-pharmacological).

only by a random study number, and data entry for all outcome measures was done by a researcher blinded to group allocation. It was impossible to blind participants or MBSR instructors to their treatment allocation.

Patient involvement

The trial protocol was prospectively reviewed by three patient members of the UK MS Society research network who provided favourable feedback for the study.

Intervention

The intervention was based on standard MBSR, including home practice materials, but without the day retreat at week six; excluded for pragmatic, space-constraint reasons, as well as empirical evidence contesting its necessity [28] (Additional file 1). All MBSR classes were led by two experienced physician facilitators and took place at the NHS Centre for Integrative Care (NHS CIC), in Glasgow.

MBSR instructors

The MBSR instructors were used to working together. Over the previous 3 years they had regularly taught weekly mindfulness groups to multimorbid people with a variety of LTCs (including MS) as part of their routine clinical responsibilities. However, neither instructor had taught groups exclusively for people with MS.

The first MBSR instructor had a clinical background in General Practice since 1983 and worked full time as a Specialty Doctor at the NHS CIC. She had completed teacher training in Mindfulness-Based Cognitive Therapy (MBCT) in 2005, via the University of Bangor, and had been teaching mindfulness regularly since then. She had also completed residential MBSR training in with Jon-Kabat-Zinn, in the USA in 2011, and regularly attended training retreats in MBCT and Vipasana meditation. She had a teaching qualification in Pranayama and Iyengar Yoga. She regularly attended one-to-one mindfulness clinical supervision and had a longstanding daily practice.

The second MBSR instructor also came from a General Practice background, completing her clinical training in 1994. She qualified as a mindfulness teacher in 2011 via the University of Bangor. She was halfway through completing an MSc in teaching mindfulness via the University of Bangor and had a longstanding daily mindfulness practice with regular clinical supervision.

Intervention fidelity

Fidelity assessment was informed by the National Institutes of Health guidance for behavioural interventions [29] (Table 2).

However, the UK Medical Research Council (MRC) guidance for developing and evaluating complex interventions [13] suggests that any such measures should be flexible during the early stages of evaluation of a novel intervention/context. For example, there was no 'reviewer' sitting in or video-recording the classes, something that would be important in a full-scale trial.

Outcome objectives

As a feasibility study, the main outcome objectives were:

1. To determine if recruitment, delivery, and retention for a RCT of MBSR was feasible
2. To determine if outcome measurement data collection was feasible
3. To assess likely effectiveness on outcome measures in a definitive trial

The primary participant-report outcomes were:

a. Perceived stress (Perceived Stress Scale-10 – PSS [30])
b. Quality of life (EQ-5D-5 L) [31].

Table 2 Treatment fidelity

Domain of fidelity	How it was met
1. Study design	A priori study protocol; fixed number/length of MBSR sessions; recording of any protocol deviations; scripted manual for course; external monitoring by research team and MBSR instructor not part of the research project; monitoring homework completion
2. Provider training	Qualified and experienced mindfulness teachers trained together using standardised MBSR treatment manuals; same instructors throughout; regular external provider debriefing and supervision; easy access to senior research staff (SM); participant exit interviews enquiring about intervention content
3. Improving delivery of MBSR	Qualitative assessment of provider 'warmth/ credibility' from participants, complaint monitoring; treatment workbook provided to all participants;
4. Improving receipt of MBSR	Providers asked for weekly participant feedback, both verbal, and in writing (embedded questionnaire – not part of study data); completion of regular activity logs; participant and provider feedback on MBSR exercises during classes; telephone follow-up with drop-outs
5. Improving MBSR skill enactment	Semi-structured participant interviews on completion; regular home practice and materials provided along with diary for adherence; in class discussion/post-interview discussion on ongoing use/application of MBSR skills in daily life

Secondary participant-report outcomes sought to:

1. Capture common MS symptoms with a MS specific measure (Multiple Sclerosis Quality of Life Inventory - MSQLI) [32]. The MSQLI includes measures of:
   a. Fatigue (cognitive, physical, psychosocial) (Modified Fatigue Impact Scale – MFIS)
   b. Mental health (anxiety, depression, behavioural control, positive affect) (Mental Health Inventory-18 - MHI)
   c. Social support (tangible, emotional, affection, positive interactions) (Modified Social Support Survey - MSSS)
   d. Cognitive function (attention, retrospective memory, prospective memory, planning) (Perceived Deficits Questionnaire - PDQ)
   e. Pain (Pain Effects Scale – PES)
   f. Visual function (Impact of Visual Impairment Scale - IVIS)
   g. Bladder function (Bladder Control Scale - BCS)
   h. Bowel function (Bowel Control Scale - BWCS)
   i. Sexual satisfaction (Sexual Satisfaction Scale – SSS)

2. Assess items measuring the putative processes of mindfulness:
   a. Mindfulness (Mindful Attention Awareness Scale – MAAS) [33].
   b. Self-compassion (Self-Compassion Scale - short form – SCS-sf) [34].

3. Measure emotional lability via the Emotional Lability Questionnaire (ELQ) [35].

For psychometric properties and justification of measures used, see Additional file 2.

A baseline participant questionnaire also recorded demographic information, including deprivation, as measured by the Scottish Index of Multiple Deprivation (SIMD) [36], number of comorbid conditions, and use of disease-modifying, antidepressant, or analgesic medications.

Statistical analysis
An a priori statistical analysis plan was developed in conjunction with a Consultant Biostatistician from the Robertson Centre for Biostatistics, University of Glasgow. This was made publicly available online, in advance of all data collection: http://www.gla.ac.uk/researchinstitutes/

healthwellbeing/research/generalpractice/research/mbsr-ms/.

Key outcomes to assess feasibility, acceptability, and accessibility included rates of recruitment and retention. These were recorded using descriptive statistics.

Baseline characteristics were summarised by intervention arm.

Differences were tested via two-sample t-tests for normally distributed variables, and chi-squared tests for categorical variables. Questionnaire outcome data were analysed relative to change from baseline via an analysis of covariance (ANCOVA) approach, where adjustments were made for the baseline score, as appropriate, including age, sex, and deprivation, as well as any other characteristics found to differ between the intervention arms at baseline. On the advice of the statistician, age, sex, and SES were included as common confounders, however, unadjusted analyses were also undertaken for comparison.

An a priori decision was made not to perform data imputation for missing values. There were no interim analyses performed. All statistical analyses were undertaken using SPSS v21.

For questionnaire data, results are reported for between group mean (standard deviation - SD) baseline scores, change scores, treatment effects (β) with 95% confidence intervals (95% CIs), significance levels, and effect sizes (ES) (Cohen's 'd') with 95% CIs.

Sample size calculation
Given the aim of this study being to assess feasibility and power estimate for a phase-3 trial, sample size was not based on a power calculation. However, based on the advice of a statistician, a working sample size of 50 people was chosen as:

1. Browne [37] has demonstrated that an 'n' of 30 is sufficient to allow estimates of sample size for an efficacy trial.
2. Pragmatic reasons including a) the MBSR instructors were used to routinely delivering groups of this size; and b) space constraints meant that a maximum of 25 participants could be accommodated in each group.

Data access
Data for the trial was accessible to all authors (RS, FM, SM), who each contributed to its interpretation.

Results
Objective 1 - To determine if recruitment, delivery, and retention for a large scale RCT of MBSR were feasible
In total, 101 patients were approached, of whom 66 (65%) contacted the researcher (RS) and were screened.

Following screening, three people were ineligible (EDSS > 7.0), and 13 declined to take part due to: difficulties securing transport ($n = 7$); difficulty getting time off work ($n = 4$); thought the course would be too tiring ($n = 1$); unclear ($n = 1$). Consent rate was thus 50/66, or 76%. Recruitment was completed within 10 weeks (out of the pre-specified 12) (Table 3).

Following randomisation, one participant assigned to MBSR could not attend the allocated dates, and thus did not receive the intervention, but continued to complete measures throughout, and another three participants withdrew due to: a) a MS symptom exacerbation (fatigue), b) family conflict, and c) becoming enrolled in a pharmacological trial. Thus, from the 25 participants originally assigned to the intervention, only 21 could attend any classes. See Fig. 1 below for a detailed CONSORT flow diagram.

Treatment adherence

Treatment adherence was assessed via attendance at the MBSR sessions, and via home practice recordings. Fifteen participants (60%) attended four or more MBSR sessions, meeting the criteria for course 'completion'. There were no significant differences in demographic factors between completers and non-completers (Additional file 3). Reasons cited for session non-attendance included inter-current illness, work commitments, being on holiday, and 'sleeping-in'. See Table 4 for details of MBSR session attendance.

Participants were asked to return a home-practice log each week, but only 16/25 (60%) people returned any data. From these, an average home practice time of 32.5 min per day was observed. Four people allocated to MBSR did not attend any sessions, and provided no data on home-practice.

Baseline participant characteristics

The sample at baseline had a mean age (SD) of 44.96 (10.90), was predominantly female (92%), and of White Scottish ethnicity (98%). Forty participants (80%) had Relapsing Remitting MS (RRMS), eight (16%) had Secondary Progressive (SPMS), and two (4%) had Primary Progressive disease (PPMS). The mean (SD) EDDS was 4.41 (1.75). After randomisation, the intervention and control groups were similar in terms of age, sex, SES, ethnicity, level of education, MS phenotype, disease duration, number of comorbidities, and EDSS score, with the only significant baseline difference relating to previous meditation/yoga experience, which by chance was higher in the intervention group. Thus, this potential confounder was controlled for in the subsequent analyses, along with age, sex, and SES. Baseline demographic and clinical data are summarised in Table 5.

Objective 2 - To determine if outcome measurement data collection was feasible

All 50 participants completed outcome measures at baseline (100%). At the post intervention point (two-months) 45/50 (90%) returned these measures, and at the final follow-up point (five-months) 44/50 (88%) were returned. Over the entire period for collecting post-intervention and follow-up measures, an average of 4.4 telephone reminders were required per participant (222 calls in total). Missing data varied considerably across the range of outcome measures. Thirty-nine out of 50 (78%) participants returned at least one item of missing data, and it was commoner among measures towards the back of the questionnaire. It was lowest on the EQ-5D-5 L (0–12%), and highest for the SCS-sf (2–22%), with 13/15 measures having less than 20% missing values. There were no significant differences in age (Mean age 47.12 [SD 10.44] vs. 44.96 [SD 10.90]; $p = 0.39$), disability level (Mean EDSS 4.51 [SD 1.77] vs. 4.41 [SD 1.75]; $p = 0.40$), or SES (Mean deprivation decile 5.08 [SD 2.64] vs. 5.22 [SD 2.71]; $p = 0.60$) between those returning missing values, and those who did not. See Additional file 4 for further details regarding missing data.

Table 3 Sources of trial recruitment and relative contributions

Source of engagement/ recruitment	Numbers known to have been approached	Numbers (known) expressing interest	Numbers recruited into trial (n/50)	Percentage of recruitment overall
MS Specialist Nurses	75	52	34	68%
MS Revive Nurse	6	6	6	12%
Integrative Medicine Specialists	9	9	5	10%
General practitioners	11	11	5	10%
Via MS Society advertisement	Freely available online	2	0	0%
Via University web (Twitter/ Facebook)	Freely available online	0	0	0%
Via protocol (clinical trials.gov)	Freely available online	5	0	0%
Total	101(+)	85	50	N/A

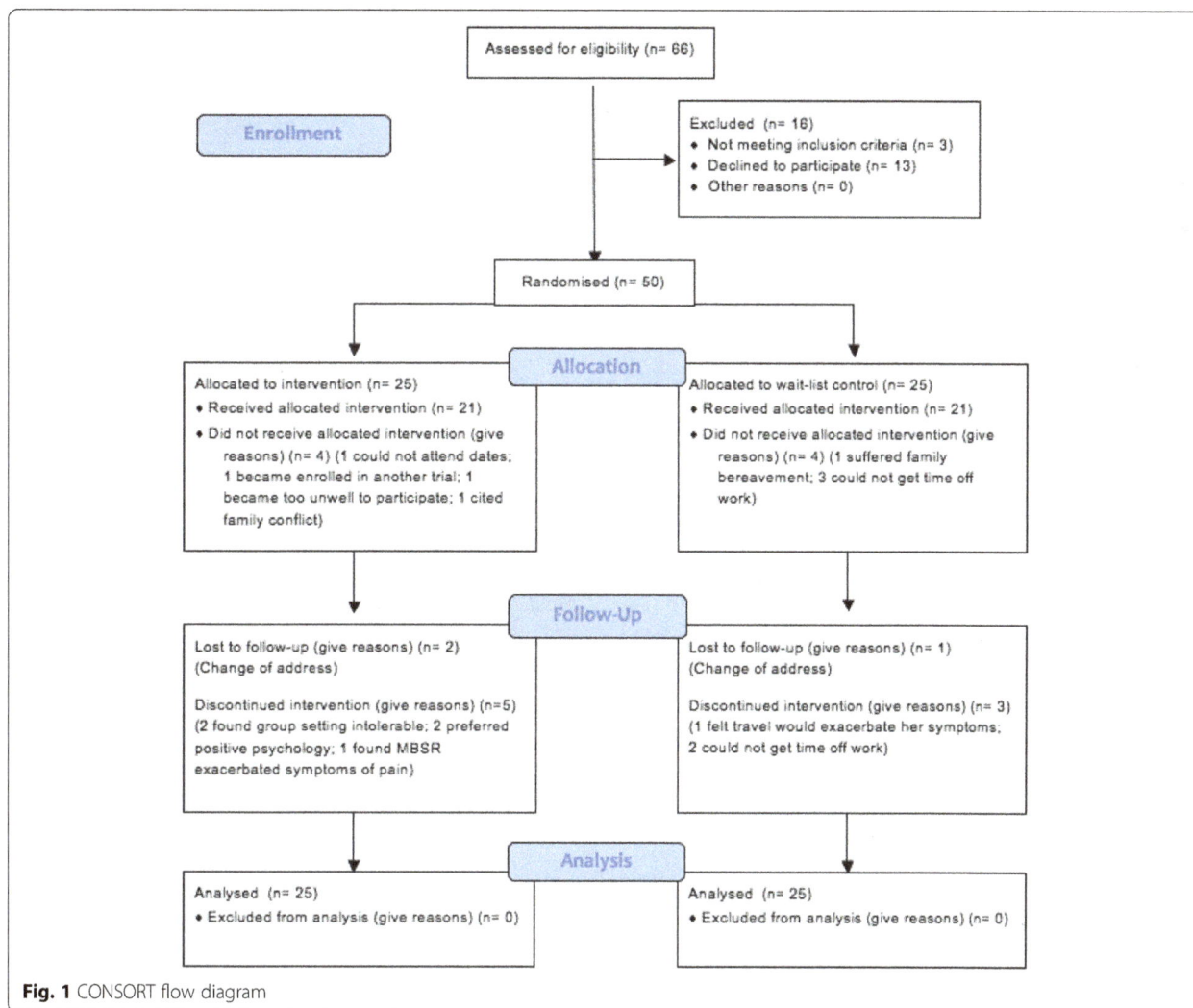

Fig. 1 CONSORT flow diagram

Objective 3 - To assess likely effectiveness on outcome measures in a definitive trial

There were no significant differences between the groups on any of the baseline outcome measures. Two models were explored in the analyses 1) a 'raw' model that made no adjustments for demographic factors; and 2)

Table 4 MBSR session attendance

MBSR sessions completed	Number of participants	Percentage (%)
All	3	12%
7	8	32%
6	3	12%
5	1	4%
4	0	0%
3	1	4%
2	1	4%
1	4	16%
0	4	16%

a model that adjusted for age, sex, SES, and previous yoga/meditation experience. There were only minor differences between the models. In the raw model beneficial effect sizes were slightly larger on all measures (Additional file 5). As such, the model presented below is that adjusted for age, sex, deprivation and previous yoga/meditation experience.

In the model adjusted for age, sex, SES, and previous meditation/yoga experience, at immediately post-MBSR, PSS scores improved with a large effect size (ES 0.93; $p < 0.05$), but EQ-5D-5 L scores showed only very small improvement (ES 0.17; $p = 0.48$). From the secondary outcomes, improvements with a large effect size were evident for depression (ES 1.35; $p < 0.05$), positive affect (ES 0.87; $p = 0.13$), anxiety (ES 0.85; $p = 0.05$), and self-compassion (ES 0.80; $p < 0.01$). Overall, 14 out of 15 of the composite outcome measures (primary and secondary) showed a positive trend for treatment effect immediately post-MBSR (Fig. 2).

Table 5 Baseline participant characteristics

	Intervention	Control	Significance p
Mean age in years (standard deviation - SD)	43.6 (10.7)	46.3 (11.1)	0.37
Sex	Female 23 (92%)	Female 22 (88%)	1.00
Ethnicity	White British 25 (100%)	White British 25 (100%)	1.00
MS phenotype RRMS – relapsing remitting; SPMS – secondary progressive; PPMS – primary progressive	RRMS 22 (88%) SPMS 1 (4%) PPMS 2 (8%)	RRMS 18 (72%) SPMS 7 (28%)	0.74
Deprivation	5.0 (2.8)	5.4 (2.6)	0.64
Education – highest level	Secondary school 3 (12%) College 7 (28%) University 15 (60%)	Secondary school 5 (20%) College 7 (28%) University 13 (52%)	0.73
Employment	Full time 4 (16%) Part time 3 (12%) Unemployed 6 (24%) Retired 5 (20%) Other 7 (28%)	Full time 7 (28%) Part time 6 (24%) Unemployed 7 (28%) Retired 3 (12%) Other 2 (8%)	0.39
Living arrangement	Lives alone 6 (24%) With partner 9 (36%) With family/friends 10 (40%)	Lives alone 3 (12%) With partner 10 (40%) With family/friends 12 (48%)	0.54
EDSS	4.5 (1.8)	4.3 (1.7)	0.64
Mean disease duration in years (SD)	8.9 (8.5)	9.6 (9.4)	0.79
Mean total comorbidity count (SD)	2.5 (2.2)	2.3 (1.9)	0.68
Mean mental health comorbidity count (SD)	0.8 (0.83)	0.7 (0.8)	0.73
• Comorbid anxiety	11 (44%)	8 (32%)	0.12
• Comorbid depression	9 (36%)	11 (44%)	0.29
Mean physical health comorbidity count (SD)	1.8 (1.5)	1.6 (1.5)	0.71
Using analgesic drugs	19 (76%)	17 (68%)	0.75
Using disease modifying drugs	14 (56%)	12 (48%)	0.78
Using antidepressant drugs	12 (48%)	11 (44%)	1.00
Previous meditation/yoga experience	17 (68%)	10 (40%)	*0.04*

*Statistically significant difference

At follow-up, 3 months following MBSR, beneficial effects on the PSS had diminished to a small effect size (ES 0.26; p = 0.39) and those for the EQ-5D-5 L were negligible (0.08; p = 0.71). From secondary outcomes, improvements with a large effect size were evident for mindfulness (ES 1.21; p < 0.001), positive affect (ES 0.90; p = 0.54), anxiety (ES 0.82; p = 0.15), prospective memory (ES 0.81; p < 0.05), and self-compassion (ES 0.80; p < 0.05). There was an overall trend towards improvement on 14 out of 15 of the composite measures (Fig. 3).

See Figs. 2 and 3 for a graphical summary of treatment effects for adjusted models covering the PSS, EQ-5D-5 L, the

MSQLI, MAAS, SCS-sf, and the ELQ. Further statistical details are outlined in Tables AF6.1–AF6.9 in Additional file 6.

Harms
One participant allocated to the intervention group reported an exacerbation in her symptoms of neuropathic pain following her first and only MBSR class.

Discussion
This study assessed the feasibility of delivering MBSR for people with MS in an exploratory phase-2 RCT. We recruited our target of 50 participants within 3 months.

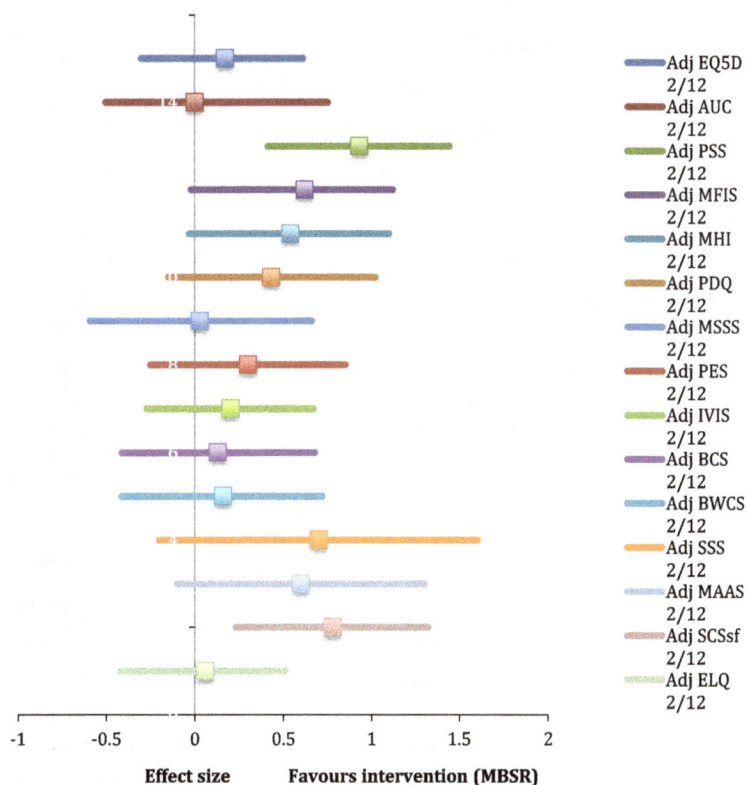

Fig. 2 Effect sizes with 95% confidence intervals immediately post-MBSR (adjusted for age/sex/SES/previous meditation/yoga): EQ5D – EuroQol QOL measure adjusted for age/sex/SES/meditation/yoga. AUC – EuroQol area under the curve adjusted for age/sex/SES/meditation/yoga. PSS – Perceived stress scale adjusted for age/sex/SES/meditation/yoga. MFIS – Modified fatigue impact scale adjusted for age/sex/SES/meditation/yoga. MHI – Mental health inventory adjusted for age/sex/SES/meditation/yoga. PDQ – Perceived deficits questionnaire adjusted for age/sex/SES/meditation/yoga. MSSS – Modified social support survey adjusted for age/sex/SES/meditation/yoga. PES – Pain effects scale adjusted for age/sex/SES/meditation/yoga. IVIS – Impact of visual impairment scale adjusted for age/sex/SES/meditation/yoga. BCS – Bladder control scale adjusted for age/sex/SES/meditation/yoga. BWCS – Bowel control scale adjusted for age/sex/SES/meditation/yoga. SSS – Sexual satisfaction scale adjusted for age/sex/SES/meditation/yoga. MAAS – Mindful attention awareness scale adjusted for age/sex/SES/meditation/yoga. SCS-sf – Self-compassion scale – short form adjusted for age/sex/SES/meditation/yoga. ELQ – Emotional lability questionnaire adjusted for age/sex/SES/meditation/yoga

Very high rates of study retention were achieved, with 45 (90%) participants completing outcome measures immediately post-intervention, and 44 (88%) at follow-up, 3 months later. Missing values were generally low. MBSR session attendance was only 60%, less than that reported in other studies of MBIs for people with MS (range 92–95%) [21, 24].

Regarding primary efficacy outcomes, large initial improvements were seen in perceived stress at post-intervention in this study, but diminished to small at three-month follow-up. Improvements in QOL were very small at post-intervention and negligible at three-month follow-up. For secondary outcomes, large improvements in depression, positive affect, anxiety, and self-compassion were apparent immediately post-MBSR, whilst at three-month follow-up large improvements were present for mindfulness, positive affect, anxiety, prospective memory, and self-compassion.

Comparison with existing literature

A large RCT testing MBSR in less disabled patients with MS that took place in a university hospital location reported a lower refusal rate (9%) than the current study (24%), but they used an advertisement-based 'opt-in' approach to recruitment, whereas the current study employed a multifaceted strategy with a greater potential to record refusal [24]. Outcome measure completion in their study was 91% at six-month follow-up, versus 88% in ours at 3 months post MBSR. They also reported much higher session attendance (92%) than the current study (60%), perhaps reflecting lower levels of disability in their participants (mean EDSS 3.0; SD 1.0 versus mean EDSS 4.41; SD 1.75), or slightly higher level of mindfulness teacher experience (>9 years versus 7.5). They delivered MBSR in smaller groups (n = 10–15 per course), versus the relatively large group size in this

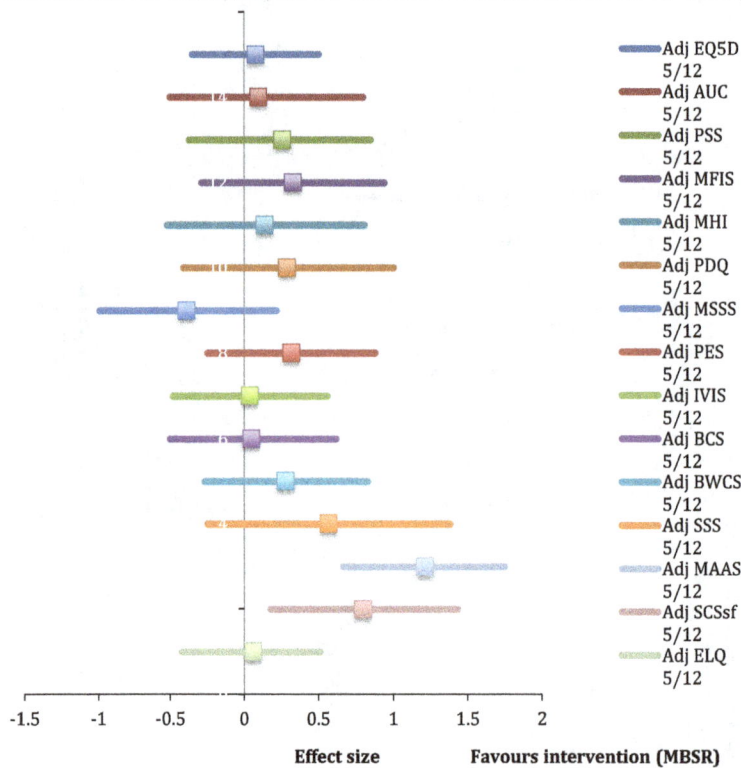

Fig. 3 Effect sizes with 95% confidence intervals 3 months post-MBSR (adjusted for age/sex/SES/previous meditation/yoga): EQ5D – EuroQol QOL measure adjusted for age/sex/SES/meditation/yoga. AUC – EuroQol area under the curve adjusted for age/sex/SES/meditation/yoga. PSS – Perceived stress scale adjusted for age/sex/SES/meditation/yoga. MFIS – Modified fatigue impact scale adjusted for age/sex/SES/meditation/yoga. MHI – Mental health inventory adjusted for age/sex/SES/meditation/yoga. PDQ – Perceived deficits questionnaire adjusted for age/sex/SES/meditation/yoga. MSSS – Modified social support survey adjusted for age/sex/SES/meditation/yoga. PES – Pain effects scale adjusted for age/sex/SES/meditation/yoga. IVIS – Impact of visual impairment scale adjusted for age/sex/SES/meditation/yoga. BCS – Bladder control scale adjusted for age/sex/SES/meditation/yoga. BWCS – Bowel control scale adjusted for age/sex/SES/meditation/yoga. SSS – Sexual satisfaction scale adjusted for age/sex/SES/meditation/yoga. MAAS – Mindful attention awareness scale adjusted for age/sex/SES/meditation/yoga. SCS-sf – Self-compassion scale – short form adjusted for age/sex/SES/meditation/yoga. ELQ – Emotional lability questionnaire adjusted for age/sex/SES/meditation/yoga

current study ($n = 25$). Average home-practice times in their study (29.2 min) were comparable to those in this current study (32.5 min).

No previous research studies have demonstrated improvements in cognitive function among MS patients following mindfulness training. With respect to mental health outcomes, a high quality powered RCT tested MBSR in people with MS, but did not control for potential confounders in their analyses [24]. The authors similarly reported improvements in mental health, with smaller beneficial effects on depression post-intervention (ES 0.65; $p < 0.001$), which diminished less than ours at six-month follow-up (ES 0.36; $p < 0.05$). They also found smaller improvements than us in anxiety post-intervention (ES 0.39; $p < 0.001$) and at six-month follow up (ES 0.36; $p < 0.05$). The authors also reported that beneficial effects on both anxiety and depression were greater when subgroup analyses focused only on those with

pre-intervention scores deemed to be of clinical significance [24].

More recently, an unpowered pilot study testing a tailored remote Skype-delivered MBCT course minus mindful-movement in people with progressive MS demonstrated preliminary evidence to suggest likely effectiveness at improving mental health. Bogosian et al. [21] included only those with levels of distress on the General Health Questionnaire (GHQ) indicative of psychiatric 'case-ness'. Improvements with a large effect size were noted in distress 3 months post MBCT (ES 0.97; $p < 0.05$); but were smaller for anxiety post intervention (ES 0.40; $p = 0.10$), increasing to large 3 months later (ES 0.86; $p < 0.05$). Improvements in depression were smaller post-intervention (ES 0.65; $p < 0.05$), but sustained 3 months later (ES 0.53; $p < 0.05$); whilst improvements in MS symptom psychological impact post-intervention were large (ES 0.99; $p < 0.001$) and sustained 3 months later (ES 1.12; $p < 0.01$).

Four other small studies have reported similar benefits in anxiety [25, 26], depression [23, 25, 26], pain [27], balance [23, 26], and QOL [23], but methodological limitations such as small sample size [26], failure to randomise [23, 27], failure to control for researcher bias [23], and selective outcome reporting [26] limit their relevance. Furthermore, modifications to their intervention approaches, such as substituting Tai Chi in place of Hatha Yoga [23, 26, 27], or not taking place in a group format [26] raise questions regarding the relevance of their findings to the current study. Nevertheless, taking the findings from the current study into account, there is now a growing body of evidence to suggest likely effectiveness of MBIs for treating anxiety in MS. The interim benefits reported on depression following MBSR in this study and one other high quality RCT [24] are also encouraging, but the decline in effect seen at study endpoints suggest that there may be scope for judicious tailoring of MBSR to render beneficial treatment effects more stable. One such measure that has worked in MBCT for depression is the provision of post-completion 'drop-in' sessions, where beneficial effects have persisted for up to 2 years [38].

We also measured mindfulness and self-compassion, thought key components in how MBIs work [15, 16, 22]. No previous studies in people with MS have assessed the impact of MBI training on levels of mindfulness. Meta-analysis suggests that improvements in mindfulness may mediate improved mental health in non-MS populations [39]. Cross-sectional analyses [40–42] (n = 69–119) support that increased mindfulness is associated with greater positive affect, improved relationship satisfaction, less anxiety, less stress, improved wellbeing and QOL, and enhanced coping in people with MS. Having more self-compassion is associated with a greater resilience to anxiety, depression and stress in other LTCs [43], and may also make a small contribution to better mental health in people with MS [22].

Strengths and limitations
We followed the MRC guidelines for developing and evaluating complex interventions [13]. The small size of the study is a limitation, but is acceptable in feasibility work. The high proportion of female patients in this study (92%) is notable when compared with previous research in this area (range 69–100% [23–27]). This could reflect the higher incidence of stress-related mental health comorbidities in women with MS in Scotland [44], a greater stigma among men towards reporting mental health concerns [45], or that men may be less willing to participate in research studies [46].

We adjusted for common confounding variables in this study, along with those found to differ significantly at baseline. As this study was not powered to detect significant baseline differences, the findings from our analyses must thus be treated with caution (for example other variables such as baseline between group differences in diagnoses of anxiety and depression, antidepressant usage, disease activity and/or disease modifying drug (DMD) therapy could conceivably also impact on stress levels and effectiveness and should thus be considered in a future definitive study, powered to detect significant differences on these variables).

Evidence of effectiveness cannot be reliably determined in a small, unpowered sample. In this scenario, significance levels are unreliable, and observed beneficial treatment effects on stress, mood, and cognition can, at best, only be seen as an indication of likely effectiveness in a future phase three trial. Further, the novel findings of subjective improvements in cognitive function could be better contextualised if combined with a more objective neuropsychological assessment. Criticisms of commonly used objective measures of cognitive function are that they are either too short, too long, too generic, fail to detect deficits, or require to be administered by an expert [47]. The Brief International Cognitive Assessment for Multiple Sclerosis (BICAMS) is an internationally validated, standardised assessment tool with good reliability and validity, with the added advantage over other neuropsychological tests that it can be administered by a non-expert and could thus be used in a definitive phase three study [48].

The follow-up period post MBSR was relatively short in this study i.e. 3 months, and a future phase three trial could assess whether MBIs might have more lasting effects. Further optimisation work will help with the creation of a bespoke MBI for people with MS, which may improve recruitment and render beneficial treatment effects more stable.

Conclusion
Delivering MBSR to people with MS in a NHS setting is feasible. We achieved our recruitment target of 50 people within the specified time limits. Levels of retention i.e. completion rates for outcome measures were good post-intervention, and at follow-up. Encouraging improvements were noted on various outcome measures, in particular anxiety, with most measures having acceptable levels of missing values. However, initial beneficial effects on stress and depression were greatly diminished at study endpoint and only 60% of participants completed MBSR, suggesting that further optimisation is required before proceeding to a phase-3 definitive trial.

Additional files

Additional file 1: – MBSR; a week-by-week class overview. **Table S1.** describes the week-by-week session content for the MBSR classes in this study.

Additional file 2: – Outcome measures tested for feasibility. **Table S2.** provides a list of the outcome measures used in the study, the justification for their use, and basic psychometric properties.

Additional file 3: – Baseline characteristics: completers versus non-completers. **Table S3** provides an overview of participant demographics comparing MBSR course completers with non-completers.

Additional file 4: – True rates for missing values for participant questionnaires. **Table S4:** provides an overview of missing data for each of the participant report outcome measures.

Additional file 5: – Unadjusted RCT patient report outcome models. **Tables S5.1–S5.5.** provide detailed statistical data for unadjusted analyses. **Figure S5.1** provides a forest plot for unadjusted treatment effects immediately post-MBSR, whilst **Figure S5.2.** provides a forest plot of unadjusted treatment effects three months post-MBSR.

Additional file 6: - Adjusted RCT patient report outcome models. **Tables S6.1–S6.9.** provide detailed statistical data for adjusted analyses (age, sex, SES, previous meditation/yoga experience).

Acknowledgements
Thank you to all those people with MS who took part in this study. Further thanks to those involved in recruitment, and in particular to those facilitating the MBSR intervention.

Funding
This project was funded by the Scottish Homeopathic Research and Educational Trust (SC006557). The funder had no role in the design of the study, collection, analysis, and interpretation of data, or in writing of the manuscript.

Authors' contributions
SM, FM, and RS conceived this study. RS carried out the literature search, data collection, and analysis, with input from all authors. RS wrote the first draft of the paper, but all authors contributed to the final version. All authors read and approved the final manuscript.

Competing interests
The authors declare that they have no competing interests.

References
1. Dennison L, Moss-Morris R, Chalder T. A review of psychological correlates of adjustment in patients with multiple sclerosis. Clin Psychol Rev. 2009; 29(2):141–53.
2. Marrie RA, et al. The incidence and prevalence of psychiatric disorders in multiple sclerosis: a systematic review. Mult Scler J. 2015;21(3):305–17.
3. Finkelsztejn A. Multiple Sclerosis: Overview of Disease-Modifying Agents. Perspectives in medicinal chemistry. 2014;6:65.
4. Mohr DC, et al. Association between stressful life events and exacerbation in multiple sclerosis: a meta-analysis. BMJ. 2004;328(7442):731.
5. Artemiadis AK, Anagnostouli MC, Alexopoulos EC. Stress as a risk factor for multiple sclerosis onset or relapse: a systematic review. Neuroepidemiology. 2011;36(2):109–20.
6. McEwen BS, Getz L. Lifetime experiences, the brain and personalized medicine: An integrative perspective. Metabolism. 2013;62:S20–6.
7. McEwen BS. Central effects of stress hormones in health and disease: Understanding the protective and damaging effects of stress and stress mediators. Eur J Pharmacol. 2008;583(2):174–85.
8. Salehpoor G, Rezaei S, Hosseininezhad M. Quality of life in multiple sclerosis (MS) and role of fatigue, depression, anxiety, and stress: A bicenter study

from north of Iran. Iranian journal of nursing and midwifery research. 2014; 19(6):593.
9. Koch MW, et al. Pharmacologic treatment of depression in multiple sclerosis. The Cochrane Library. 20112011 Feb 16;(2):CD007295. doi:10.1002/ 14651858.CD007295.pub210.1002/14651858.CD007295.pub2
10. Fiest K, et al. Systematic review and meta-analysis of interventions for depression and anxiety in persons with multiple sclerosis. Multiple Sclerosis and Related Disorders. 2016;5:12–26.
11. Reynard AK, Sullivan AB, Rae-Grant A. A Systematic Review of Stress-Management Interventions for Multiple Sclerosis Patients. International journal of MS care. 2014;16(3):140–4.
12. Goyal M, et al. Meditation programs for psychological stress and well-being: a systematic review and meta-analysis. JAMA Intern Med. 2014; 174(3):357–68.
13. MRC U. Developing and evaluating complex interventions: new guidance. London: Medical Research Council; 2008.
14. Kabat-Zinn J. Wherever you go, there you are: Mindfulness meditation in everyday life. Hyperion. 1994;4.
15. Tang Y-Y, Hölzel BK, Posner MI. The neuroscience of mindfulness meditation. Nat Rev Neurosci. 2015;16(4):213–25.
16. Hölzel BK, et al. How does mindfulness meditation work? Proposing mechanisms of action from a conceptual and neural perspective. Perspect Psychol Sci. 2011;6(6):537–59.
17. Kabat-Zinn J. An outpatient program in behavioral medicine for chronic pain patients based on the practice of mindfulness meditation: Theoretical considerations and preliminary results. Gen Hosp Psychiatry. 1982;4(1):33–47.
18. Fjorback L, et al. Mindfulness-Based Stress Reduction and Mindfulness-Based Cognitive Therapy–a systematic review of randomized controlled trials. Acta Psychiatr Scand. 2011;124(2):102–19.
19. Lakhan SE, Schofield KL. Mindfulness-based therapies in the treatment of somatization disorders: a systematic review and meta-analysis. PLoS One. 2013;8(8):e71834.
20. Simpson R, et al. Mindfulness based interventions in multiple sclerosis-a systematic review. BMC Neurol. 2014;14(1):15.
21. Bogosian A, et al. Distress improves after mindfulness training for progressive MS: A pilot randomised trial. Mult Scler J. 2015;21(9):1184–94.
22. Bogosian A, et al. Potential treatment mechanisms in a mindfulness based intervention for people with progressive multiple sclerosis. Br J Health Psychol. 2016;21(4):859–80.
23. Burschka JM, et al. Mindfulness-based interventions in multiple sclerosis: beneficial effects of Tai Chi on balance, coordination, fatigue and depression. BMC Neurol. 2014;14(1):165.
24. Grossman P, et al. MS quality of life, depression, and fatigue improve after mindfulness training A randomized trial. Neurology. 2010;75(13):1141–9.
25. Kolahkaj B, Zargar F. Effect of Mindfulness-Based Stress Reduction on Anxiety, Depression and Stress in Women With Multiple Sclerosis. Nursing and Midwifery Studies. 2015;4(4).
26. Mills N, Allen J. Mindfulness of movement as a coping strategy in multiple sclerosis: a pilot study. Gen Hosp Psychiatry. 2000;22(6):425–31.
27. Tavee J, et al. Effects of meditation on pain and quality of life in multiple sclerosis and peripheral neuropathy: A pilot study. International journal of MS care. 2011;13(4):163–8.
28. Carmody J, Baer RA. How long does a mindfulness-based stress reduction program need to be? A review of class contact hours and effect sizes for psychological distress. J Clin Psychol. 2009;65(6):627–38.
29. Bellg AJ, et al. Enhancing treatment fidelity in health behavior change studies: best practices and recommendations from the NIH Behavior Change Consortium. Health Psychol. 2004;23(5):443.
30. Cohen S, Kamarck T, Mermelstein R. A global measure of perceived stress. J Health Soc Behav. 1983:385–96.
31. Janssen M, et al. Measurement properties of the EQ-5D-5L compared to the EQ-5D-3L across eight patient groups: a multi-country study. Qual Life Res. 2013;22(7):1717–27.
32. Ritvo P, et al. MSQLI—Multiple Sclerosis Quality of Life Inventory, A user's manual. New York: National MS Society; 1997.
33. Brown KW, Ryan RM. The benefits of being present: mindfulness and its role in psychological well-being. J Pers Soc Psychol. 2003;84(4):822.
34. Raes F, et al. Construction and factorial validation of a short form of the self-compassion scale. Clinical psychology & psychotherapy. 2011;18(3):250–5.
35. Newsom-Davis I, et al. The emotional lability questionnaire: a new measure of emotional lability in amyotrophic lateral sclerosis. J Neurol Sci. 1999;169(1):22–5.

36. Carstairs V, Morris R. Deprivation and health in Scotland. Health Bull. 1990; 48(4):162–75.

37. Browne RH. On the use of a pilot sample for sample size determination. Stat Med. 1995;14(17):1933–40.

38. Mathew KL, et al. The long-term effects of mindfulness-based cognitive therapy as a relapse prevention treatment for major depressive disorder. Behav Cogn Psychother. 2010;38(5):561–76.

39. Gu J, et al. How do mindfulness-based cognitive therapy and mindfulness-based stress reduction improve mental health and wellbeing? A systematic review and meta-analysis of mediation studies. Clin Psychol Rev. 2015;37:1–12.

40. Schirda, B., J.A. Nicholas, and R.S. Prakash, Examining Trait Mindfulness, Emotion Dysregulation, and Quality of Life in Multiple Sclerosis. 2015.

41. Senders A, et al. Perceived Stress in Multiple Sclerosis The Potential Role of Mindfulness in Health and Well-Being. Journal of evidence-based complementary & alternative medicine. 2014;19(2):104–11.

42. Pakenham KI, Samios C. Couples coping with multiple sclerosis: A dyadic perspective on the roles of mindfulness and acceptance. J Behav Med. 2013;36(4):389–400.

43. Sirois FM, Molnar DS, Hirsch JK. Self-Compassion, Stress, and Coping in the Context of Chronic Illness. Self Identity. 2015;14(3):334–47.

44. Simpson RJ, et al. Physical and mental health comorbidity is common in people with multiple sclerosis: nationally representative cross-sectional population database analysis. BMC Neurol. 2014;14(1):128.

45. Mackenzie C, Gekoski W, Knox V. Age, gender, and the underutilization of mental health services: the influence of help-seeking attitudes. Aging and Mental Health. 2006;10(6):574–82.

46. Markanday S, et al. Sex-differences in reasons for non-participation at recruitment: Geelong Osteoporosis Study. BMC research notes. 2013;6(1):104.

47. Chiaravalloti ND, DeLuca J. Cognitive impairment in multiple sclerosis. The Lancet Neurology. 2008;7(12):1139–51.

48. Benedict RH, et al. Brief International Cognitive Assessment for MS (BICAMS): international standards for validation. BMC Neurol. 2012;12(1):55.

49. Kurtzke, J.F., Rating neurologic impairment in multiple sclerosis an expanded disability status scale (EDSS). Neurology, 1983. 33(11): p. 1444–4.

14

Caught in a no-win situation: discussions about CCSVI between persons with multiple sclerosis and their neurologists

S. Michelle Driedger[1*], Ryan Maier[1], Ruth Ann Marrie[2] and Melissa Brouwers[3]

Abstract

Background: In recent years, shared decision making (SDM) has been promoted as a model to guide interactions between persons with MS and their neurologists to reach mutually satisfying decisions about disease management – generally about deciding treatment courses of prevailing disease modifying therapies. In 2009, Dr. Paolo Zamboni introduced the world to his hypothesis of Chronic Cerebrospinal Venous Insufficiency (CCSVI) as a cause of MS and proposed venous angioplasty ('liberation therapy') as a potential therapy. This study explores the discussions that took place between persons with MS (PwMS) and their neurologists about CCSVI against the backdrop of the recent calls for the use of SDM to guide clinical conversations.

Methods: In 2012, study researchers conducted focus groups with PwMS ($n = 69$) in Winnipeg, Canada. Interviews with key informants were also carried out with 15 participants across Canada who were stakeholders in the MS community: advocacy organizations, MS clinicians (i.e. neurologists, nurses), clinical researchers, and government health policy makers.

Results: PwMS reported a variety of experiences when attempting to discuss CCSVI with their neurologist. Some found that there was little effort to engage in desired discussions or were dissatisfied with critical or cautious stances of their neurologist. This led to communication breakdowns, broken relationships, and decisions to autonomously access alternative opinions or liberation therapy. Other participants were appreciative when clinicians engaged them in discussions and were more receptive to more critical appraisals of the evidence. Key informants reported that they too had heard of neurologists who refused to discuss CCSVI with patients and that neurology as a whole had been particularly vilified for their response to the hypothesis. Clinicians indicated that they had shared information as best they could but recommended against seeking liberation therapy. They noted that being respectful of patient emotions, values, and hope were also key to maintaining good relationships.

Conclusions: While CCSVI proved a challenging context to carry out patient-physician discussions and brought numerous tensions to the surface, following the approach of SDM can minimize the potential for unfortunate outcomes as much as possible because it is based on principles of respect and more two-way communication.

Keywords: Chronic disease, Communication, Chronic Cerebrospinal Venous Insufficiency, Liberation therapy, Canada, Clinical interactions, Venous angioplasty

* Correspondence: michelle.driedger@umanitoba.ca
[1]Department of Community Health Sciences, Max Rady College of Medicine, Rady Faculty of Health Sciences, University of Manitoba, Winnipeg, MB, Canada
Full list of author information is available at the end of the article

Background

The nature of multiple sclerosis

Canada has among the highest prevalence of multiple sclerosis (MS) in the world, with an estimated prevalence of over 250 per 100,000 of the population [1]. This translates into approximately 100,000 Canadians living with the disease [2]. MS is an incurable chronic immune-mediated disease which affects the brain, optic nerves, and spinal cord [3]. Symptoms vary from person to person [4], and while the clinical course can be broadly classified into several groups [5], the progression of MS is unique for each individual, and typically worsens over time. In terms of disease management, there is an increasing array of disease modifying therapies (DMTs) that partially reduce the risk of relapses and slow disease progression, but they have varying benefit-risk profiles [6, 7]. The inherent uncertainty of MS outcomes and its treatments, plus its chronic and degenerative nature, make living with MS an emotional experience for persons with MS (PwMS) and their families [8].

MS care in Canada

Canada has a universal, publicly funded health system which provides access to medically necessary hospital and physician services [9]. Health services delivery is the responsibility of Canada's provinces and territories. Specialized MS Clinics exist across the country. These clinics offer expertise in the diagnosis and treatment of MS. Care is delivered by teams involving neurologists, nurses, and allied health professionals such as occupational therapists and physical therapists; the specific resources available and roles of specific professionals may differ somewhat from one clinic to another. In Manitoba, the Winnipeg MS Clinic is the sole clinic providing specialized MS care, and provides access to neurologists, nurses, a physiotherapist, occupational therapist, social worker and dietitian. In most provinces, prescription of disease-modifying therapies is limited to neurologists with specific expertise in MS. Provincial programs provide coverage for these disease-modifying therapies; however, criteria for accessing these therapies and residual out of pocket costs vary from one province to another [10].

Recommendations for shared decision making (SDM) in the MS context

The relationship that PwMS have with their MS specialist, typically their neurologist, is a core foundation for MS disease management. Indeed, many PwMS have reported having good confidence in their neurologist's care and that their concerns are being heard and addressed [11]. However, these often long-term relationships have also been shown to be sources of considerable conflict and dissatisfaction for many other PwMS, where sub-optimal perceptions of communication and information exchange have been most commonly identified problem areas [12–14]. PwMS have expressed their desire for more active or autonomous roles in making decisions about disease management and therapies arising from perceptions that some clinicians had often taken a paternalistic approach and gave limited or selective information while still expecting PwMS to adhere to physician recommendations [14–18]. Furthermore, some MS doctors overlook the emotional cues (e.g. worry, anxiety) of their MS patients [8].

In 2007, Heesen et al. [19] declared that MS was a "prototypic condition" (and later, a "paradigmatic disease" [20]) for using a shared decision making (SDM) process between PwMS and their neurologists to reach mutually satisfying decisions about disease management – generally about deciding on which DMTs to use. To address the sources of conflict noted above, SDM promotes a more egalitarian relationship, an openness of dialogue, and a dedication to fulsome information exchange. Both parties bring to the discussion their own set of required competencies. Clinicians are to present a set of options for DMTs, detailing their respective profiles of benefits and risks that have been established through randomized control trials (RCTs). PwMS are to share their values and risk sensibilities [19]. Both then discuss these factors while weighing the options to assist PwMS in deciding ultimately what is best for them at the time. By fostering this dialogical approach, a key aspect of SDM is that it intends to create the space for greater patient input and autonomy in decision making [21], while also impressing on doctors the need to be more empathetic to the values and personal inclinations of their patient [8]. SDM may also help to foster trust between a patient and their doctor [22–24], the loss of which could lead to a troubling breakdown of communication. The consequences of a communication breakdown could be especially problematic if PwMS then feel compelled to make decisions about disease management without consulting their neurologist, such as stopping or altering their treatment courses of DMTs or accessing alternative therapies. Altogether, the ideal outcomes of SDM are not dependent on the specific option chosen, but that decisions satisfy all parties and build trust and mutual understanding.

Chronic Cerebrospinal Venous Insufficiency (CCSVI) and venous angioplasty

In 2009, Dr. Paolo Zamboni introduced the world to his hypothesis of CCSVI as a cause of MS and proposed venous angioplasty as a potential therapy [25, 26]. Although Zamboni's research was based on a non-randomized small sample of PwMS, and subsequent evidence was purely anecdotal at the time, the possibility that a cause and even a cure had been found for MS gave considerable hope to many PwMS and their families. The surprising news attracted the immediate attention of Canadian media, who played a key role in raising the profile of Zamboni's hypothesis and in highlighting the anecdotal success stories – often at the expense of more critical or scientifically rigorous perspectives (and is the subject of forthcoming papers related to this study) [27–29].

The earliest news media dubbed MS-related venous angioplasty the "liberation treatment" or "liberation therapy" [29]. While the term "liberation" can refer in a technical sense to the medical procedure of venous angioplasty proposed to restore blood flow through stenosed jugular veins, it may also (intentionally or not) bring with it emotionally charged, hope-driven desires for freedom – in this case, for a person to be "liberated" from their MS to some degree. Thereafter, in traditional media, but also especially in new forms of social media (blogs, networking sites), issues often became framed in normative terms of rights (for PwMS who were being 'denied' a breakthrough therapy) and in journalistic narrative tropes as 'good guys' and 'underdogs' (PwMS and advocates for CCSVI and liberation therapy) versus the 'bad guys' and 'villains' (scientists and MS clinicians who were cautious about the hypothesis) [27, 30–34]. Moreover, the quality and reliability of evidence for CCSVI and liberation therapy found on the internet and social media is not always self-apparent or easy to contextualize, which often helped to blur the lines between anecdotal and scientifically validated kinds of evidence [33].

PwMS have been recognized as highly interested, sophisticated, and resourceful information seekers and informal researchers about their disease as they follow the latest research to assess what might be useful for their disease management [35–39]. Although Zamboni's treatment still required extensive clinical trials to investigate its efficacy and safety (and a link between CCSVI and MS and in the efficacy of venous angioplasty still remains to be proven even after a number of follow-up studies [40–42]), many Canadian PwMS became immediately interested in the potential breakthrough and began demanding domestic access to this as a publicly funded treatment or at least access to diagnostic testing for 'collapsed veins.' However, without the necessary evidence base to demonstrate substantial positive benefit, the publically funded Canadian health system could not justify supporting a hypothetical treatment as an insured service [27]. Facing a seemingly recalcitrant or indifferent health system, and despite a lack of evidence, many PwMS felt compelled by their hope to travel abroad to have their veins tested and receive venous angioplasty, often paying large sums of money as 'medical tourists' [43].

This paper explores the discussions that took place between PwMS and their neurologists following the release of news of Zamboni's hypothesis. We investigate these conversations about CCSVI against the backdrop of the recent calls for SDM to improve communicating and decision making about therapeutic options. However, it is crucial to recognize that the contexts of CCSVI and Canada's healthcare system represent potential confounders for considering this a 'prototypical' or 'paradigmatic' situation for following a SDM approach in the MS clinical setting. Notably, SDM was proposed for scenarios of DMTs that had much more clearly defined risk-benefit profiles and evidence bases derived from prevailing scientific standards of RCTs. Furthermore, testing and treatment for CCSVI was not available to PwMS in Canada, and therefore it was not even a potential domestic option for clinical recommendations. Nevertheless, it is precisely with these confounders in mind that we will examine the appropriateness, applicability, and suitability of following the general principles of SDM in this context – because regardless of the state of the evidence or the unavailability of the treatment in Canada – PwMS still went to their neurologists to discuss CCSVI and many still wanted access to its testing and treatment. We are interested in the consequences for patient-physician dynamics, relationships, and outcomes, if neurologists reported they attempted to apply principles of SDM during this controversial time – and, conversely, the repercussions if they did not. Investigating a scenario where the issue in question and the SDM approach do not fit together cleanly (or as ideally intended) is important and still timely, because a debate over a potentially 'breakthrough' therapy, procedure, drug, etc. – whether for MS or some other disease – is certainly a situation likely to happen again in the future. Under such circumstances, clinicians and patients (and other stakeholders) will have to grapple with how to make decisions when the evidence is lacking, uncertain, or contested, and yet people may still demand access (at the most) or more information (at the least) from their health care provider and the health system. This study thus holds some potential to provide some insights into how to better navigate such scenarios.

While there have been some explorations into the broader public discourse among the MS community and other media stakeholders when news of CCSVI went public, there has yet to be a critical examination of conversations between PwMS and their physicians that the controversial treatment engendered. This study seeks to fill this gap by investigating the perspectives a variety of MS stakeholders, including PwMS, MS clinicians, advocacy organizations, researchers, and government health policy makers. While this study is focused largely on the interactions between PwMS and their neurologist, relevant non-neurologist key informant perspectives are also included as they were also part of, or privy to, the broader clinical and popular discourses within which these relationships were embedded.

Methods

For this study, in 2012 researchers conducted seven focus groups with 69 PwMS in Winnipeg, Manitoba, who were recruited from the local MS clinic. Focus groups were made up of people with different types of MS (relapsing-remitting, and primary or secondary progressive) who had lived with their diagnoses for different lengths of time ranging from less than 5 years, 10 to 19 years, to over 20 years (due to scheduling and availability, sometimes a participant had to join a focus group that was outside of their own disease duration range). Focus groups lasted approximately 2 h. The interview guide was pilot tested with the first focus group (with participants of varying disease type and duration). As no changes were required, findings from the pilot test were included in the analysis. Some participants were accompanied by their spouse who also contributed to the discussions to aid with communication as well as to reflect on the impact of MS for the entire family. All participants gave informed consent and PwMS were given an honorarium of $60 for participating in the research project. Discussions were semi-structured and participants were asked to give their thoughts on a variety of MS-related issues, including their information-seeking behaviors and information sources consulted, the CCSVI hypothesis and venous angioplasty, and their communication interactions with their doctors about MS.

Between 2012 and 2014, researchers also conducted key informant interviews with 15 participants who were stakeholders in the MS community when the CCSVI theory emerged. Seven neurologists were interviewed and the rest were members of advocacy organizations, other types of clinicians who worked primarily in the MS field (i.e. nurse clinicians, physiatrists, psychiatrists), clinical researchers, and government health policy makers. Interviews lasted one to two hours and were semi-structured. Participants were asked about their views on CCSVI and venous angioplasty, and clinicians were asked about the discussions they had with their patients about CCSVI. Non-clinicians were also asked about their second-hand impressions of doctor-patient interactions of that time. In neither the focus group interviews nor the key informant interviews were participants asked explicitly about shared decision making. Rather, participants self-reported on the nature of the discussions they had with health care providers and/or PwMS regarding MS care and the issue of CCSVI.

Following data collection, recorded interviews were transcribed, audio-verified and imported into NVivo10, a qualitative data analysis software. Coding schemes were developed by SMD and three research assistants by using an iterative process of reviewing transcripts and identifying key themes (e.g. doctor-patient communication) in the data using constant comparative and concept-development approaches [44]. Data were coded and a sample inter-coder reliability test achieved 86% Kappa scores, well above recommended levels [45]. In the results that follow, key issues around doctor-patient communication in the context of CCSVI and venous angioplasty will be presented and representative quotes will be used to illustrate common themes that were raised during the conversations. To protect anonymity, PwMS (and their spouses) are given a pseudonym and key informants are referred to only by their status as a neurologist or a non-neurologist MS clinician, or by their associated organization.

An additional file provides a more detailed methods description, with a particular emphasis on the analysis process (see Additional file 1) as well as copies of the focus group (see Additional file 2) and key informant (see Additional file 3) interview guides. Also included with this article is a checklist of consolidated criteria for reporting qualitative research (COREQ). This checklist is used when reporting qualitative research to ensure greater transparency around data collection, analysis, and reporting processes (see Additional file 4).

Results

PwMS: Description of focus group participants

Twelve participants had elected to travel out of Canada and already received the liberation therapy at the time the focus groups were conducted (June 2012). All but one who had sought out the treatment had lived with the disease for more than 10 years, and 8 had the most debilitating form of MS: primary or secondary progressive. There existed a spectrum among all participants in their opinions about CCSVI and liberation therapy. Some were very skeptical about it, some wanted to wait to see what research would show, and others were much more supportive of it – including those who had gotten the treatment. Despite some skepticism that existed among participants in all focus groups, there tended to be a common motivation to positively view the potential of the CCSVI hypothesis – at the time it gave many PwMS and their families a source of much needed hope for a better future. This positive perception of CCSVI was more general to PwMS who had MS for a long period of time and who had more debilitating progressive forms of the disease – although some still expressed skepticism or even pessimism towards it. On the other hand, while patients with a recent diagnosis and with little progression of their MS were more likely to view the new hypothesis cautiously, there were also some who were more enthusiastic about the treatment's potential.

Most of the participants had done at least some of their own independent research into CCSVI and venous angioplasty. Some participants reported that they sought out information from traditional mainstream media sources (television, newspaper), and others went to greater lengths to find information, whether doing Google searches, or looking to websites of MS stakeholders (eg. MS Society, Dr. Paolo Zamboni's website, advocate or community-driven websites or blogs, social media sites like Facebook, etc.), or consulting academic journals. Nevertheless, with as much information they could locate from their own research, many participants went to their MS clinician and asked them about the hypothesis and the treatment.

Focus group participants' perspectives of their discussions with their doctors about CCSVI and venous angioplasty – communication breakdowns

In all focus groups, many PwMS recalled their experiences with their neurologists with a tone of discouragement when they had attempted to discuss CCSVI and venous angioplasty. While we found that some participants shared positive remarks about their conversations with neurologists (see below), those voices were often overwhelmed by other negative comments. Some PwMS indicated that their neurologist was not even willing to indulge in a conversation about CCSVI and venous angioplasty. For other participants, they felt that the information that they got from their neurologist about liberation therapy was decidedly negative. They felt that their desire to discuss CCSVI was met with immediate skepticism, derision of the hypothesis, or prompt recommendations against seeking venous angioplasty without any further discussion. For many of these participants, such responses from their MS clinician all fed into a generalized view that neurologists seemed disinterested in, totally opposed to, or implicitly biased against a new therapy that already looked like it was producing positive results. The field of neurology as a whole was similarly characterized in negative tones.

But [my neurologist] doesn't even want to talk about it [CCSVI]. It's just like it's taboo. [Barbara, 20+ years]

They [healthcare providers] are all comfortable [talking about CCSVI and venous angioplasty] except the neurologists. [Leo, husband of Elaine, 20+ years]

They [the neurologists] were the naysayers [about Zamboni's hypothesis]. [Gord, husband of Lisa, 20+ years]

All [neurologists were] negative. [Clint, husband of Martha, 10-19 years]

Refused a discussion of the new hypothesis, PwMS became frustrated because they desperately wanted any or as much information they could get. This frustration often became directed at their neurologists, who were seen as gatekeepers to more information about CCSVI as well as to potential access to testing and treatment. Many simply wanted some support or respectful dialogue in whether they should be making a decision about whether to travel to get venous angioplasty.

CCSVI as a source of hope for PwMS

At times, PwMS linked their dissatisfaction about their discussions with their neurologists about CCSVI with broader concerns they had about communication with, and the care by, their neurologists.

My neurologist told me they didn't agree with the CCSVI treatment. But then in the next breath told me that I'd be blind in a wheelchair. And I think, I personally feel a lot—I'm not saying all—a lot of neurologists are very negative when they speak to MS patients and they give you no hope, no hope. I've seen three neurologists since 19 and a half years ago and the first one told me the same thing that I'd be blind in a wheelchair. And I never went back to them. I find a lot of neurologists aren't supportive. [Pat, 10-19 years]

The sense of hope that the prospective hypothesis offered was often more pronounced for those PwMS who had lived with MS for many years or who saw themselves as further along on an irreversible downward slope of MS progression. For them, venous angioplasty seemed to offer the last chance to potentially halt or reverse some of the symptoms of their disease and to reclaim lost or cherished abilities. Instead, they felt that not even the hope of a potential new understanding of their disease and its treatment was being afforded to them or even acknowledged by their care providers. For these participants, it did not bother them that there was some risk or possible lack of effectiveness to the unproven therapy. In fact, for some the uncertainty surrounding venous angioplasty was in the same vein as that which also characterizes the uncertain efficacy of approved and available DMTs.

I'm progressive and every year I'm going down that ramp. And pretty soon I'm not going to be able to do the things ... I can't get down on my hands and knees and play with my grandson. [Hank, 10-19 years]

I really want to have [venous angioplasty] done regardless of the outcome. I'll try anything to be able to walk. My big thing in life is to get into my son's house, get up the stairs, and see my grandchildren's bedrooms. I can't do any of that. That's my aim. So I definitely want to have [liberation therapy] done. [Wanda, 7 years]

I had one friend of mine that went and [venous angioplasty] did absolutely nothing. I had another friend and they're improving all the time. So it's one of those things you take. Betaseron doesn't help you or it does help. [Liberation therapy] might help you, it might not. The last time I saw my doctor I said my right hand is getting worse, now I don't have a lot of function left. And they said, 'Well, can't do nothing for you.' I said, 'do you want me to just sit here and watch it happen?' And they said, 'yeah, basically.' So I decided I'm going for liberation [therapy]. I wouldn't mind getting back a little balance and stability. I wouldn't mind anything because there's so many symptoms that I have that even if two out of 100 get better I'm willing to go. [Hannah, less than 5 years]

This sense of hope, and lack of results from existing therapies, led many participants to wish that their neurologist would be more open to discussing or exploring new or unorthodox hypotheses like CCSVI. Sometimes they referred to particular neurologists who they felt were more 'open-minded' or who seemed more empathetic to the plights of their patients. Many were also adamant that they did not see venous angioplasty as a cure for their disease, but as a promising means to achieve some relief or respite from at least some of their MS symptoms or progression. Many acknowledged that there was still much more to be learned about CCSVI and that there were risks, but the positive anecdotal reports of symptom relief – even if however temporary – should be enough to prove to neurologists and the scientific community that some kind of connection existed between CCSVI and MS symptoms and that this warranted a more open-minded approach.

Our best neurologist was [Dr. X]. [They] looked like they wanted to open the door to try something. [They] had compassion, and I've never met a better neurologist. All the other ones are so closed-minded. [Lynn, 10-19 years]

I think [CCSVI and venous angioplasty] is phenomenal, it is going in the right direction. No, it isn't the cure; there is still a lot of grey area. [Nina, 10-19 years]

While many participants felt that their hope was being unjustly disregarded, others who were actually comfortable with their neurologist's skepticism of the new hypothesis agreed that a core problem was that neurologists just generally lack a capacity for good communication and compassionate care. This is also illustrative of the complexity and dynamics inherent in these relationships that debates like CCSVI can bring to the fore. People may still (have to) trust their clinician, but an underlying issue is reaffirmed.

They [neurologists] are not "people" people. I mean my neurologist is an excellent [physician] and I wouldn't want anyone else handling my brain. [Their] bedside manner is – I mean this [referencing a soft drink can] has got a better bedside manner than my neurologist so someone has to do more. The skills they have are not [bedside manner]. [Perry, unknown years]

Fallout from communication breakdowns

Without their MS clinician's desired support in providing information (at the least) or endorsing the therapy (at the most), many PwMS saw these as ultimate signs that their MS clinician did not care about their concerns. Some participants simply began avoiding talking about the new research with their neurologist and sought information elsewhere. Other participants noted that they found a more receptive medical opinion when they talked to their general practitioner rather than a MS clinician. Some also wished that their own neurologists would share the same openness and willingness to talk about a new therapy that other doctors had – even other neurologists about which they heard – seemed to offer.

I've never talked to [the neurologist at the MS clinic] about it [CCSVI and venous angioplasty] because I already knew where [they] stood ... I had done my own research. [Marge, unknown years]

I know what you guys are saying about the neurologist. I took all the information that I had compiled through friends and family, that entire shoebox. And I took it in and tried to go through it with my neurologist at the MS clinic. And as soon as [they] saw what was contained in that shoebox [they] almost pushed it off the desk back into my lap. They said, "I don't want to deal with this." It upset me a lot. Whereas when I took it to my GP he went through it with me. [June, 20+ years]

My [general practitioner] said "you get the information and come to me and we'll go through it and I'll give you the medical perspective and then we can make the decision." And it's, that's the kind of doctor we need to have. I was very, very fortunate. [Sue, 20+ years]

Some PwMS then felt compelled to then take matters into their own hands and make decisions about their MS care completely on their own. Some of those who opted to seek venous angioplasty outside of Canada – as well as many of those considering it – indicated that they did not discuss any of their independent research about it or their related decisions with their MS clinician. In some cases, if PwMS disagreed with the stance that their neurologist had, those participants simply did not tell them about their decision to attempt a major act of autonomous disease management.

But we said to the neurologist that we were seeing at the time, "What would you do?" And [they] said "I'd wait" [to get venous angioplasty] and I said "We don't have five or seven years to wait anymore and if there is a very slim or slight [chance that it could help]." I never did tell them that we were already in the process of scheduling the trip. I just wanted their opinion what they thought about it. [Leo, husband of Elaine, 20+ years]

Some participants chose to keep their decisions to travel for venous angioplasty a secret lest it garner disapproval from their neurologist who had recommended against it. They worried that sharing their decision to get the treatment would negatively influence their relationships with their neurologist before and after they got back and that their doctors would make them feel guilty or treat them worse. Participants also expressed worry that their neurologist would no longer want to continue care for them upon their return.

In some cases, the perceived mismatch between the wishes of PwMS and the lack of desired engagement by MS clinicians led to other drastic actions with long term and significant implications. If PwMS no longer trusted their MS clinician to act in their best interest, it affected other (non-CCSVI) aspects of care, such as decisions to remain on current disease management strategies and medications. Or, going to greater lengths, some participants indicated that they may no longer want the care of a neurologist.

My doctor refused to do any testing on the veins for me and with the MS Clinic I've been on every kind of needle they've had. The pain got so severe I was on morphine. I was a drug addict for a couple of years and missed a couple of years of my life. And then when they refused to do testing on

my veins I just stopped everything, I stopped everything. I said no more needles for MS, no more morphine, no more anything. No more, I want to live my life. [Clair, 20+ years]

I don't know that I'm going to continue going to a neurologist. [Leigh, 20+ years]

Rationale for clinicians' opinions

Many participants shared reasons why they thought that their neurologists were dismissive of CCSVI and venous angioplasty or why they were so unwilling to discuss or endorse it. Some attributed it to pre-existing communication problems that they had with their doctors, to a lack of empathy, or to paternalistic or patronizing indifference. Many others felt that their neurologists were against any new kinds of treatment or were inappropriately dismissive of a potentially promising new way of viewing MS and its treatment. Some PwMS believed that certain younger neurologists seemed more receptive or open to discussing the hypothesis, while older ones who had practiced a long time had perhaps become too set in their ways and were not interested in anything that challenged the status quo. More commonly, some participants noted that because CCSVI is more within the realm of vascular science, neurologists would naturally dismiss or challenge the hypothesis because MS had been traditionally thought of as a purely neurological disease. This notion fed suspicions that the CCSVI debate exposed a kind of 'turf war' between specialists, with neurologists trying to shut down any potential opposition to their traditional professional primacy in MS care. Some PwMS also expressed worry that neurologists may have conflicts of interests in being too involved with, or receiving financial incentives from, the pharmaceutical companies that make DMTs.

I mean, how is a neurologist going to be involved with this, it's not their field. You need the cardiovascular surgeons and specialists involved with this because that's their field. [June, 20+ years]

But I read that Maclean's I think it's May or June 2010 where they really make a case that neurologists are in league with Big Pharma. [Heather, 10-19 years]]

And [my neurologist] was dead set against it [venous angioplasty]. So, like that said a lot of things like that [my neurologist] didn't want something that wasn't pharmaceutically financed. [Seth, 20+ years]

Positive impressions of their discussions with MS clinicians

Not all of the participants' neurologists were evasive about discussing the prospective treatment and not all

PwMS were displeased with a more skeptical view of CCSVI that their neurologists shared. On the contrary, some participants pointed out that while their neurologists did not endorse or recommend venous angioplasty, they provided a more balanced scientific perspective about the existing evidence, or had at least pointed to where one could find it, and had affirmed their patient's right to make their own decision. Many times such efforts to engage with PwMS' concerns were generally welcomed and well received. Further, while some participants agreed with their clinician to wait for further evidence, others who still wanted venous angioplasty appreciated that their doctors were understanding enough to provide information and support them in their decision no matter which way they chose. Some participants noted that their neurologists' skepticism was more indicative of due diligence in being cautious due to the lack of evidence – all that their doctors could really do was to recommend a 'wait and see' with respect to future research.

I asked my neurologist and was told it's my choice if I want to go with it. [My neurologist] said, "Information is out there. It's your decision. I'm not going to tell you which way to go." [Allen, less than 5 years]

[T]here was one other MS doctor I talked to who said 'we don't see it [the evidence] and we're not here to do any harm; we don't want to hurt anyone, we're not trying to stop people.' And I think this person's take on it made sense to me too because they care about the patients and I didn't think that they were saying they're opposed to it because they didn't want you to get better. I think they were cautious. But I think everybody had to look at it on their own and do their own research and go with what they felt. [Helene, 6 years]

I actually had to bring copies of all my paperwork from both neurologists when I went to Egypt and I read what was said. [My neurologist] said "she is informed of all the pros and cons and potential risks and, while I can't support her decision, I certainly acknowledge she has the right to make that decision and that she's informed and, you know, all the power to her, make your own decision." [Danielle, unknown years]

Another participant argued that neurologists were undeserving of scorn just for being skeptical about the new theory, because it should not discount the fact that they have been consistently working and researching towards finding better therapies for their patients for years.

Key informant interviews
All key informants, notably all neurologists and clinicians at MS clinics, reported that the year that followed the media releases about Dr. Zamboni's research was the one of the most difficult that they experienced in their professional lives in terms of doctor-patient interactions. They commonly noted that the first media releases framed the CCSVI hypothesis and venous angioplasty as a disease breakthrough that could signal the discovery of a cause and a cure for MS. They agreed that the stories contained limited evidence and lacked a more critical – and thus balanced – perspective. Due to limited evidence supporting CCSVI, neurologists said they were compelled to take a cautious and critical approach and preferred to 'wait and see' what future research would hold. Yet it was with these first news stories in mind (and ensuing social media advocacy) that PwMS came to their doctors desperate for information and possibly for help with accessing the new therapy. And so it fell to the PwMS' usual MS clinicians to attempt to answer those questions with the very little information that they had – since they were essentially hearing about new developments at the same time as the public – and try to provide the more balanced evaluation of the issues. Furthermore, they also had to then inform their patients that testing and treatment for CCSVI would not be available in Canada until there was clear evidence to validate the hypothesis – something that might take years to complete or might never even happen.

Hostility towards MS clinicians
As key informants noted, this more critical stance was not very well received by many PwMS and their families. They saw that while many PwMS accepted the more cautious approach recommended by their neurologists, others saw it as dismissiveness or inappropriate 'gatekeeping' of patients from a potentially revolutionary treatment. MS clinicians felt that they became the "demonized" specialty and many neurologists reported being on the receiving end of considerable hostility, and some even reported receiving death threats.

The media told them there was a treatment that would help them. But they couldn't have it. And it was primarily the people who cared for them that were creating the barrier for them to get this treatment. So during that time we were threatened. Hate mail was sent. Death threats were sent to physicians. [Non-neurologist MS clinician]

The MS public and the general public weren't ready for that critical appraisal of it. It was almost too much like cold-water-in-the-face, I suppose, to people. Initially, I had some very angry people who demanded the treatment and demanded that I make it happen. [Neurologist]

It was remarkable how many patients were very, very angry at neurology, yeah. [Non-neurologist MS clinician]

MS clinicians' perspectives of their discussions with PwMS about CCSVI and venous angioplasty

All of the MS clinicians interviewed for this study indicated that they had done their best to share what information they could about CCSVI or had directed patients to where they might be able to find reliable information. They all described how they had told PwMS that there was little evidence to support the hypothesis of a link between CCSVI and MS, and that the best course that they could recommend at the time was to wait and see what future research will show. As for venous angioplasty, they generally acknowledged to their patients that there seemed to be some anecdotal indications of some symptom relief, but there was no evidence yet in terms of the actual efficacy of therapy, of success rates (including long term versus short term), and of the safety of using angioplasty – a treatment developed for arteries – on jugular veins. In addressing PwMS' wishes to access therapy, clinicians often claimed that while they could not recommend or endorse venous angioplasty, they recognized the right of their patients to make their own decisions. Most said that they had indicated support for their patients' decision making by sharing the current state of benefits and risks and by continuing their care afterwards if they chose to seek treatment. As clinicians pointed out, some PwMS received the more critical appraisal of CCSVI positively, while others did not, and some PwMS said they were going to go for treatment anyway.

I would give them the information that I had [about CCSVI], which developed as research developed in the field. There are some people who will hear this information and say "oh my goodness, this is not for me, this is so experimental, I kinda want to see where this goes." But there are some people who say to me "you know what, I kinda want to try it anyways." I don't think that's wrong; you're just trying to do the best that you can for your disease and I think that if you hear this information and you still want to do it, well then you've educated yourself as much as you can about the situation, make sure you try and go to a place that has a good track record and things. So I found that most people, when I would say that to them beforehand, you know, we're going to discuss

CCSVI, you're going to hear some of my views, but ultimately it comes down to your decision, everybody responded to that in the end, almost universally. [Neurologist]

Some key informants concurred with what the focus group participants reported above that they too had heard that some neurologists were refusing to even discuss CCSVI-related issues at all. However, rather than attribute the lack of discussion to outright dismissal of patient concerns, one key informant noted that one possible reason for that was due to the practical rules and ethics that a neurologist may feel bound to, including time constraints but also the need to attend to the ongoing disease and symptom management that is necessary. CCSVI was an unproven theory and discussing it took time away from other pressing matters.

They have a very short period of time that they have to see patients. And often these patients would come and didn't want to talk about what was going on that needed attending, that the physician was worried about. They [patients] went straight into CCSVI. And in a 30-minute appointment [CCSVI took up all the time]. And then the patient left without addressing any of their concerns about frequent falls, about UTIs that could kill them if they developed urosepsis, aspiration issues. So the things that they were trained to assess for and treat the patient wouldn't address, and so they had to be very structured, the conversation, in a very organized manner. [Non-neurologist MS clinician]

Nevertheless, if a PwMS saw that their neurologist did not want to discuss CCSVI, most key informants conceded that patients could understandably interpret such treatment as a dismissal of their concerns – an egregious one if the PwMS sees the potential for a cure or more effective treatment at stake.

Communication breakdowns and other fallout

Whether by refusing to talk about CCSVI, informing about lack of evidence and uncertainties in risks and benefits as well as the lack of domestic access to venous angioplasty, or recommending against accessing venous angioplasty as a medical tourist, all key informants had reported that they too had experienced or heard about particular consequences when PwMS did not hear what they wanted to hear. Commonly, they noted that PwMS would often not tell their neurologist that they were going out of country to receive venous angioplasty, and their doctor would only find out after the fact, if they found out at all. They speculated that given the cautious and more critical stance neurologists had about CCSVI, PwMS did not want to be embarrassed in admitting that they went (especially if the therapy was unsuccessful, or less successful than anticipated), or did not want to risk the (perceived) anticipated ire of their clinician, who could potentially castigate them for their decisions (whether before or after they decided to access treatment). Other clinicians reported that they knew of or had patients who no longer went to their neurologist, or who switched to one that they perceived as more open-minded:

So no, they didn't advertise their intent before and I think in some ways they knew that the neurologist thought that this was a load of nonsense and so they didn't quite believe the neurologist so they thought they were going to do it anyway. And some of them, I almost had a sense that they slunk away to get it done, you know. [Non-neurologist MS clinician]

A lot of people, they really did sever their relationship with their neurologist. [Neurologist]

I know a lot of patients who went and had it done who claim they never told their neurologist. Because they *assumed* how their neurologist would act, right? Or react. Probably they wouldn't, but they kept hearing stories from other people that oh, my neurologist got mad at me. When we were given the opportunity, to try to show the pros and cons, I think partly what happened is that people who really wanted to have it done stopped talking to us. Because they didn't like our perspective that we needed to wait for the research, so they essentially stopped and started talking to people who were providing the other side of the story. [MS advocacy organization]

Many key informants lamented the breakdown of communication and relationships between PwMS and their clinicians, given the crucial role that the doctor-patient relationship plays in managing a chronic and progressively debilitating disease like MS. Even some seemingly ideal doctor-patient relationships did not withstand the wedge that the issue thrust between them.

Like I felt patients who had very strong, really positive trust and clinical relationships with their neurologist who didn't trust their neurologist anymore, because the neurologist was telling them "don't go for CCSVI, we don't have enough information." [Non-neurologist MS clinician]

However, following the early period of hype, media intensity, and controversy about CCSVI, clinicians noted that some of the interest and discussion of the therapy had gradually died down, along with some of the animosity towards neurology. Many PwMS had also since been returning to their usual routines of care. Nevertheless, that time was not without its consequences, both short and long-term. Some communication breakdowns may take time to repair, while some may never recover. Key informants noted that many MS clinicians and nurses had seriously contemplated leaving the field of MS care, due to the intense pressure and negativity that they had endured. Some neurologists also indicated that since the CCSVI debate cast such public ire on neurologists, few neurologists are now looking to specialize in MS.

And I was really quite shocked by the negativity toward neurologists, I have to say. And it has had a negative impact, because we have not had anybody new... none of our grads have gone into MS since. [Neurologist]

Bedside manners – empathy, respect, and hope

Inevitably, some PwMS would not agree with the more critical stance towards the CCSVI hypothesis. While all clinicians agreed that they had done their best with what little information they had in providing a more critical assessment of the unproven hypothesis, a subset of those interviewed indicated that the crucial aspect in getting this information across to PwMS was not solely *what* was being said, but also *how* one was saying it. Two key informants used the term of having good "bedside manners" to describe what others also recounted as empathy, respect, and a willingness to acknowledge the perspectives of PwMS. This, they maintained, was the best way to increase the odds that a breakdown of communication did not occur and that a positive relationship could be continued no matter what their patient decided to do. Many key informants indicated that they recognized that PwMS were a particularly vulnerable population, frustrated by the lack of knowledge over a cause or cure for their disease, and facing an uncertain yet progressive disease. Against this prognosis, PwMS are understandably desperate for, as one interviewee said, "a new ray of hope."

If people feel that you have already made up your mind and you're not as impartial as you think to the new notions, they will not like you. And especially when you just erase their hope, and you offer nothing else. Put yourself in the patient's shoes -you have an untreatable disease, and you're looking desperately for hope, and some new things emerge, a little bit of hope, very little, and the doctor says no, it doesn't work, it doesn't work. Okay, what do you have to offer instead? [Neurologist]

A clinician who has a rigid mind with the blinders on, no it doesn't work, no it doesn't-, okay it doesn't work, but say it differently so people can digest it and can realize that you're on their side, but you don't recommend it. [If] you have this oppositional strategy, in practice, that's the source of all the problems. [Neurologist]

Participants agreed that to be dismissive of PwMS' interests and perspectives towards CCSVI was to take away their hope and potentially signal an adversarial posture. Moreover, appreciating the sense of hope that the unproven and risky therapy offered was also a way to understand the high risk tolerance that PwMS exhibited when they opted for liberation therapy even though they had been apprised of its uncertain benefits and potential for risks.

Participants noted that many PwMS likely would not have switched or severed their relationship with their neurologist if they had been treated in a more empathetic fashion. Listening to their patients and being open and willing to engage with the concerns of PwMS were keys to maintaining a good relationship. Even if PwMS chose to go against their doctor's recommendation, they would feel that at least they had been heard, had their concerns validated, and know that they would still have the support of their healthcare provider if they chose to be a medical tourist. One doctor noted that approaching their patients in this way actually saved time during appointments, as it prevented more adversarial postures that could grind conversations to a halt or a stalemate, and it facilitated outcomes that were more agreeable to all if PwMS were set on seeking treatment.

So I think it has to do with listening. And being open. And sometimes if they want to take you in a particular direction, it might not take very long to talk about that direction, but to just have an openness of thought, that actually it saves time in the appointment overall....But it's so easy to do. [...] The trick is to not spend a lot of time with people but to make them think that they've spent a lot of time with you. I think that you can spend a very little amount of time with a person yet make it really count in some way or another, but it has to be real. It's about validating, it's about empathizing. And all it takes is a simple sentence of "yeah, I can see how you would see it that way" [Neurologist].

Several clinicians added that increased training should be given to MS physicians to help them to "put yourself in the patient's shoes" to more sensitively navigate difficult conversations they will inevitably have with their patients. On the other hand, some key informants also hoped that in situations such as the CCSVI debates, some PwMS and their advocates also needed to reciprocate those sentiments of empathy and openness in kind, and that the hostility that existed towards neurologists was not necessary or helpful – as understandable as it may have been.

Conspiracy theories and turf wars

Most key informants also mentioned that they had heard about particular conspiratorial theories that purportedly explained neurologists' skepticism or lack of endorsement of CCSVI. Echoing the focus group participants, the most common suspicion they heard concerned perceptions about neurologists' relationships with pharmaceutical companies and that there was too much money being made by "Big Pharma" from DMTs. They also heard related criticism that livelihoods would be lost if CCSVI was indeed a cure, and hence any perceived skepticism was actually viewed as professional self-preservation.

Like a conspiracy theory that, you know, the drug companies were fuelling this [skepticism of CCSVI] and all the disease modifying companies don't want people going through the surgery because it will take away the money from their drug. [Non-neurologist MS clinician]

[Many patients] regarded many of us as withholding a therapy that would make them better and therefore not need our services and so therefore we were sort of protecting our livelihoods and maybe we were being paid off by pharma and so that's why we weren't offering those therapies. [Neurologist]

One neurologist countered such claims by stating that MS-related work funds so little of their practice that it was impossible that pharmaceutical companies or any financial benefits were influencing their lack of immediate advocacy for CCSVI.

It was so ironic. They're saying well, MS neurologists are making too much money treating MS, and I thought, you know what, MS is my charity work; you know, I have another half of my practice – it funds my practice. MS does not pay, you know, you specialize in MS for different reasons....that kind of got lost. You're either for it or against it [CCSVI and liberation therapy], that if you weren't lobbying for immediate access, you were against it. [Neurologist]

Clinicians who were interviewed also flatly denied any suspicions that there was a kind of 'turf war' between neurologists and the specialties associated with CCSVI – radiologists and vascular surgeons. Key informants repeatedly claimed that MS care is multi-disciplinary and that neurology often collaborates with other specialties, and did so again when learning about CCSVI.

> I disagree with that 100 percent [that there was a turf war]. There was some mutual discussion within the vascular arena. There were physicians who we brought in to give us some help with this. There was a lot of collaborative work that went on during this crisis so that neurologists could help understand, the vascular people could help understand, that if they looked at techniques how would this work. They really worked collaboratively. They really did try and help each other out because both had pressure from different world views of medicine. [Non-neurologist MS clinician]

CCSVI-induced changes in MS advocacy and communication

Some key informants shared that they thought that amidst all the challenges that the CCSVI debates created between them and PwMS, the situation had also stimulated some necessary changes and realizations. They noted that PwMS and their advocates had found a new voice for themselves and that the relationship dynamics between PwMS and clinicians had likely been changed irrevocably – changes that may be difficult, but could also be for the greater good. Many clinicians agreed that, in the end, open and collaborative communication with PwMS needs to be improved.

> It galvanized a whole group of people to act out in a certain kind of way and advocate for their illness, which I think has been good in the end. And it's made neurologists approach their patients differently. I think that it should be a collaborative discussion; I think it should be a discussion over how much do you know about this, what don't you know about it. You know, bring stuff in from the internet and show it to me and if I don't know about it we'll look at it together on the internet and we'll try and figure it out together and I will just be honest with what I know and don't know. [Neurologist]

> And I hope that [what] comes out of this whole issue in Canada, is how should we – as the scientific, academic, clinical community – communicate better with patients. Because, you know, let's say... there's different scenarios that can come out of the CCSVI thing. Let's say the predicted scenario, is that it ends up just being noise. Just a fad. It was weak science

and it can't be reproduced. So let's say if that is the scenario, are people going to remember this five years from now? All the money that was spent, all the emotions that were hurt and bruised? Or is it just going to be forgotten and something else is going to go through the same process again? The other is I think it's created dialogue; dialogue that hasn't happened before. It's made people more aware of the power of the internet, the social community, how well aware MS patients are of the issues, how well educated they are. I think it's forcing us clinicians to be better communicators. We still... We gotta listen to our patients. It's tough sometimes, right? Like I don't want to spend my whole clinic talking about CCSVI. I'd rather talk about some other things. But it's forced dialogue. [Neurologist]

As described in the above comments, there are clearly lessons that stakeholders want to draw from this experience. The controversy and its consequences forced some key informants to reflect on their experiences and use them as a guide to improve doctor-patient communication.

Discussion

Could a clinical dynamic guided by principles of SDM still prove amenable to a highly controversial context like CCSVI? The spectrum of perspectives found in our results point to both the potential and limitations of SDM when faced with a controversial new hypothesis and a public debate being played out in real time. The neurologists we interviewed all described their CCSVI-related discussions with PwMS in ways that aligned closely with SDM – although only one key informant actually used that term to describe their approach and several others used the term "informed decision making" (and both have been used synonymously in the MS context [19]). They all self-reported that they had openly discussed the state of limited evidence about CCSVI and risks and benefits of venous angioplasty, encouraged patient inquiry, and with each of these factors in mind felt compelled to recommend against seeking treatment of this kind or waiting for more evidence. Further, they all noted that they left the ultimate decision to seek venous angioplasty to their patients and that they would continue to support them if they did so. Key informant clinicians indicated that this approach was crucial in maintaining their responsibilities to the evidence as well as to the good care of their patients. Of course, it may be possible that a clinician's self-assessment of their own actions may tend towards the positive, and these more benign perceptions should be contrasted with the widespread negative characterizations that PwMS participating in this study shared regarding their interactions with their own clinicians about CCSVI. Outside of the MS context, research has shown that despite doctors' claims to be adhering to SDM, surveys of patients have claimed otherwise [46]. After reviewing our results, it is not possible to make a judgment about whether the neurologists we interviewed simply over-represented those who exhibited good 'bedside manners' or were assessing their own practices in a more favorable light. Nevertheless, it should be taken as a positive sign that all MS clinicians we interviewed described their experiences in ways that modeled SDM principles and believed that it was due to this patient-centered approach that they had many positive or satisfactory responses from their patients, and minimized as best as possible the potential for a breakdown of trust and communication.

Some PwMS participating in this study also shared positive experiences they had with their doctors when they wanted to discuss CCSVI and venous angioplasty. They appreciated their neurologists' efforts to be open and hear their concerns, to provide them with what information that they could, and to support them even if they sought out liberation therapy. These perspectives lend further support to the value of the SDM approach when discussing even novel, uncertain, or controversial therapies. These participants were freely able to inquire about their concerns, feel reassured that their opinions and values were validated and respected, and could be certain that they could maintain the continuity of specialist care that is crucial to optimal MS disease management [47, 48]. These positive outcomes are valuable even in light of the fact that not all facets of SDM could be present in their ideal form (i.e. where there is a much stronger evidence base (at the time), the availability of patient decision-aids, etc). Even though the evidence base was lacking on which to make decisions about CCSVI and its testing and treatment were not accessible therapy options in Canada, the crucial point is that in many cases even when it is only possible to affirm the values of the patient, that alone may be all that is necessary for relationships to be maintained and prevent breakdowns of communication.

Although these positive results are encouraging, we also found many examples where the perceptions of PwMS of their clinical discussions of CCSVI were decidedly negative, and these too can be analyzed on the basis of the SDM model. Further, they illuminate the rationale behind some of the unfortunate consequences of those perceptions, whether being communication breakdowns, loss of trust (and having to rebuild it), severing of relationships, independently altering/ceasing existing treatment courses, or hiding decisions to seek venous angioplasty.

Some PwMS reported that their neurologist had refused to talk about CCSVI and saw this as a trend associated with all neurologists – or the field of neurology – more generally. This left focus group participants with many of their questions unanswered and the perception that their neurologist was preemptively dismissing their pressing concerns amidst a time of widespread public controversy and interest. While all neurologists in this study maintained that they had not done so, our key informants also corroborated that they too had heard of neurologists who had refused to discuss CCSVI with their patients. These reports stand in stark contrast to SDM's promotion of an open and two-way exchange between physicians and patients [19]. Of course, SDM is premised on the sufficient exchange of risk and benefit information about treatment options – which for CCSVI and liberation therapy was insufficient at the time. Nevertheless, simply avoiding the topic – however valid or practical the reasons on the part of the clinicians – was viewed by MS participants as a significant rebuff of their concerns and could feed and nurture existing adversarial narratives in the media or already existing discontent that PwMS had with their neurologist. Refusal to engage with their concerns were the key factors behind PwMS making drastic decisions to quit their neurologist or heed the advice of those more likely to listen to them or to be supportive of CCSVI. Thus, even if a therapeutic option does not fit the profile of an established DMT or deviates from matters of importance from a clinician's perspective, to prevent a breakdown of communication, care must be taken not to be insensitive or indifferent to discussing matters of importance from the perspectives of PwMS.

Not all neurologists were dismissive of CCSVI if PwMS wanted to discuss it. All of the key informant clinicians interviewed indicated that they engaged in related dialogues with their patients and shared information as they could. As noted above, many focus group participants responded positively to this more critical approach, but as was also found in our results, it was not what some wanted to hear and could also engender a breakdown in communication. As a result, some clinicians noted that they still had patients who sought venous angioplasty and who did not tell them about it. Some PwMS also shared that because once they knew (or perceived to know) where their neurologist stood on the issue, they saw no further point in belaboring it or in discussing their private decision to seek liberation therapy. While being open and collegial about patient concerns fulfills an aspect of SDM and can be sufficient for some PwMS in making a decision based on what is or is not known about a novel hypothesis, it may not satisfy others who approach their condition differently and may have differing preferences or levels of risk tolerance – tolerances that reflect the length of time they have had MS or their level of disease progression [21, 49].

This last point bridges onto another facet of SDM that is also of critical importance for health decision making: the opportunity for the patient to share their values [19]. Indeed, patients bring preferences and personal values to many kinds of clinical contexts, but they likely obtain greater salience – and emotional gravitas – in the case of a progressive disease like MS or other physically debilitating chronic diseases with few therapeutic options. SDM involves conversations that seek to balance the evidence of known benefits and risks with a patient's preferences and values – that is, what patients want to achieve and how much risk they want to tolerate in turn [21, 50]. For the case of CCSVI, it was not just an unproven hypothesis that PwMS wanted to discuss with their physicians, but what it also represented – hope [51, 52]. Indeed many focus group participants spoke in emotionally laden terms while describing the hypothesis as finally finding a "ray of hope," where historically none have existed – let alone been offered. Participants processed information about CCSVI in such an intensely emotional way that it may have drowned out or overrode more critical or analytical rationale [53–55]. Even if neurologists offered a more balanced illustration of the evidence, they could still overlook what even a weak hypothesis meant to PwMS suffering from a progressive disease with (hitherto) no known cause or cure [41]. Facing this prognosis and given even a remote chance of a better life, many PwMS were willing to forgo their neurologists recommendations and take the risk. Notably, and in keeping with recent research [49, 56], most focus group participants who sought out venous angioplasty had more progressive forms of the disease and consequently felt they had less to lose and potentially the most to (hopefully) gain by taking on the increased risk of an unknown therapy. Furthermore, any frustrations of their hope or desire for more information would likely come to be directed at those who seemed to stand in the way – their neurologists. PwMS with an unsatisfactory relationship with their neurologist would have seen this as just another disappointment among others.

As noted by key informant clinicians, PwMS responded best to their more critical discussions when doctors invited and validated the values and emotions (hope, desperation, etc.) of their patients. Therefore, clinicians who ignore or dismiss the emotional cues (e.g. hope, worry, desperation) of PwMS do so at the risk of missing a crucial part of how patients understand a new hypothesis as well as their disease [8], and as illustrated in our results, the unfortunate possible consequences when patient values or preferences are ignored. Many key informant neurologists described how they tried to put themselves "in their patients' shoes" or assume a more empathetic "bedside manner" in their discussions

of CCSVI. They noted that assuming this kind of posture was a key reason why their relationships with many of their patients were able to endure through such a stressful time and that this element was likely missing for PwMS who severed their connections with their neurologist or lost trust. Some focus group participants also reported a desire for their clinician to exhibit better "bedside manners," meaning better communication skills and respect for the hopes and values of PwMS. Such an approach is in keeping with SDM and its commitment to mutual trust, creating shared understandings, and respect for more autonomous patient decision making – even when that decision may be contrary to the clinical recommendation presented. This highlights the importance of actively eliciting the values of the patient, and validating their emotions in addition to presenting the scientifically-based perspective of an unproven hypothesis. Indeed, it may well be better to consider addressing the former with PwMS even before presenting the latter – in fact, it may be the only facet of SDM that is possible in a situation where a clinician may themselves not even know what evidence exists. Admittedly, if a clinician avoids discussion of a topic because they too lack knowledge about it, it could be potentially perceived as a rebuff of patient concerns as well. In other words, before an MS clinician tells their patients what they know (or what is known or not known), they should first identify with how PwMS feels and connect with those values, which may in turn create a more respectful discussion of the state of the evidence [57]. This may form a basis of trust that may make more biomedical discussions of practice or evidence more acceptable to PwMS [58–60], and further build a stronger foundation that can help all parties weather these inevitable challenges. As was suggested by some key informant neurologists, further training in such approaches of good "bedside manners" may be necessary for MS clinicians when facing such highly emotional contexts.

Nonetheless, even with greater emphasis on good "bedside manners" or with heeding the call of SDM for greater integration of exchange of information and values between doctors and patients, there still existed the potential for misattributions of intentions that flowed from both directions – from perspectives of clinicians and PwMS. Of course, there were instances where PwMS and their neurologists found their opinions to be well-received and acknowledged by each other. However, in many other instances neurologists may not have believed that they were being unduly negative or dismissive by giving little time or a more balanced view to CCSVI, but rather that they were just exhibiting the necessary caution for an unproven hypothesis. On the other hand, PwMS may believe that their inquiries about CCSVI are of critical relevance to their care, but may indeed misattribute clinical caution as undue negativity or dismissal of concerns. Regardless of the intention of either side, PwMS can be left feeling as though they are not being heard, and clinicians can be left feeling unfairly characterized as "villains" or as indifferent. These kinds of disconnects may prove a foil at times even for the SDM approach, especially in this particularly media-driven and emotionally charged context where there were spectrums of perspectives and expectations on both the patients' and clinicians' sides. In the end both sides need to be effective communicators with each other; SDM may be the leading model for minimizing breakdowns of communication between PwMS and their clinicians. At the same time, the dialogical approach of SDM is always subject to prevailing expectations and biases of either side, which may always hold the potential for a misalignment of intentions, perceptions, and understandings. Furthermore, while SDM is modeled on participants co-creating mutually satisfying outcomes, the context of CCSVI shows that it may not be so straightforward a goal. In fact, in situations where a person believes that their last hope for improving their quality of life is at stake, the satisfaction of a patient's desired outcome may move to the forefront from the patients' perspective. This case study therefore also sheds light on these particular tensions – among others noted above – and the challenges they can pose to the SDM type of approach in specific clinical contexts. Such tensions are sure to come to the fore again in future scenarios where a 'breakthrough' hypothesis (whether for MS or other diseases) forces stakeholders to navigate unique and complex decision making processes when the stakes are high but the evidence is lacking or uncertain.

Limitations

There are some specific limitations to this research worth noting. First, we did not conduct paired interviews with the health professionals of our focus group participants of PwMS but rather reported the general statements made by PwMS in only one city as compared to the reflections of other key informant participants (neurologists, other health professionals, advocacy organizations) from across Canada. Second, the general tendency to present oneself in the best possible light is a characteristic concern of any research that relies on self-report; but it is even potentially more relevant when examining statements within a highly controversial public debate such that participants may not have accurately represented their actions. However, the similarity of the groups in the reported challenges in how PwMS discussed CCSVI with their clinicians (whether from their own experiences or others they had heard about) do overall substantiate each other's testimonies. Third, while this case study focuses particularly on the doctor-patient discussion

of CCSVI, the views that PwMS had of those discussions were not in a relational vacuum, but were part of a context of care that may or may not have preceded the emergence of the CCSVI debate. Thus, PwMS interpreted their discussions (or lack thereof) within the context of their overall care of their neurologist such that particular broader issues may have influenced participant responses to the research questions that were central to this study. Fourth, it is possible that the experiences reported here may not be generalizable to other countries given how the CCSVI/liberation therapy issue was handled by our news media as well as by the shifting policy responses of different levels of government. Last, there was a considerable time-lag between when the research was carried out (especially for focus groups held in 2012) and the study's publication. Nevertheless, the results of the study are still instructive for the inevitable 'next time'.

Conclusion

SDM was initially recommended for MS doctor-patient relationships to improve communication and decision making with respect to prevailing MS therapies, or DMTs. However, when a controversial hypothesis arises, it can put those relationships and principles of SDM to the test and force new or latent challenges to the surface. Within the context of this research, even though the CCSVI debate was not the ideal setting for SDM, when its core elements of dialogue promotion and values acknowledgement were present it decreased the likelihood of breakdowns of communication. Instructively, there exist patient decision aids for more general health screening, testing, and treatment services for improving decision-making in the clinical context. These decision aids also emphasize the importance of clarifying patient values for medical "grey areas" where the status of evidence is conflicting, or at least not entirely conclusive [50].

The CCSVI debates exposed and at times amplified communication problems between PwMS and their neurologists. While some of those relationships coped well enough, many others were left broken or bruised with struggles that continue to this day [61]. It also gave PwMS an opportunity to gain more of a voice for themselves in the management of their disease. To fix existing problems and to accommodate the values of PwMS as well as the recommendations of their clinician – even in the context of a new and controversial hypothesis – incorporating the principles of SDM even into uncharted and unanticipated areas of MS disease management can be part of the ongoing efforts toward making necessary improvements in MS doctor-patient communication and care.

Additional files

Additional file 1: Detailed Methods for "Caught in a no-win situation: Discussions about CCSVI between persons with multiple sclerosis and their neurologists – a qualitative study". This document provides a much more detailed of the study's methods, with particular close attention to the process of data collection and analysis.

Additional file 2: CCSVI Focus Group Interview Guide. This document contains the semi-structured focus group instrument that guided discussions with people with MS regarding the CCSVI issue.

Additional file 3: Key Informant (MS) Interview Questions. This document contains the semi-structured key informant interview guide used for clinicians, researchers, health policy makers, and advocacy organizations. Various individual tailoring for specific groups are represented in this document, but as interviews progressed, further tailoring was undertaken as most relevant for that key informant stakeholder group.

Additional file 4: Consolidated criteria for reporting qualitative research (COREQ) – Checklist. This document contains a checklist used when reporting qualitative research to ensure greater transparency around data collection, analysis, and reporting processes.

Abbreviations
CCSVI: Chronic Cerebrospinal Venous Insufficiency; DMT: Disease modifying therapy; MS: Multiple sclerosis; PwMS: Persons with multiple sclerosis; RCT: Randomized control trial; SDM: Shared decision making

Acknowledgements
We would like to sincerely thank all the participants who participated in the focus group for sharing their valuable time and opinions with the study researchers. We also wish to thank all the key informants for their time and thoughts. We express our gratitude to Gary Annable and Christine Mazur for their assistance in data collection and analysis.

Funding
Funding for this study was provided by the Multiple Sclerosis Society of Canada and Research Manitoba (EGID 1261). The funders had no role in designing the study, or in collection, analysis, and interpretation of data, or in writing the manuscript.

Authors' contributions
SDM, RAM, and MB conceived of the study. SDM, RM and other affiliated study staff collected the data. SDM and RM drafted the manuscript, and RAM and MB provided comments on the draft. All authors approved of the final manuscript.

Competing interests
S. Michelle Driedger receives research funding from Canadian Institutes of Health Research, Research Manitoba, Multiple Sclerosis Society of Canada, Canadian Cancer Society Research Institute, Canada Research Chair, Canadian Immunization Research Network.
Ruth Ann Marrie receives research funding from Canadian Institutes of Health Research, Research Manitoba, Multiple Sclerosis Society of Canada, Multiple Sclerosis Scientific Foundation, National Multiple Sclerosis Society, Rx & D Health Research Foundation, the Waugh Family Chair in Multiple Sclerosis, Crohn's and Colitis Canada, and has conducted clinical trials funded by Sanofi-Aventis.
Melissa Brouwers receives research funding from Canadian Institutes of Health Research, Cancer Care Ontario, the Ontario Institute of Cancer Research, and Hamilton Health Sciences.

Author details
[1]Department of Community Health Sciences, Max Rady College of Medicine, Rady Faculty of Health Sciences, University of Manitoba, Winnipeg, MB, Canada. [2]Departments of Internal Medicine and Community Health Sciences, Max Rady College of Medicine, Rady Faculty of Health Sciences, University of Manitoba, Winnipeg, MB, Canada. [3]Department of Oncology, McMaster University, Hamilton, ON, Canada.

References
1. Browne P, Chandraratna D, Angood C, Tremlett H, Baker C, Taylor BV, Thompson AJ. Atlas of multiple sclerosis 2013: a growing global problem with widespread inequity. Neurology. 2014;83(11):1022–4. doi:10.1212/WNL. 0000000000000768.
2. About MS. n.d. https://mssociety.ca/about-ms. Accessed 13 Feb 2017.
3. Compston A, McDonald I, Noseworthy J, Lassmann H, Miller D, Smith K. McAlpine's multiple sclerosis. 4th ed. London: Churchill Livingstone Elsevier; 2006.
4. Noseworthy JH, Lucchinetti C, Rodriguez M, Weinshenker BG. Multiple sclerosis. N Engl J Med. 2000;343:938–52.
5. Zwibel HL, Smrtka J. Improving quality of life in multiple sclerosis: an unmet need. Am J Man Care. 2011;17(Suppl 5):S139–45.
6. Marrie RA, Rudick RA. Drug insight: interferon treatment in multiple sclerosis. Nat Clin Pract Neurol. 2006;2:34–44. doi:10.1038/ncpneuro0088.
7. Salter AR, Marrie RA, Agashivala N, Belletti DA, Kim E, Cutter GR, Cofield SS, Tyry T. Patient perspectives on switching disease-modifying therapies in the NARCOMS registry. Patient Prefer Adher. 2014;8:971–9. doi:10.2147/PPA.S49903.
8. Del Piccolo L, Pietrolongo E, Radice D, Tortorella C, Confalonieri P, Pugliatti M, Lugaresi A, Giordano A, Heesen C, Solari A, et al. Patient expression of emotions and neurologist responses in first multiple sclerosis consultations. PLoS One. 2015;10(6):e0127734. doi:10.1371/journal.pone.0127734.
9. Canada's health care system. n.d. https://www.canada.ca/en/health-canada/services/canada-health-care-system.html. Accessed 4 July 2017.
10. Disease-modifying therapies. 2017. https://mssociety.ca/managing-ms/treatments/medications/disease-modifying-therapies-dmts. Accessed 4 July 2017.
11. Vickrey BG, Edmonds ZV, Shatin D, Shapiro MF, Delrahim S, Belin TR, Ellison GW, Myers LW. General neurologist and subspecialist care for multiple sclerosis: patients' perceptions. Neurology. 1999;53(6):1190–7.
12. Wollin J, Dale H, Spencer N, Walsh A. What people with newly diagnosed MS (and their families and friends) need to know. Int J MS Care. 2000;2(3):4–14.
13. Vickrey BG, Shatin D, Wolf SM, Myers LW, Belin TR, Hanson RA, Shapiro MF, Beckstrand M, Edmonds ZV, Delrahim S, et al. Management of multiple sclerosis across managed care and fee-for-service systems. Neurology. 2000;55(9):1341–9.
14. Heesen C, Kolbeck J, Gold SM, Schulz H, Schulz KH. Delivering the diagnosis of MS–results of a survey among patients and neurologists. Acta Neurol Scand. 2003;107(5):363–8.
15. Heesen C, Kasper J, Segal J, Kopke S, Muhlhauser I. Decisional role preferences, risk knowledge and information interests in patients with multiple sclerosis. Mult Scler. 2004;10(6):643–50.
16. Burnfield A. Doctor-patient dilemmas in multiple sclerosis. J Med Ethics. 1984;10(1):21–6.
17. Elian M, Dean G. To tell or not to tell the diagnosis of multiple sclerosis. Lancet. 1985;2(8445):27–8.
18. Thorne S, Con A, McGuinness L, McPherson G, Harris SR. Health care communication issues in multiple sclerosis: an interpretive description. Qual Health Res. 2004;14(1):5–22. doi:10.1177/1049732303259618.
19. Heesen C, Kasper J, Köpke S, Richter T, Segal J, Mühlhauser I. Informed shared decision making in multiple sclerosis - inevitable or impossible? J Neurol Sci. 2007;259(1–2):109–17. doi:10.1016/j.jns.2006.05.074.
20. Heesen C, Solari A, Giordano A, Kasper J, Kopke S. Decisions on multiple sclerosis immunotherapy: new treatment complexities urge patient engagement. J Neurol Sci. 2011;306(1–2):192–7. doi:10.1016/j.jns.2010.09.012.
21. Clanet MC, Wolinsky JS, Ashton RJ, Hartung H-P, Reingold SC. Risk evaluation and monitoring in multiple sclerosis therapeutics. Mult Scler. 2014;20(10):1306–11. doi:10.1177/1352458513513207.
22. Thom DH, Campbell B. Patient-physician trust: an exploratory study. J Fam Pract. 1997;44(2):169–76.
23. Entwistle V. Trust and shared decision-making: an emerging research agenda. Health Expect. 2004;7(4):271–3. doi:10.1111/j.1369-7625.2004.00304.x.

24. Peek ME, Gorawara-Bhat R, Quinn MT, Odoms-Young A, Wilson SC, Chin MH. Patient trust in physicians and shared decision-making among African-Americans with diabetes. Health Commun. 2013;28(6):616–23. doi:10.1080/10410236.2012.710873.

25. Zamboni P, Galeotti R, Menegatti E, Malagoni AM, Gianesini S, Bartolomei I, Mascoli F, Salvi F. A prospective open-label study of endovascular treatment of chronic cerebrospinal venous insufficiency. J Vasc Surg. 2009;50(6):1348–1358.e1–3. doi:10.1016/j.jvs.2009.07.096.

26. Zamboni P, Galeotti R, Menegatti E, et al. Chronic cerebrospinal venous insufficiency in patients with multiple sclerosis. J Neurol Neurosurg Psychiatry. 2009;80(4):392–9. doi:10.1136/jnnp.2008.157164.

27. Pullman D, Zarzeczny A, Picard A. Media, politics and science policy: MS and evidence from the CCSVI trenches. BMC Med Ethics. 2013;14(1) doi:10.1186/1472-6939-14-6.

28. Favaro A, Picard A. The Globe and Mail. In: A cure in sight. Toronto, Phillip Crawley; 2009. 1 and 10.

29. Favaro A, St. Philip E. The liberation treatment: a whole new approach to MS. Toronto: CTV News; 2009. http://www.ctvnews.ca/the-liberation-treatment-a-whole-new-approach-to-ms.1.456617. Accessed 15 Feb 2017

30. Tulk B. Constructing scientific controversy: framing liberation therapy for multiple sclerosis in Canadian mainstream press. Masters thesis. Ottawa: University of Ottawa; 2013.

31. Reekers JA. CCSVI and MS: a never-ending story. Eur J Vasc Endovasc Surg. 2012;43(1):127–8. doi:10.1016/j.ejvs.2011.09.019.

32. Ogilvie M, Smith J. MS doctors attacked for their skepticism. Toronto: Toronto Star Newspapers; 2010. https://www.thestar.com/life/health_wellness/2010/09/24/ms_doctors_attacked_for_their_skepticism.html. Accessed 13 Feb 2017

33. Mazanderani F, O'Neill B, Powell J. "People power" or "pester power"? YouTube as a forum for the generation of evidence and patient advocacy. Patient Educ Couns. 2013;93(3):420–5. doi:10.1016/j.pec.2013.06.006..

34. Chafe R, Born KB, Slutsky AS, Laupacis A. The rise of people power. Nature. 2011;472(7344):410–1. doi:10.1038/472410a.

35. Hay MC, Strathmann C, Lieber E, Wick K, Giesser B. Why patients go online: multiple sclerosis, the internet, and physician-patient communication. Neurologist. 2008;14(6):374–81. doi:10.1097/NRL.0b013e31817709bb.

36. Baker LM. Sense making in multiple sclerosis: the information needs of people during an acute exacerbation. Qual Health Res. 1998;8(1):106–20. doi:10.1177/104973239800800108.

37. Brooks NA, Matson RR. Social-psychological adjustment to multiple sclerosis. A longitudinal study. Soc Sci Med. 1982;16(24):2129–35.

38. Lejbkowicz I, Paperna T, Stein N, Dishon S, Miller A. Internet usage by patients with multiple sclerosis: implications to participatory medicine and personalized heatlhcare. Mult Scler Int. 2010;2010:–640749. doi:10.1155/2010/640749.

39. Marrie RA, Salter AR, Tyry T, Fox RJ, Cutter GR. Preferred sources of health information in persons with multiple sclerosis: degree of trust and information sought. J Med Internet Res. 2013;15(4):–e67. doi:10.2196/jmir.2466.

40. Alroughani R, Lamdhade S, Thussu A. Endovascular treatment of chronic cerebrospinal venous insufficiency in multiple sclerosis: a retrospective study. Int J Neurosci. 2013;123(5):324–8. doi:10.3109/00207454.2012.759569.

41. Baracchini C, Perini P, Calabrese M, Causin F, Rinaldi F, Gallo P. No evidence of chronic cerebrospinal venous insufficiency at multiple sclerosis onset. Ann Neurol. 2011;69(1):90–9. doi:10.1002/ana.22228.

42. Baracchini C, Perini P, Causin F, Calabrese M, Rinaldi F, Gallo P. Progressive multiple sclerosis is not associated with chronic cerebrospinal venous insufficiency. Neurology. 2011;77(9):844–50. doi:10.1212/WNL.0b013e31822c6208.

43. Snyder J, Adams K, Crooks VA, Whitehurst D, Vallee J. "I knew what was going to happen if I did nothing and so I was going to do something": faith, hope, and trust in the decisions of Canadians with multiple sclerosis to seek unproven interventions abroad. BMC Health Serv Res. 2014;14:445. doi:10.1186/1472-6963-14-445.

44. Strauss AL, Corbin J. Basics of qualitative research: techniques and procedures for developing grounded theory. Thousand Oaks, CA: Sage Publications Inc.; 1998.

45. Miles MB, Huberman AM. Qualitative data analysis: an expanded sourceboook. 2nd ed. Thousand Oaks, CA: Sage Publications; 1994.

46. Elwyn G, Frosch D, Thomson R, Joseph-Williams N, Lloyd A, Kinnersley P, et al. Shared decision making: a model for clinical practice. J Gen Intern Med. 2012;27:1361-7.

47. Freeman J, Langdon D, Hobart J, Thompson A. Inpatient rehabilitation in multiple sclerosis. Neurology. 1999;52(1):50–6.

48. Edmonds P, Vivat B, Burman R, Silber E, Higginson IJ. Fighting for everything': service experiences of people severely affected by multiple sclerosis. Mult Scler. 2007;13(5):660–7. doi:10.1177/1352458506071789.

49. Fox RJ, Salter A, Alster JM, Dawson NV, Kattan MW, Miller D, Ramesh S, Tyry T, Wells BW, Cutter G. Risk tolerance to MS therapies: survey results from the NARCOMS registry. Mult Scler Relat Disord. 2015;4(3):241–9. doi:10.1016/j.msard.2015.03.003.

50. Légaré F, Hébert J, Goh L, Lewis KB, Leiva Portocarrero ME, Robitaille H, Stacey D. Do choosing wisely tools meet criteria for patient decision aids? A descriptive analysis of patient materials. BMJ Open. 2016;6:e011918. doi:10.1136/bmjopen-2016-011918.

51. Ploughman M, Manning OJ, Beaulieu S, Harris C, Hogan SH, Mayo N, Fisk JD, Sadovnick AD, O'Connor P, Morrow SA, et al. Predictors of chronic cerebrospinal venous insufficiency procedure use among older people with multiple sclerosis: a national case–control study. BMC Health Serv Res. 2015;15:161. doi:10.1186/s12913-015-0835-y.

52. Murray CL, Ploughman M, Harris C, Hogan S, Murdoch M, Stefanelli M. The liberation procedure decision-making experience for people with multiple sclerosis. Glob Qual Nurs Res. 2014;1 doi:10.1177/2333393614551413.

53. Kahneman D. Thinking, fast and slow. Toronto: Anchor Canada; 2013.

54. Slovic P. Trust, emotion, sex, politics, and science: surveying the risk-assessment battlefield. Risk Anal. 1999;19(4):689–701.

55. Slovic P, Finucane ML, Peters E, MacGregor DG. Risk as analysis and risk as feelings: some thoughts about affect, reason, risk, and rationality. Risk Anal. 2004;24(2):311–22. doi:10.1111/j.0272-4332.2004.00433.x.

56. Metz LM, Greenfield J, Marrie RA, Jette N, Blevins G, Svenson LW, Alikhani K, Wall W, Dhaliwal R, Suchowersky O. Medical tourism for CCSVI procedures in people with multiple sclerosis: an observational study. Can J Neurol Sci. 2016;43(3):360–7.

57. Stone L, Baker D, Lee R, Hartman F, Ortega J, Sáenz C, Sanchez M, Todini N, Frankenberger T, Starr L, et al. Tool 12: fundamentals of communication during crises and emergencies. In: leadership during a pandemic: what your municipality can do. US Agency for international. Development. 2009;1–8. http://iptk.moh.gov.my/doc/Tool%20of%20Communication%20During%20Crises%20and%20Emergencies.pdf. Accessed 6 Sept 2017.

58. Siegrist M, Earle T, Gutscher H. Test of a trust and confidence model in the applied context of electromagnetic field risks (EMF). Risk Anal. 2003;23:705–16.

59. Siegrist M, Gutscher H, Earle TC. Perception of risk: the influence of general trust, and general confidence. J Risk Res. 2005;8(2):145–56. doi:10.1080/1366987032000105315.

60. Earle T, Siegrist M. Trust, confidence and cooperation model: a framework for understanding the relation between trust and risk perception. International Journal of Global Environmental Issues. 2008;8(1):17–29. doi:10.1504/IJGENVI.2008.017257.

61. Johnstone H. Years after MS liberation therapy discredited, patients, doctors struggle with its legacy. Ottawa: CBCNews; 2016. http://www.cbc.ca/news/canada/ottawa/discredited-ms-treatment-patient-researcher-impact-1.3809026. Accessed 15 Feb 2017.

15

Effect of exercising at minimum recommendations of the multiple sclerosis exercise guideline combined with structured education or attention control education

Susan Coote[1,2]* iD, Marcin Uszynski[1,3], Matthew P. Herring[2,4], Sara Hayes[1,2], Carl Scarrott[5,6], John Newell[5,7], Stephen Gallagher[2,8], Aidan Larkin[3] and Robert W Motl[9]

Abstract

Background: Recent exercise guidelines for people with multiple sclerosis (MS) recommend a minimum of 30 min moderate intensity aerobic exercise and resistance exercise twice per week. This trial compared the secondary outcomes of a combined 10-week guideline based intervention and a Social Cognitive Theory (SCT) education programme with the same exercise intervention involving an attention control education.

Methods: Physically inactive people with MS, scoring 0–3 on Patient Determined Disease Steps Scale, with no MS relapse or change in MS medication, were randomised to 10-week exercise plus SCT education or exercise plus attention control education conditions. Outcomes included fatigue, depression, anxiety, strength, physical activity, SCT constructs and impact of MS and were measured by a blinded assessor pre and post-intervention and 3 and 6 month follow up.

Results: One hundred and seventy-four expressed interest, 92 were eligible and 65 enrolled. Using linear mixed effects models, the differences between groups on all secondary measures post-intervention and at follow-up were not significant. Post-hoc, exploratory, within group analysis identified improvements in both groups post intervention in fatigue (mean Δ(95% CI) SCT -4.99(−9.87, −0.21), $p = 0.04$, Control −7.68(−12.13, −3.23), $p = 0.00$), strength (SCT -1.51(−2.41, −0.60), $p < 0.01$, Control −1.55(−2.30, −0.79), $p < 0.01$), physical activity (SCT 9.85(5.45, 14.23), $p < 0.01$, Control 12.92(4.69, 20.89)), goal setting (SCT 7.30(4.19, 10.4), $p < 0.01$, Control 5.96(2.92, 9.01), $p < 0.01$) and exercise planning (SCT 5.88(3.37, 8.39), $p < 0.01$, Control 3.76(1.27, 6.25), $p < 0.01$) that were maintained above baseline at 3 and 6 month follow up (all $p < 0.05$). Only the SCT group improved at 3 and 6 month follow up in physical impact of MS(−4.45(−8.68, −0.22), −4.12(−8.25, 0.01), anxiety(−1.76(−3.20, −0.31), −1.99(−3.28, −0.71), depression(−1.51(−2.89, −0.13), −1.02(−2.05, 0.01)) and cognition(5.04(2.51, 7.57), 3.05(0.81, 5.28), with a medium effect for cognition and fitness (Hedges' g 0.75(0.24, 1.25), 0.51(0.01, 1.00) at 3 month follow up.

(Continued on next page)

* Correspondence: susan.coote@ul.ie
[1]Department of Clinical Therapies, University of Limerick, Limerick, Ireland
[2]Health Research Institute, University of Limerick, Limerick, Ireland
Full list of author information is available at the end of the article

(Continued from previous page)

Conclusions: There were no statistically significant differences between groups for the secondary outcomes once age, gender, time since diagnosis and type of MS were accounted for. However, within the SCT group only there were improvements in anxiety, depression, cognition and physical impact of MS. Exercising at the minimum guideline amount has a positive effect on fatigue, strength and PA that is sustained at 3 and 6 months following the cessation of the program.

Keywords: Multiple sclerosis, Exercise, Fatigue, Cognition, Behaviour change techniques, Social cognitive theory, Randomised controlled trial

Background

Multiple sclerosis (MS) is a chronic and often progressive condition affecting the central nervous system. MS has many consequences, including impaired strength, fitness, mood, fatigue and cognition, along with limitations of activities such as walking that impact on quality of life. Available evidence supports the beneficial effects of exercise on fatigue [1, 2], depression [3] fitness [4], walking mobility [5, 6], in addition to quality of life [7]. Indeed, this evidence has led to the development of the MS Exercise guideline [8, 9] which recommends moderate intensity aerobic exercise for 30 min and resistance training involving major muscle groups twice weekly.

We are not aware of a single trial that has actually documented the benefits of the exercise guidelines in MS. Of further concern, there are few studies in the MS exercise literature that have evaluated the long-term benefits of exercise interventions, and the results are mixed. For example, we reported positive improvements from a combined aerobic and resistance exercise programme in the community [10]; however, the improvements generally were not maintained 12 weeks post-intervention [11], suggesting that additional measures are required to enable sustained increases in physical activity behaviour among PwMS. This need to foster long-term exercise participation is not unique to PwMS and authors have highlighted the need to include theory-based behaviour change interventions [12]. Social cognitive theory has been extensively investigated among PwMS, and exercise self-efficacy and goal setting are consistently associated with [13] and predictive of [14] physical activity behaviour. Indeed a recent meta-analysis demonstrated significant associations of these constructs and outcome expectancies with physical activity [15].

We have conducted a series of clinical trials (i.e., Phase I and II) with relatively small samples for examining the efficacy of an Internet-delivered behavioural intervention based on social cognitive theory (SCT) for increasing physical activity among ambulatory persons with MS [16–19]. Our most recent trial included the website and one-one-one video coaching and demonstrated moderate to large improvements in

minutes/day of moderate/vigorous physical activity, endurance walking performance, information processing speed, symptoms of fatigue, depression, anxiety, and pain, and quality of life (QOL) over a six-month period [20]. Collectively, such data support the efficacy of the behavioural intervention for increasing and sustaining physical activity in PwMS and possibly improving walking, cognition, symptoms, and QOL outcomes.

The Step it Up study [21] combined the collective knowledge and expertise gained from the Irish community exercise programme with the U.S. online intervention. The 10-week programme firstly aimed to enable inactive PwMS to reach the recently published aerobic and resistance exercise guidelines. We further investigated how embedding this exercise programme in a structured SCT-based education intervention compared to an attention-control education intervention. The current paper reports the results for the secondary outcomes of MS symptoms, physical activity, and SCT constructs. The primary outcome and feasibility metrics, presented elsewhere (Hayes et al. in press) demonstrated that both groups improved significantly in the primary outcome, the six minute walk test (6MWT), and this improvement was maintained at 6 month follow-up. An exploratory analysis of those with three of four assessments demonstrated that the SCT group had a ~ 40 m greater improvement in 6MWT than the control group post-intervention and at 6-month follow up ($p = 0.04$ for both).

Methods

Design

This was a multicentre, double blind, randomised controlled trial (RCT).

Setting and participants

Participants were recruited through the MS Society of Ireland, and via neurology clinics in three urban locations in the Republic of Ireland. Details of the recruitment process are further detailed in the protocol paper [21]. Inclusion criteria were: (1) physician-confirmed formal diagnosis of MS, (2) aged 18 years or more, (3) Patient Determined Disease Steps (PDDS) scale score of

0–3, (4) a sedentary lifestyle (<30 min of moderate to strenuous exercise one day or more per week over the last six months) and (5) willing to give written informed consent. Exclusion criteria were: (1) pregnancy, (2) MS relapse in the previous 12 weeks and (3) changes to MS medication or steroid treatment in the previous 12 weeks. Participants were sent the consent form in advance of the baseline assessment, and written consent was obtained in person by a blinded assessor.

Randomisation and blinding

Participants were randomly allocated into the exercise plus SCT-based intervention or the exercise plus attention control education intervention. Random allocation procedures have been previously outlined [21] and were adhered to. JN generated the random allocation sequence, SH enrolled participants, and SC assigned participants to interventions. The outcome assessor (SH) was blind to allocation throughout the study as were the statisticians (CS, JN). All participants were informed that the study aimed to examine the effect of combining exercise and education, and therefore were blinded regarding group allocation.

Screening questionnaire

Potential participants were screened for eligibility for this study using a questionnaire that included the Patient Determined Disease Steps (PDDS) scale [22], confirmation from participant of MS diagnosis and questions regarding PA levels that have been detailed elsewhere [21].

Outcomes

Outcome measures were conducted pre-intervention post-intervention and at 3 and 6 month follow-up.

At baseline, participants provided demographic details and a researcher formally trained in the use of the Expanded Disability Status Scale (EDSS [23]) (SH) administered the EDSS to all participants at baseline. MS diagnosis according to the McDonald or Poser criteria was confirmed in writing from the participant's consultant neurologist.

The SenseWear Arm band (SWA) provided an objective estimate of PA [24] using both mean daily step count and mean daily energy expenditure estimates over a 7-day period. The 5 times sit to stand test (5xSTS) [25], the Modified Canadian Aerobic Fitness Test (mCAFT) [26] and the Godin Health Index of the Godin Leisure-Time Exercise Questionnaire (GLTEQ) [27] measured lower extremity muscle strength, aerobic capacity and PA behaviour, respectively. The Hospital Anxiety and Depression Scale (HADS) [28], Symbol Digit Modalities Test (SDMT) [29], Multiple Sclerosis Impact Scale 29 (MSIS-29) [30], and Modified Fatigue Impact Scale (MFIS) [31] measured depression, anxiety, cognitive processing speed, impact of

MS and fatigue, respectively. Five questionnaires were implemented to measure SCT domains. These included the Exercise Self-Efficacy Scale (EXSE) [32], Exercise Goal Setting (EGS) scale [33], Multidimensional Outcomes Expectations for Exercise Scale (MOEES) [34], Social Provisions Scale (SPS) [35], and Exercise Benefits and Barriers questionnaire [36]. These measures and associated psychometric properties have been described in the trial protocol [21].

Interventions

The exercise intervention was common to both groups and was delivered by physiotherapists. The aim of the exercise component was to progressively increase the intensity of both aerobic and strengthening exercise to enable the participants to reach the published exercise guidelines for people with mild-to-moderate MS [37], and has been previously described in detail [21]. Over the 10-week programme participants attended the group exercise class on six occasions, supplemented with a telephone coaching call in the weeks without classes (intervention weeks 4, 6, 7 and 9). After each of the group exercise classes the attention control group received an education session about topics unrelated to PA behaviour, e.g. diet, vitamin D, sleep, temperature and hydration, and immunisations and vaccinations. The exercise plus SCT-based intervention group received a similar duration of education based on the principles of SCT for health behaviour change, namely: self-efficacy, outcome expectations, goal-setting, barriers and benefits and has been previously described [21].

Analysis

The study was powered for the primary outcome, 6MWT and consistent with data from a large international study [38], it was assumed that the effect of the intervention would yield an average improvement in 6MWT distance of 36 m with an estimated standard deviation of 48.2 m. In order to have 80% power (at the 5% significance level) to detect such a difference in mean improvement in 6MWT over the study period between groups, a sample of size 62 randomised equally to two arms (i.e. 31 per arm) was needed.

Suitable numerical statistics and graphical summaries were used to describe characteristics of the sample at baseline and to assess the validity of any distributional assumptions needed for the formal analysis. All tests of significance were two-sided and conducted at an alpha = 0.05 level of statistical significance.

The statistical modelling compared differences in the longitudinal response variables between the two intervention arms at each of the three post-intervention follow-ups while correcting for the baseline measurements for each participant. A linear mixed model for a continuous response over time due to the two interventions, whilst adjusting for participant-specific covariates and factors; namely the response of interest at baseline, age, gender, time since diagnosis and MS type (i.e. benign, primary progressive and relapsing-remitting) was developed. Treatment and time (and their interaction) were specified as fixed effects, centre (three levels) and participant (nested in centre) as random effects in order to account for homogeneity within centre and within participant correlation over time. Initially a model containing the main effects of the treatment, time and a treatment-by-time interaction was specified in order to test whether there is evidence that the treatment effects varies over time. If the interaction was deemed unnecessary (using a likelihood ratio test) the model was refitted excluding the interaction term, so the treatment effect was then constant over time. All analyses were carried out using all available measurements. All models were fitted in R 3.2.0 using the lme4

and lmerTest packages. Model diagnostics involved suitable plots of the residuals.

Given increased calls across the literature to move beyond null-hypothesis significance testing in favour of effect sizes and confidence intervals [39] we also quantified and compared the magnitude of change in secondary outcomes using Hedges' g effect sizes and associated 95% confidence intervals (95%CI) using Cohen's conventions for effect sizes (0.2 small, 0.5 moderate, 0.8 large). For each outcome measure, the mean baseline to post intervention and 3 and 6 month change for the control condition was subtracted from the mean baseline to post intervention and 3 and 6 month change for the intervention condition and divided by the pooled baseline standard deviation [40]. Effect sizes were calculated such that greater improvements in outcomes in the intervention group compared to the control group resulted in positive effect sizes.

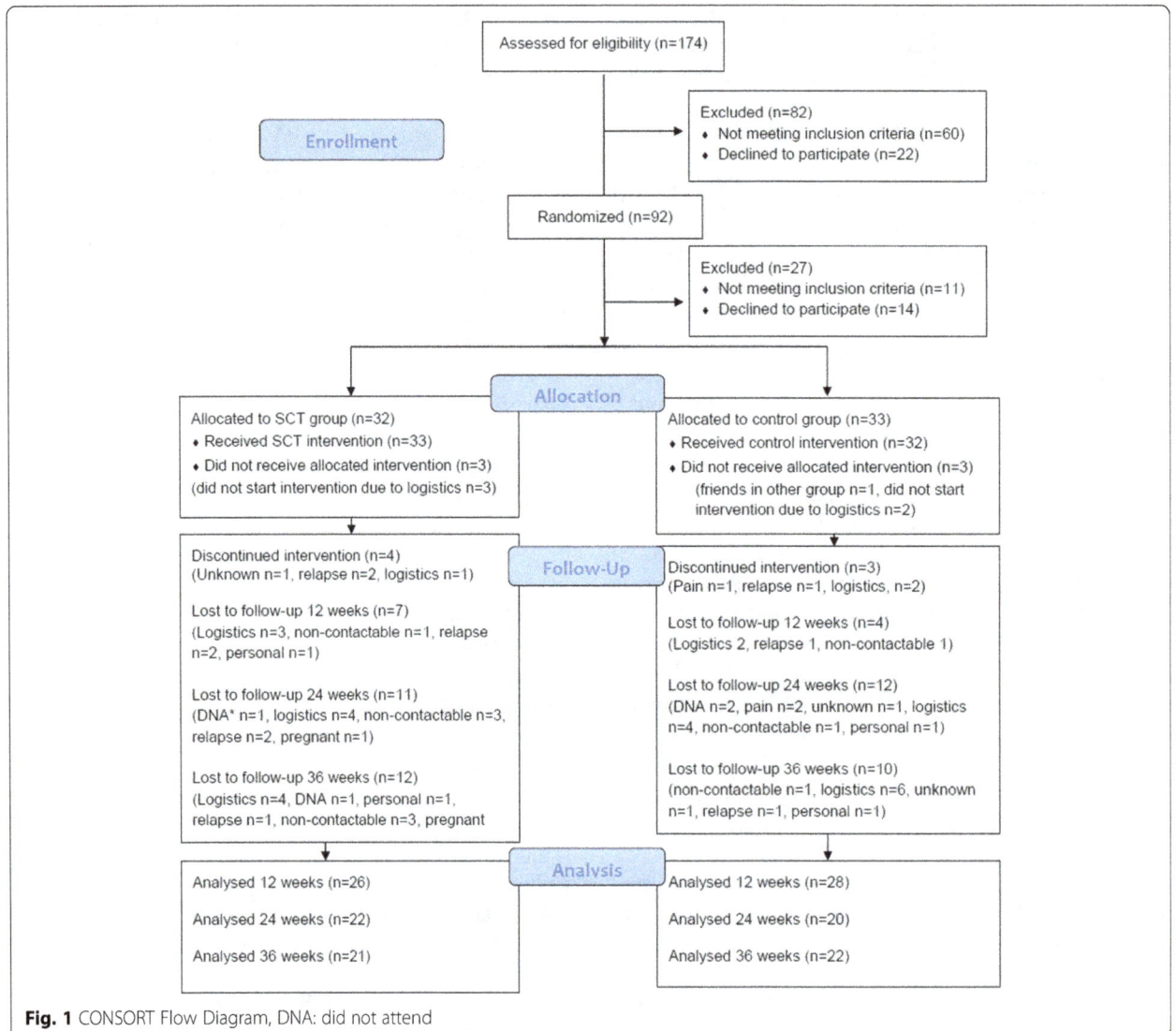

Fig. 1 CONSORT Flow Diagram, DNA: did not attend

An exploratory paired t-test between baseline post intervention and 3- and 6- month follow-ups was also conducted. This provides a summary of the effects of the estimated treatment and control from the raw data. These "unadjusted" results do not account for the patient covariates and repeated measurements.

Results

One hundred and seventy-four PwMS contacted the trial centre and were screened for inclusion over the phone between September 2013 and May 2014. Figure 1 illustrates the flow through the trial, including reasons for loss to follow-up and discontinuation of intervention. We randomised 92 individual participants and waited for 6 participants in a region to run a group before baseline assessment. While waiting for others to be randomised, 27 people became ineligible or declined to participate. One participant was not treated as randomised (two acquaintances had been randomised to the other group and the participant wanted to exercise with them). Sixty-five participants were assessed at baseline and commenced the intervention (intervention group $n = 33$, control group $n = 32$). Baseline demographics are presented in Table 1; the groups were similar at baseline. Feasibility, fidelity and adherence metrics are published elsewhere (Hayes et al. in press).

The raw data at each time point is presented in Table 2. Linear mixed effects models showed no statistically significant differences between the SCT and control groups for any secondary outcome at post intervention and at 3 and 6 month follow up assessment points

Table 1 Clinical baseline characteristics of those receiving exercise plus SCT (SCT) and exercise plus control education (CON)

	SCT ($n = 33$)	CON ($n = 32$)
MS type		
Benign	3	1
Primary progressive	1	0
Relapsing-remitting	27	27
Secondary progressive	0	1
Not reported	2	3
EDSS (mean, SD)	3.3 (0.7)	3.3 (0.7)
Years since diagnosis (mean, SD)	6.7 (5.7)	7.0 (6.1)
Centre (n)s		
Cork	10	9
Galway	8	10
Limerick	15	13
Age (years)	43.3 (9.9)	41.9 (9.3)
Gender (n)		
Male	4	6
Female	29	26

(Table 2). Hedges' g effect sizes and associated 95% CIs are also presented for each group in Table 3. At three month follow up, compared to the control group, the exercise and SCT education resulted in statistically significant moderate-to-large improvements in cognitive processing speed (SDMT: $g = 0.75$, 95% CI: 0.24, 1.25) and aerobic capacity (mCAFT: $g = 0.51$, 95% CI: 0.01, 1.00). Though not statistically significant, compared to control post intervention, the SCT group had small-to-moderate improvements in the perceived psychological impact of MS ($g = 0.25$), anxiety symptoms ($g = 0.34$), estimated energy expenditure ($g = 0.39$), exercise planning ($g = 0.34$), and social support ($g = 0.40$). Compared to control at three month follow-up, the SCT group had nonsignificant, small-to-moderate improvements in the perceived psychological impact of MS ($g = 0.34$), anxiety ($g = 0.37$) and depressive ($g = 0.20$) symptoms, lower extremity muscle strength ($g = 0.41$), estimated energy expenditure ($g = 0.40$), exercise planning ($g = 0.31$), exercise self-efficacy ($g = 0.33$), and social support ($g = 0.49$). At six month follow-up, compared to control the intervention showed nonsignificant small-to-moderate improvements in anxiety ($g = 0.17$) and depressive ($g = 0.23$) symptoms, cognitive processing speed ($g = 0.15$), lower extremity muscle strength ($g = 0.49$), aerobic capacity ($g = 0.34$), exercise planning ($g = 0.17$), exercise self-efficacy ($g = 0.28$), and social support ($g = 0.45$).

Within-group outcome changes, including the unadjusted, unstandardized mean changes from baseline, associated 95%CIs, and paired t-test results for both groups, are presented in Table 4. Both groups demonstrated significant improvements from baseline following the 10-week intervention in the perceived impact of fatigue (MFIS), lower extremity muscle strength (5xSTS), self-reported PA (Godin Health Index), exercise goal setting, and exercise planning that are maintained above baseline at three and six month follow-up. Only the SCT group had significant improvements in perceived physical impact of MS (MSIS-29 physical), anxiety (HADS-A) and depressive (HADS-D) symptoms, and cognitive processing speed (SDMT) at three and six month follow-up. There was no significant change in objectively-measured PA using the outputs of steps and energy expenditure, and no significant change in exercise self-efficacy in either group across time points.

Discussion

This paper presents the secondary outcome results from an intervention designed to enable inactive people with MS to reach the minimum recommendation of the MS Exercise Guidelines and further compared the effect of a structured SCT-based education to an attention-control education intervention. Null hypothesis testing

Table 2 Mean (SD) for secondary outcome measures at each time point

Variables	Baseline mean (SD)		Post Intervention mean (SD)		Three month follow up mean (SD)		Six month follow up mean (SD)	
	EXE + SCT	Control	EXE + SCT	Control	EXE + SCT	Control	EXE + SCT	Control
Modified Fatigue Impact Scale	43.6 (17.7)	46.1 (14.3)	37.2 (14.5)	37.7 (12.9)	35.7 (15.5)	37.6 (13.4)	37.9 (15.3)	36.4 (14.3)
Multiple Sclerosis Impact Scale29 - physical	29.6 (21.8)	30.0 (18.9)	25.6 (17.6)	27.2 (15.0)	24.3 (18.5)	24.4 (13.5)	25.8 (18.7)	25.8 (17.4)
Multiple Sclerosis Impact Scale29 psychological	39.8 (23.9)	36.1 (17.8)	29.4 (16.7)	30.9 (20.2)	29.7 (25.2)	33.1 (22.3)	35.3 (22.9)	29.2 (18.9)
Hospital Anxiety Depression Scale-Anxiety	8.2 (4.4)	7.3 (3.7)	6.6 (4.4)	7.1 (3.7)	6.2 (4.3)	6.8 (3.4)	6.4 (3.7)	6.2 (3.5)
Hospital Anxiety Depression Scale-Depression	5.9 (3.3)	5.5 (3.6)	4.9 (3.4)	4.9 (4.1)	4.1 (3.7)	4.4 (4.5)	4.8 (3.2)	5.2 (3.6)
Symbol Digit Modality Test	46.0 (10.2)	51.2 (14.2)	49.8 (9.1)	55.6 (12.6)	52.4 (7.5)	48.4 (14.1)	49.2 (9.5)	52.6 (15.8)
5xSit To Stand	11.5 (2.7)	10.8 (2.6)	9.8 (2.2)	9.4 (1.9)	9.9 (1.9)	10.3 (2.3)	9.3 (2.4)	9.9 (2.4)
Modified Canadian Aerobic Fitness Test	295.7 (54.6)	313.6 (59.0)	309.1 (53.8)	331.3 (51.6)	301.6 (50.2)	292.5 (53.5)	308.0 (51.5)	307.7 (51.9)
Godin Leisure Time Exercise Questionnaire – Health Index	3.0 (6.2)	2.8 (9.1)	13.8 (11.7)	16.1 (21.1)	15.2 13.9	16.0 (16.7)	15.7 (14.8)	15.0 20.9
Mean steps per day	6098.4 (2362.7)	7222.6 (2694.5)	6107.7 (3304.9)	7582.1 (2372.3)	6429.0 (2447.6)	7396.5 (2611.9)	6558.3 (3059.4)	7450.3 (3099.5)
Mean Energy Expenditure per day	1908.9 (299.8)	2031.6 (382.5)	1908.6 (372.4)	1897.4 (426.5)	1866.2 (407.7)	1851.5 (368.4)	1822.5 (348.16)	1899.7 (355.4)
Exercise Benefits Questionnaire	88.9 (9.1)	88.2 (8.4)	90.4 (12.1)	90.6 (11.2)	89.8 (12.6)	90.1 (11.7)	90.6 (12.5)	91.6 (11.8)
Exercise Barriers Questionnaire	29.8 (5.8)	29.8 (4.0)	28.1 (4.1)	28.5 (4.1)	28.7 (6.6)	27.5 (4.2)	28.7 (5.8)	28.0 (4.7)
Multidimensional Outcomes Expectations for Exercise Scale total	60.9 (6.9)	60.2 (5.9)	60.5 (7.4)	61.0 (7.3)	61.3 (7.0)	60.4 (6.0)	61.2 (7.9)	60.4 (6.9)
Exercise Goal setting Questionnaire	17.2 (7.9)	13.8 (6.6)	24.1 (10.2)	20.2 (7.7)	23.0 (10.5)	21.1 (7.8)	21.4 (10.1)	20.0 (9.9)
Exercise Planning Questionnaire	19.6 (6.3)	19.7 (5.3)	25.6 (6.7)	23.7 (7.4)	26.7(8.1)	25.0 (7.3)	24.9 (8.2)	24.0 (7.5)
Exercise Self-efficacy	66.3 (21.9)	69.2 (25.9)	66.0 (26.3)	70.5 (27.5)	69.0 (19.3)	63.9 (27.2)	68.7 (30.0)	64.9 (23.7)
Social Provisions Scale total	74.9 (9.7)	78.1 (9.1)	77.9 (8.3)	77.3 (9.0)	77.9 (10.2)	76.5 (10.6)	78.7 (9.6)	77.7 (10.1)

Table 3 Estimated treatment effects for secondary outcomes at each time point from linear mixed effects model and effect sizes

		Estimate of difference between SCT and Control	Standard error	95% CI	p-value	Hedges' g (95% CI)
Modified Fatigue Impact Scale	Post Intervention	1.05	3.32	(-5.56, 7.65)	0.75	-0.12 (-0.61, 0.36)
	Three month follow up	-0.11	3.49	(-7.05, 6.82)	0.97	-0.04 (-0.52, 0.45)
	Six month follow up	4.39	3.41	(-2.38, 11.17)	0.20	-0.25 (-0.74, 0.24)
Multiple Sclerosis Impact Scale29 - physical	Post Intervention	-2.58	3.26	(-9.06, 3.89)	0.43	0.06 (-0.43, 0.55)
	Three month follow up	-2.34	3.45	(-9.19, 4.51)	0.50	-0.01 (-0.50, 0.47)
	Six month follow up	-0.54	3.35	(-7.19, 6.10)	0.87	-0.02 (-0.51, 0.47)
Multiple Sclerosis Impact Scale29 - psychological	Post Intervention	-3.01	4.39	(-11.71, 5.70)	0.50	0.25 (-0.24, 0.73)
	Three month follow up	-5.26	4.71	(-14.59, 4.06)	0.27	0.34 (-0.15, 0.83)
	Six month follow up	3.90	4.54	(-5.09, 12.90)	0.39	-0.11 (-0.60, 0.37)
Hospital Anxiety Depression Scale-Anxiety	Post Intervention	-0.92	0.91	(-2.72, 0.88)	0.31	0.34 (-0.15, 0.83)
	Three month follow up	-0.93	0.95	(-2.81, 0.92)	0.33	0.37 (-0.12, 0.86)
	Six month follow up	0.01	0.93	(-1.83, 1.86)	0.99	0.17 (-0.32, 0.66)
Hospital Anxiety Depression Scale-Depression	Post Intervention	0.45	0.77	(-1.08, 1.97)	0.56	0.12 (-0.37, 0.60)
	Three month follow up	0.43	0.81	(-1.18, 2.03)	0.60	0.20 (-0.28, 0.69)
	Six month follow up	0.10	0.79	(-1.46, 1.66)	0.90	0.23 (-0.26, 0.72)
Symbol Digit Modality Test	Post Intervention	-3.03	2.34	(-7.70, 1.64)	0.20	0.06 (-0.42, 0.55)
	Three month follow up	4.93	2.49	(-0.02, 9.87)	0.05	**0.75 (0.24, 1.25)**
	Six month follow up	-0.55	2.51	(-5.54, 4.44)	0.83	0.15 (-0.34, 0.63)
5xSit To Stand	Post Intervention	0.06	0.45	(-0.84, 0.97)	0.89	0.11 (-0.37, 0.60)
	Three month follow up	-0.09	0.48	(-1.10, 0.86)	0.85	0.41 (-0.08, 0.91)
	Six month follow up	-0.62	0.48	(-1.60, 0.33)	0.20	0.49 (-0.003, 0.98)
Modified Canadian Aerobic Fitness Test	Post Intervention	-7.02	9.75	(-26.45, 12.41)	0.47	-0.08 (-0.57, 0.40)
	Three month follow up	16.12	10.63	(-5.03, 37.26)	0.13	**0.51 (0.01, 1.00)**
	Six month follow up	10.53	10.90	(-11.13, 32.19)	0.34	0.34 (-0.15, 0.83)
Godin Leisure Time Exercise Questionnaire – Health Index	Post Intervention	-2.24	4.55	(-11.30, 6.82)	0.62	-0.32 (-0.81, 0.17)
	Three month follow up	0.42	4.75	(-9.02, 9.87)	0.93	-0.13 (-0.62, 0.36)
	Six month follow up	0.11	4.64	(-9.12, 9.34)	0.98	0.06 (-0.42, 0.55)
Mean steps per day	Post Intervention	-163.35	696.12	(-1552.20, 1225.50)	0.81	-0.14 (-0.63, 0.35)
	Three month follow up	-439.08	703.49	(-1842.34, 964.19)	0.53	0.06 (-0.42, 0.55)
	Six month follow up	448.87	737.27	(-1020.74, 1918.48)	0.54	0.08 (-0.57, 0.40)
Mean Energy Expenditure per day	Post Intervention	114.42	95.05	(-74.65, 303.48)	0.23	0.39 (-0.10, 0.88)
	Three month follow up	53.61	98.07	(-141.39, 248.61)	0.59	0.40 (-0.09, 0.89)
	Six month follow up	63.47	103.30	(-141.84, 268.78)	0.54	0.12 (-0.36, 0.61)
Exercise Benefits Questionnaire	Post Intervention	0.311	3.01	(-5.34, 6.23)	0.84	-0.10 (-0.59, 0.38)
	Three month follow up	1.01	3.09	(-5.16, 7.19)	0.74	-0.11 (-0.60, 0.37)
	Six month follow up	0.11	3.05	(-5.98, 6.20)	0.97	-0.19 (-0.68, 0.29)
Exercise Barriers Questionnaire	Post Intervention	-0.24	1.07	(-2.37, 1.88)	0.82	0.08 (-0.41, 0.57)
	Three month follow up	0.73	1.12	(-1.50, 2.96)	0.52	-0.24 (-0.73, 0.25)
	Six month follow up	0.67	1.09	(-1.50, 2.85)	0.54	-0.14 (-0.63, 0.35)
Multidimensional Outcomes Expectations for Exercise Scale total	Post Intervention	-0.42	1.56	(-3.52, 2.68)	0.79	-0.18 (-0.67, 0.30)
	Three month follow up	1.31	1.63	(-1.93, 4.55)	0.42	0.03 (-0.46, 0.52)
	Six month follow up	1.13	1.59	(-2.03, 4.30)	0.48	0.02 (-0.47, 0.50)

Table 3 Estimated treatment effects for secondary outcomes at each time point from linear mixed effects model and effect sizes (Continued)

Exercise Goal setting Questionnaire	Post Intervention	2.03	(−2.24, 6.30)	2.15	0.35	0.07 (−0.42, 0.56)
	Three month follow up	−0.50	(−5.05, 4.06)	2.30	0.83	−0.21 (−0.69, 0.28)
	Six month follow up	−0.26	(−4.65, 4.13)	2.21	0.91	−0.27 (−0.76, 0.21)
Exercise Planning Questionnaire	Post Intervention	2.08	(−1.38, 5.34)	1.74	0.24	0.34 (−0.15, 0.83)
	Three month follow up	1.86	(−1.78, 5.51)	1.84	0.31	0.31 (−0.18, 0.80)
	Six month follow up	0.77	(−2.77, 4.32)	1.79	0.67	0.17 (−0.32, 0.66)
Exercise Self-efficacy	Post Intervention	−3.89	(−18.15, 10.38)	7.17	0.59	−0.07 (−0.55, 0.42)
	Three month follow up	3.01	(−11.86, 17.88)	7.48	0.69	0.33 (−0.16, 0.82)
	Six month follow up	1.66	(−12.88, 16.20)	7.31	0.82	0.28 (−0.21, 0.77)
Social Provisions Scale total	Post Intervention	1.69	(−1.94, 5.32)	1.82	0.36	0.40 (−0.09, 0.90)
	Three month follow up	2.79	(−0.10, 6.58)	1.91	0.15	0.49 (−0.005, 0.98)
	Six month follow up	1.15	(−2.55, 4.85)	1.86	0.54	0.45 (−0.05, 0.94)

Bold text indicates moderate effect (Heges G > 0.5)

Table 4 Unadjusted comparisons of change in secondary outcome measures in each group at each time point

Variables	Mean change Baseline to Post Intervention (95% CI) p-value		Mean change Baseline to three month follow up (95% CI) p-value		Mean change baseline to six month follow up (95% CI) p-value	
	Intervention	Control	Intervention	Control	Intervention	Control
Modified Fatigue Impact Scale	**-4.99** (**-9.78, -0.21**) **p = 0.04**	**-7.68** (**-12.13, -3.23**) **p = 0.01**	**-8.09** (**-13.97, -2.20**) **p < 0.01**	**-7.41** (**-12.77, -2.04**) **p < 0.01**	-5.22 (-10.99, 0.55) p = 0.07	**-10.35** (**-16.43, -4.27**) **p < 0.01**
Multiple Sclerosis Impact Scale29 - physical	-2.06 (-6.36, 2.23) p = 0.33	-0.13 (-5.63, 5.37) p = 0.96	**-4.45** (**-8.68, -0.22**) **p = 0.04**	-1.42 (-7.69, 4.84) p = 0.64	**-4.12** (**-8.25, 0.01**) **p = 0.05**	-3.61 (-9.83, 2.62) p = 0.24
Multiple Sclerosis Impact Scale29 psychological	**-7.54** (**-13.28, -1.81**) **p = 0.01**	-4.22 (-11.19, 2.76) p = 0.22	**-8.37** (**-15.85, -0.89**) **p = 0.03**	-2.02 (-8.11, 4.07) p = 0.50	-4.94 (-12.84, 2.98) p = 0.21	**-7.60** (**-13.71, -1.49**) **p = 0.02**
Hospital Anxiety Depression Scale-Anxiety	-1.60 (-2.50, 0.30) p = 0.12	-0.35 (-1.61, 0.90) p = 0.57	**-1.76** (**-3.20, -0.31**) **p = 0.02**	-0.51 (-1.94, 0.92) p = 0.47	**-1.99** (**-3.28, -0.71**) **p < 0.01**	-1.26 (-2.67, 0.15) p = 0.08
Hospital Anxiety Depression Scale-Depression	-0.76 (-1.54, 0.33) p = 0.20	-0.61 (-1.54, 0.33) p = 0.19	**-1.51** (**-2.89, -0.13**) **p = 0.03**	-1.02 (-2.50, 0.47) p = 0.17	**-1.02** (**-2.05, 0.01**) **p = 0.05**	-0.37 (-1.35, 0.61) p = 0.44
Symbol Digit Modality Test	1.65 (-1.68, 4.99) p = 0.32	3.43 (-1.01, 7.87) p = 0.12	**5.04** (**2.51, 7.57**) **p < 0.01**	0.24 (-3.71, 4.18) p = 0.90	**3.05** (**0.81, 5.28**) **p < 0.01**	2.56 (0.07, 5.06) p = 0.04
5xSit To Stand	**-1.51** (**-2.41, -0.60**) **p < 0.01**	**-1.55** (**-2.30, -0.79**) **p < 0.01**	**-2.13** (**-3.00, -1.26**) **p < 0.01**	**-1.49** (**-2.32, -0.65**) **p < 0.01**	**-2.29** (**-3.20, -1.39**) **p < 0.01**	**-1.19** (**-1.97, -0.40**) **p < 0.01**
Modified Canadian Aerobic Fitness Test	8.56 (-6.86, 23.98) p = 0.26	10.54 (-6.29, 27.37) p = 0.21	3.40 (-14.07, 20.87) p = 0.69	-11.97 (-33.02, 9.08) p = 0.25	2.87 (-7.18, 13.54) p = 0.58	-11.54 (-27.67, 4.59) p = 0.15
Godin Leisure Time Exercise Questionnaire – Health Index	**9.85** (**5.46, 14.23**) **p < 0.01**	**12.92** (**4.69, 20.89**) **p < 0.01**	**10.87** (**4.20, 17.53**) **p < 0.01**	**12.35** (**5.63, 19.07**) **p < 0.01**	**10.65** (**4.18, 17.12**) **p < 0.01**	**11.67** (**5.67, 17.67**) **p < 0.01**
Mean steps per day	118.67 (-1002.54, 1239.87) p = 0.83	30.38 (-1116.58, 1177.34) p = 0.96	-5.88 (-940.73, 928.97) p = 0.99	96.85 (-621.18, 814.88) p = 0.78	756.92 (-440.88, 1954.73) p = 0.19	86.28 (-849.85, 1022.42) p = 0.85
Mean Energy Expenditure per day	46.22 (-119.73, 212.17) p = 0.56	-72.90 (-224.14, 78.33) p = 0.33	-58.18 (-162.68, 46.33) p = 0.25	**-182.5** (**-335.03, -29.97**) **p = 0.02**	6.61 (-140.78, 154.01) p = 0.92	-66.76 (-212.64, 79.12) p = 0.35
Exercise Benefits Questionnaire	2.64 (-0.53, 5.80) p = 0.09	2.08 (-2.31, 6.48) p = 0.34	2.18 (-2.41, 6.78) p = 0.33	1.83 (-3.21, 6.87) p = 0.46	3.38 (-0.59, 7.35) p = 0.09	2.39 (-2.33, 7.12) p = 0.31

Table 4 Unadjusted comparisons of change in secondary outcome measures in each group at each time point (*Continued*)

Exercise Barriers Questionnaire	**-1.51** **(-2.86, -0.17)** **p = 0.03**	-1.09 (-2.41, 0.24) p = 0.10	-1.27 (-3.35, 0.82) p = 0.22	-1.51 (-3.40, 0.37) p = 0.11	-1.57 (-3.22, 0.07) p = 0.06	-2.11 (-4.24, 0.02) p = 0.05
Multidimensional Outcomes Expectations for Exercise Scale total	1.17 (-0.87, 3.21) p = 0.25	0.86 (-1.46, 3.19) p = 0.45	1.84 (-0.24, 3.93) p = 0.08	-0.21 (-2.87, 2.44) p = 0.87	1.84 (-0.35, 4.04) p = 0.10	-0.70 (-3.09, 1.68) p = 0.55
Exercise Goal setting Questionnaire	**7.30** **(4.19, 10.4)** **p < 0.01**	**5.96** **(2.92, 9.01)** **p < 0.01**	**5.44** **(2.14, 8.74)** **p < 0.01**	**6.38** **(2.76, 10.0)** **p < 0.01**	**4.88** **(2.01, 7.76)** **p < 0.01**	**5.51** **(1.89, 9.13)** **p < 0.01**
Exercise Planning Questionnaire	**5.88** **(3.37, 8.39)** **p < 0.01**	**3.76** **(1.27, 6.25)** **p < 0.01**	**6.42** **(3.89, 8.96)** **p < 0.01**	**4.68** **(1.76, 7.61)** **p < 0.01**	**4.86** **(2.63, 7.09)** **p < 0.01**	**4.20** **(1.55, 6.86)** **p < 0.01**
Exercise Self-efficacy	-0.06 (-12.20, 12.07) p = 0.99	0.52 (-11.75, 12.79) p = 0.93	1.32 (-10.62, 13.26) p = 0.82	-9.42 (-24.03, 5.19) p = 0.19	4.24 (-7.78, 16.25) p = 0.47	-5.62 (-15.65, 4.42) p = 0.26
Social Provisions Scale total	1.66 (-1.13, 4.44) p = 0.23	-0.20 (-2.65, 2.25) p = 0.86	2.29 (-0.08, 4.65) p = 0.06	-0.66 (-4.61, 3.29) p = 0.73	**3.13** **(0.35, 5.90)** **p = 0.03**	0.77 (-2.18, 3.72) p = 0.60

Bold text indicates statistical significance p < 0.05

demonstrated no statistically significant between-group differences for any secondary outcome over time. However, examination of the magnitude of change quantified by Hedges' *g* effect sizes illustrated potentially important differences between exercise plus SCT compared to the attention control condition, including significant moderate-to-large improvements in cognitive processing speed and aerobic capacity at three month follow-up. Additionally, though not statistically significant, compared to the attention-control condition, exercise plus SCT resulted in small-to-moderate improvements of ¼ to ½ standard deviation in anxiety and depressive symptoms, the perceived psychological impact of MS, cognitive processing speed, aerobic capacity, estimated energy expenditure, exercise planning, and social support, and the magnitude of many of these improvements persisted at 24- and 36-week follow-up. The magnitude of improvements in these outcomes is consistent with previous reports of the positive effects of exercise training on symptoms among PwMS, including fatigue [1], anxiety [41], depression [42, 43], quality of life [7, 44], and mobility [5], and highlights the potential additive benefit of combined SCT-based education and exercise training.

The finding that both groups improved in strength and physical activity is not surprising given the content of the intervention. Participants completed twice weekly resistance exercise and moderate intensity walking exercise. The changes in lower extremity muscle strength 6 months post intervention, measured with the 5xSTS test, are in line broadly with previously reported changes using that measure [45], providing support for the fidelity of the current intervention to enhance strength. The Health Index score of the GLTEQ also increased in both groups, confirming the exercise log data which indicated that SCT and the CON group groups completed an average of 33.2 of 44 available sessions (75.5%) and 32.0 sessions (72.6%), respectively (Hayes et al. in press). Of note, the objective measure of PA, mean steps/day and mean energy expenditure/day did not change in line with the positive effects on walking mobility and the increase in PA reported in the exercise logs and the GLTEQ Health Index. This may be due to reduced non-exercise physical activity, such that participants reduced leisure, transport and occupational PA in order to engage in exercise training, thereby maintaining, or even decreasing, their overall PA levels. There has been some support in the literature for initial decreases in non-exercise physical activity when beginning an exercise training intervention, though the available evidence suggests that decreased activity dissipates with continued training [46]. It is also possible that the arm worn accelerometer did not capture the changes in PA or that an alternative output, such as increased mild/moderate PA specifically or a reduction in sedentary behaviour, may capture the changes due to the intervention.

Importantly, the results of within-group changes confirmed the positive effect of exercise on fatigue for people with MS [1, 2]. The included sample of PwMS started with scores on the MFIS greater than 38 [47], indicative of clinically meaningful fatigue, and both groups improved, reporting scores below 38 at three and 6 month follow up. To the authors' knowledge, this is the first study to confirm that exercising at the minimum recommendations of the Canadian MS Exercise guideline [9] has a positive effect on fatigue for inactive people with MS with mild-moderate disability.

Both groups also improved in exercise goal setting and planning and these improvements were maintained at both follow-up assessments. This was expected in the SCT group because the structured education intervention specifically addressed these and other SCT domains. The improvement in the control group was unexpected as they engaged in didactic education on topics unrelated to exercise. On reflection, in our efforts to document adherence and fidelity to the intervention, we inadvertently provided the control group with several physical activity behaviour change techniques (BCT's) [12]. This involved exercising in a group setting, advice on the guideline amount and its benefits, recording exercise in a log, seeing personal improvements and monitoring step count on a pedometer. Participants further reported in our qualitative data that knowing they were going to be assessed at 3- and 6-months further served as a motivator to keep exercising. These, somewhat "simple", BCT's warrant consideration for inclusion in interventions that aim to enable long term exercise behaviour and its benefits though we note that there was a greater improvement in the SCT group for the primary outcome of walking endurance seen in a per protocol analysis (Hayes et al. in press). Adding a booster session with both assessment and intervention in the follow up periods may further maintain exercise behaviour and its associated outcomes and is in line with a recent systematic review [48] and reports from participants in this study.

Interestingly exercise self efficacy did not change neither did outcome expectancies or exercise benefits. Notably, compared to the control condition, exercise plus SCT resulted in small, nonsignificant improvements in self-efficacy and exercise plus SCT also resulted in near half-standard deviation improvements in social support, measured with the Social Provisions Scale, at all time points. Though the objective of the current study was not to examine plausible mediators of the effects of exercise plus SCT on outcomes, given previous evidence of the potential intermediary role of social support in the effects of physical activity and exercise among PwMS [49], the ability of exercise to concurrently improve social support and symptoms may be particularly important.

Interestingly only the SCT group demonstrated improvements in physical impact of MS, anxiety, depression and cognition. Compared to the attention-control condition, the exercise plus SCT group showed small-to-moderate improvements in anxiety and depressive symptoms, the perceived psychological impact of MS, and cognitive processing speed. These findings warrant further focused examination but may be due in part to the greater change in walking mobility seen in the exercise plus SCT group (Hayes et al. in press). Both groups improved significantly in six minute walk test (6MWT) distance after treatment and at 3- and 6-month follow-up, and using intention-to-treat analysis the SCT group demonstrated 22.70 m, 11.80 m and 27.42 m greater improvements in this measure. Data suggest that a 21 m change is clinically meaningful to participants, supporting the hypothesis that the SCT group had more meaningful changes in 6MWT distance at 3- and 6-month follow-up that may have resulted in reduced physical impact of MS. More of the SCT group reached the guideline and they reported completing more sessions. This increased "total exercise dose" and the resulting change in depression is supported by our recent systematic review and meta-regression analysis [42], which found increased frequency of exercise was associated with greater reductions of depression. There is limited specific information on the dose/response relationship of exercise for MS and this warrants consideration in trials designed specifically to address this question.

Strengths and limitations

The main strength of this study is that we purposely recruited inactive people with MS and engaged them in a 10-week exercise and education programme with the aim of enabling long-term physical activity engagement and its associated benefits. A weakness is that we did not power the study for these secondary outcomes; nonetheless, the preliminary findings presented in the current paper, particularly the magnitude of improvements in fatigue, anxiety and depressive symptoms, the perceived impact of MS, strength and aerobic capacity, and cognitive processing speed, will inform future trials and targeted analyses of these important factors. A further strength is that we measured a broad range of MS symptoms, and reported the effect of the resistance and aerobic exercise programme on strength, fitness, and subjectively and objectively measured PA. A limitation is that the measures of objective PA and fitness did not change and a more direct measure of fitness, such as cycle ergometry to determine VO^2 max, is recommended [50]. Participants reported some dissatisfaction with the SWA arm band; therefore, alternative tools for objectively measuring PA among PwMS are warranted. A further strength

is that we used exercise logs to capture intensity of aerobic exercise using steps from a pedometer, but a limitation is that we did not record heart rate and this is recommended in future trials.

Conclusion

This paper presents data to suggest that enabling inactive people with mild-moderate disability due to MS to exercise at the minimum suggested by the exercise guideline results in a range of benefits. Improvements in fatigue, strength, goal setting and planning were seen in both the structured SCT and attention control groups and were maintained at 3 and 6 month follow up. The similar responses in both groups for these secondary outcomes can be explained as they both had the same exercise intervention and by the inadvertent inclusion of several behaviour change techniques for the control group through our adherence logging and trial structure.

The results of this pilot trial for the secondary outcome measures suggest that the SCT group had greater improvements in cognitive processing and aerobic capacity at 3 month follow up. This paper further presents preliminary evidence for improvements in physical impact of MS, anxiety, depression and cognition in the exercise plus SCT group alone. This may in part be due to the greater improvements in walking mobility reported elsewhere or due to the content of the education element and therefore further testing of the intervention model is warranted. These findings, in combination with the effects for the primary outcome measure, warrant progression to a definitive RCT and suggest the importance of studies directly investigating the dose-response relationship with focal outcomes.

Abbreviations

5xSTS: 5 times sit to stand test; 6MWT: Six minute walk test; BCT: Behaviour change technique; EDSS: Expanded disability status scale; EXSE: Exercise self-efficacy scale; GLTEQ: Godin leisure-time exercise questionnaire; HADS: Hospital anxiety and depression scale; mCAFT: Modified Canadian aerobic fitness test; MFIS: Modified fatigue impact scale; MOEES: Multidimensional outcomes expectations for exercise scale; MS: Multiple sclerosis; MSIS-29: Multiple sclerosis impact scale 29; PDDS: Patient determined disease steps; PwMS: People with multiple sclerosis; QOL: Quality of life; RCT: Randomised controlled trial; SCT: Social cognitive theory; SDMT: Symbol digit modalities test; SPS: Social provisions scale; SWA: SenseWear Armband

Acknowledgements

We would like to thank MS Ireland Southern, Mid-Western and Western regional offices for their assistance in recruiting participants for this trial.

Funding

This work is supported by the Irish Health Research Board Health Research Award, grant number: HRA_PHR/2013–264. The funding body had no role in the design of the study and collection, analysis, and interpretation of data and in writing the manuscript.

Authors' contributions

SC was the principal investigator for the study, co-initiated the project, contributed to the design of the trial, drafted the paper and approved the final version. MU was a post-doctoral researcher on the trial, commented on drafts of the paper and approved the final version. MH contributed to the conceptualization of the paper, analysis of data, including Hedge's g effect size calculation, provided critical revisions to the paper, and approved the final version. SH was a post-doctoral researcher on the trial, contributed to the design of the study, collected data, commented on drafts of the paper, and approved the final version. SG contributed to the design and evaluation of the trial, commented on drafts of the paper, and approved the final version. AL contributed to the recruitment strategy employed, commented on drafts of the paper, and approved the final version. JN and CS were the statisticians on the trial, cleaned and analysed the data, provided most of the statistics presented, commented on drafts of the paper, and approved the final version. RM co-initiated the project and contributed to the design of the trial, drafted the paper, and approved the final version.

Competing interests

The authors declare that they have no competing interests.

Author details

[1]Department of Clinical Therapies, University of Limerick, Limerick, Ireland. [2]Health Research Institute, University of Limerick, Limerick, Ireland. [3]Multiple Sclerosis Society of Ireland, Western office, Galway, Ireland. [4]Department of Physical Education and Sports Science, University of Limerick, Limerick, Ireland. [5]HRB Clinical Research Facility, National University of Ireland, Galway, Ireland. [6]School of Mathematics and Statistics, University of Canterbury, Christchurch, New Zealand. [7]School of Mathematics, Statistics and Applied Mathematics, National University of Ireland, Galway, Ireland. [8]Department of Psychology, University of Limerick, Limerick, Ireland. [9]Department of Physical Therapy, School of Health Professions, University of Alabama at Birmingham, Birmingham, USA.

References

1. Pilutti LA, Greenlee TA, Motl RW, Nickrent MS, Petruzzello SJ. Effects of exercise training on fatigue in multiple sclerosis: a meta-analysis. Psychosom Med. 2013;75(6):575–80.
2. Andreasen A, Stenager E, Dalgas U. The effect of exercise therapy on fatigue in multiple sclerosis. Mult Scler J. 2011;17(9):1041–54.
3. Ensari I, Motl RW, Pilutti LA. Exercise training improves depressive symptoms in people with multiple sclerosis: results of a meta-analysis. J Psychosom Res. 2014;76(6):465–71.
4. Platta ME, Ensari I, Motl RW, Pilutti LA. Effect of exercise training on fitness in multiple sclerosis: a meta-analysis. Arch Phys Med Rehabil. 2016;97(9):1564–72.
5. Pearson M, Dieberg G, Smart N: Exercise as a Therapy for Improvement of Walking Ability in Adults With Multiple Sclerosis: A Meta-Analysis. *Archives of Physical Medicine and Rehabilitation* 2015, 96(7):1339–1348.e1337.
6. Learmonth YC, Ensari I, Motl RW. Physiotherapy and walking outcomes in adults with multiple sclerosis: systematic review and meta-analysis. Phys Ther Rev. 2016:1–13.
7. Kuspinar A, Rodriguez AM, Mayo NE: The effects of clinical interventions on health-related quality of life in multiple sclerosis: a meta-analysis. *Multiple Sclerosis (Houndmills, Basingstoke, England)* 2012, 18(12):1686–1704.
8. Latimer-Cheung AE, Pilutti LA, Hicks AL, Martin Ginis KA, Fenuta AM, MacKibbon KA, et al. Effects of exercise training on fitness, mobility, fatigue, and health-related quality of life among adults with multiple sclerosis: a systematic review to inform guideline development. Arch Phys Med Rehabil. 2013;94(9):1800–28.
9. Latimer-Cheung AE, Ginis KAM, Hicks AL, Motl RW, Pilutti LA, Duggan M, Wheeler G, Persad R, Smith KM: Development of evidence-informed physical activity guidelines for adults with multiple sclerosis. *Archives of physical medicine and rehabilitation* 2013, 94(9):1829–1836. e1827.
10. Garrett M, Hogan N, Larkin A, Saunders J, Jakeman P, Coote S. Exercise in the community for people with minimal gait impairment due to MS: an assessor-blind randomized controlled trial. Mult Scler J. 2013;19(6):782–9.
11. Garrett M, Hogan N, Larkin A, Saunders J, Jakeman P, Coote S. Exercise in the community for people with multiple sclerosis - a follow-up of people with minimal gait impairment. Mult Scler J. 2013;19(6):790–8.
12. Michie S, Ashford S, Sniehotta FF, Dombrowski SU, Bishop A, French DP. A refined taxonomy of behaviour change techniques to help people change their physical activity and healthy eating behaviours: the CALO-RE taxonomy. Psychol Health. 2011;26(11):1479–98.
13. Streber R, Peters S, Pfeifer K: Systematic review of correlates and determinants of physical activity in persons with multiple sclerosis. *Archives of physical medicine and rehabilitation* 2016, 97(4):633–645. e629.
14. Motl RW, McAuley E, Sandroff BM. Longitudinal change in physical activity and its correlates in relapsing-remitting multiple sclerosis. Phys Ther. 2013;93(8):1037.
15. Casey B, Coote S, Shirazipour C, Hannigan A, Motl R, Martin-Ginis C, et al. Modifiable psychosocial constructs associated with physical activity participation in people with multiple sclerosis: a systematic review and meta-analysis. Arch Phys Med Rehabil. 2017; in press
16. Motl RW, Dlugonski D, Wojcicki TR, McAuley E, Mohr DC. Internet intervention for increasing physical activity in persons with multiple sclerosis. Mult Scler. 2011;17(1):116–28.
17. Dlugonski D, Motl RW, McAuley E. Increasing physical activity in multiple sclerosis: replicating Internet intervention effects using objective and self-report outcomes. Journal of Rehabilitation Research & Development. 2011;48(9):1129–35.
18. Dlugonski D, Motl RW, Mohr DC, Sandroff BM. Internet-delivered behavioral intervention to increase physical activity in persons with multiple sclerosis: sustainability and secondary outcomes. Psychology, Health & Medicine. 2012;17(6):636–51.
19. Motl RW, Dlugonski D. Increasing physical activity in multiple sclerosis using a behavioral intervention. Behav Med. 2011;37(4):125–31.
20. Pilutti L, Dlugonski D, Sandroff B, Klaren RE, RW M: Randomized controlled trial of a behavioral intervention targeting symptoms and physical activity in mutliple sclerosis. *Mult Scler* In press.
21. Coote S, Gallagher S, Msetfi R, Larkin A, Newell J, Motl RW, et al. A randomised controlled trial of an exercise plus behaviour change intervention in people with multiple sclerosis: the step it up study protocol. BMC Neurol. 2014;14(1):241.
22. Hadjimichael O, Kerns RD, Rizzo MA, Cutter G, Vollmer T. Persistent pain and uncomfortable sensations in persons with multiple sclerosis. Pain. 2007;127(1–2):35–41.
23. Goldman MD, Motl RW, Rudick RA. Possible clinical outcome measures for clinical trials in patients with multiple sclerosis. Ther Adv Neurol Disord. 2010;3(4):229–39.
24. Coote S, O'Dwyer C. Comparative validity of accelerometer-based measures of physical activity for people with multiple sclerosis. Arch Phys Med Rehabil. 2012;93(11):2022–8.
25. Csuka M, McCarty DJ. Simple method for measurement of lower extremity muscle strength. Am J Med. 1985;78(1):77–81.
26. Kuspinar A, Andersen RE, Teng SY, Asano M, Mayo NE. Predicting exercise capacity through submaximal fitness tests in persons with multiple sclerosis. Arch Phys Med Rehabil. 2010;91(9):1410–7.
27. Godin G, Shephard RJ. A simple method to assess exercise behavior in the community. Can J Appl Sport Sci. 1985;10(3):141–6.
28. Zigmond AS, Snaith RP. The hospital anxiety and depression scale. Acta Psychiatr Scand. 1983;67(6):361–70.
29. Smith A. Symbol digit modalities test (SDMT) manual (revised) Western psychological services. Los Angeles. 1982;
30. Hobart J LD, Fitzpatrick R, Riazi A, Thompson A.: The Multiple Sclerosis Impact Scale (MSIS-29): a new patient-based outcome measure. In., vol. 124(Part 5). Brain.; 2001: 962–973.
31. Fisk JD, Ritvo PG, Ross L, Haase DA, Marrie TJ, Schlech WF: Measuring the functional impact of fatigue: initial validation of the fatigue impact scale. *Clinical Infectious Diseases* 1994, 18(Supplement 1):S79-S83.
32. McAuley E. Self-efficacy and the maintenance of exercise participation in older adults. J Behav Med. 1993;16:103–13.
33. Rovniak LS, Anderson ES, Winett RA, Stephens RS. Social cognitive determinants of physical activity in young adults: a prospective structural equation analysis. Ann Behav Med. 2002;24(2):149–56.
34. McAuley E, Motl RW, White SM, Wójcicki TR. Validation of the multidimensional outcome expectations for exercise scale in ambulatory, symptom-free persons with multiple sclerosis. Arch Phys Med Rehabil. 2010;91(1):100–5.

35. Cutrona CE, Russell DW. The provisions of social relationships and adaptation to stress. Advances in personal relationships. 1987;1(1):37–67.

36. Sechrist KR, Walker SN, Pender NJ. Development and psychometric evaluation of the exercise benefits/barriers scale. Research in nursing & health. 1987;10(6):357–65.

37. Latimer-Cheung AE, Martin Ginis KA, Hicks AL, Motl RW, Pilutti LA, Duggan M, et al. Development of evidence-informed physical activity guidelines for adults with multiple sclerosis. Arch Phys Med Rehabil. 2013;94(9):1829–36.

38. Baert I, Freeman J, Smedal T, Dalgas U, Romberg A, Kalron A, et al. Responsiveness and clinically meaningful improvement, according to disability level, of five walking measures after rehabilitation in multiple sclerosis a European multicenter study. Neurorehabil Neural Repair. 2014; 1545968314521010

39. Cumming G. The new statistics why and how. Psychol Sci. 2013; 0956797613504966

40. Hedges LV. Advances in statistical methods for meta-analysis. N Dir Eval. 1984;1984(24):25–42.

41. Herring MP, O'connor PJ, Dishman RK. The effect of exercise training on anxiety symptoms among patients: a systematic review. Arch Intern Med. 2010;170(4):321–31.

42. Herring M, Fleming K, Hayes S, Motl R, Coote S. Moderators of exercise training effects on depressive symptoms in multiple sclerosis: a systematic review and meta-regression analysis. *Am J Prev Med* in review.

43. Herring MP, Puetz TW, O'Connor PJ, Dishman RK. Effect of exercise training on depressive symptoms among patients with a chronic illness: a systematic review and meta-analysis of randomized controlled trials. Arch Intern Med. 2012;172(2):101–11.

44. Motl R, Gosney J. Effect of exercise training on quality of life in multiple sclerosis: a meta-analysis. Mult Scler. 2008;14(1):129–35.

45. Kjølhede T, Vissing K, de Place L, Pedersen BG, Ringgaard S, Stenager E, et al. Neuromuscular adaptations to long-term progressive resistance training translates to improved functional capacity for people with multiple sclerosis and is maintained at follow-up. Mult Scler J. 2015;21(5):599–611.

46. Fedewa MV, Hathaway ED, Williams TD, Schmidt MD. Effect of exercise training on non-exercise physical activity: a systematic review and meta-analysis of randomized controlled trials. Sports Med. 2016:1–12.

47. Flachenecker P, Kumpfel T, Kallmann B, Gottschalk M, Grauer O, Rieckmann P, et al. Fatigue in multiple sclerosis: a comparison of different rating scales and correlation to clinical parameters. Mult Scler. 2002;8(6):523–6.

48. Nicolson PJ, Bennell KL, Dobson FL, Van Ginckel A, Holden MA, Hinman RS: Interventions to increase adherence to therapeutic exercise in older adults with low back pain and/or hip/knee osteoarthritis: a systematic review and meta-analysis. *British Journal of Sports Medicine* 2017:bjsports-2016-096458.

49. Motl RW, McAuley E, Snook EM, Gliottoni RC. Physical activity and quality of life in multiple sclerosis: intermediary roles of disability, fatigue, mood, pain, self-efficacy and social support. Psychology, health & medicine. 2009;14(1):111–24.

50. Van Den Akker LE, Heine M, van der Veldt N, Dekker J, de Groot V, Beckerman H. Feasibility and safety of cardiopulmonary exercise testing in multiple sclerosis: a systematic review. Arch Phys Med Rehabil. 2015;96(11):2055–66.

Sleep quality, daytime sleepiness, fatigue, and quality of life in patients with multiple sclerosis treated with interferon beta-1b

Sylvia Kotterba[1], Thomas Neusser[2], Christiane Norenberg[3], Patrick Bussfeld[4], Thomas Glaser[2], Martin Dörner[2] and Markus Schürks[2*] (iD)

Abstract

Background: Sleep disorders and fatigue are common in multiple sclerosis (MS). The underlying causes are not fully understood, and prospective studies are lacking. Therefore, we conducted a prospective, observational cohort study investigating sleep quality, fatigue, quality of life, and comorbidities in patients with MS.

Methods: Patients with relapsing-remitting MS or clinically isolated syndrome treated with interferon beta-1b were followed over two years. The primary objective was to investigate correlations between sleep quality (PSQI), fatigue (MFIS), and functional health status (SF-36). Secondary objectives were to investigate correlations of sleep quality and daytime sleepiness (ESS), depression (HADS-D), anxiety (HADS-A), pain (HSAL), and restless legs syndrome (RLS). We applied descriptive statistics, correlation and regression analyses.

Results: 139 patients were enrolled, 128 were available for full analysis. The proportion of poor sleepers (PSQI≥5) was 55.47% at the beginning and 37.70% by the end of the study (106 and 41 evaluable questionnaires, respectively). Poor sleepers performed worse in MFIS, SF-36, ESS, HADS-D, and HADS-A scores. The prevalence of patients with RLS was low (4.5%) and all were poor sleepers. Poor sleep quality was positively correlated with fatigue and low functional health status. These relationships were corroborated by multivariable-adjusted regression analyses. ESS values and poor sleep quality at baseline seem to predict sleep quality at the one-year follow-up. No variable predicted sleep quality at the two-year follow-up.

Conclusions: Our results confirm the high prevalence of poor sleep quality among patients with MS and its persistent correlation with fatigue and reduced quality of life over time. They highlight the importance of interventions to improve sleep quality.

Keywords: Multiple sclerosis, Interferon beta-1b, Sleep quality, Fatigue, Functional health status, Real world

* Correspondence: markus.schuerks@bayer.com
[2]Bayer Vital GmbH, Leverkusen, Germany
Full list of author information is available at the end of the article

Background

Multiple sclerosis (MS) is a chronic inflammatory and degenerative autoimmune disorder affecting more than two million people worldwide [1]. The prevalence is higher in women than in men. MS is a frequent cause of nontraumatic neurological disability in young adults [1].

Comorbid conditions are common in MS and may contribute to disability. Many patients with MS report sleep disorders [2], more frequently than in the general population, with prevalence estimates ranging from 25 to 54% [3]. Poor sleep quality in MS has been associated with negative outcomes, such as decreased quality of life [4], exacerbation rate and disease severity [5], and with other comorbidities such as fatigue, depression, anxiety, and pain [6, 7].

Fatigue is another common symptom in patients with MS and is closely connected with sleep disorders [3, 8]. Treatment of sleep disorders may have the potential to improve fatigue [9–11].

The underlying causes of poor sleep quality and fatigue are not fully understood. Restless legs syndrome (RLS) appears to play an important role since it has consistently been shown to be more common in patients with MS [2, 9, 12] and is associated with poor sleep [8, 13, 14]. The type of MS treatment may also impact sleep and fatigue. Disease-modifying drugs (DMD), such as interferon beta-1b, might affect sleep quality and fatigue, but results in this connection are ambiguous [8, 13, 14].

Available studies are small and have included cohorts of patients on various treatments. Prospective studies on sleep quality and fatigue are lacking.

Hence, we conducted a prospective study investigating sleep quality, fatigue, quality of life, and comorbidities in patients with MS in a real-world setting over the course of two years. In order to exclude influence of various disease modifying drugs, only patients with interferon beta-1b were included.

Methods

Study design

The BETASLEEP study (NCT01766063) was a prospective, observational cohort study in Germany sponsored by Bayer Vital GmbH. Patients were recruited from 35 neurological offices and clinics specializing in the treatment of MS between December 2012 and January 2015. Patients were followed up for a total of 24 months, with documented visits at baseline, 6, 12, 18, and 24 months. Detailed information about the data collection process and training of investigators is provided in the Additional file 1.

Eligibility

Eligible patients had relapsing-remitting MS (RRMS) or clinically isolated syndrome (CIS), were at least 18 years

old, and had an EDSS (expanded disability status scale) score ≤ 5. Furthermore, patients had to be on treatment with interferon beta-1b. Treatment duration was to be not more than six months and the treatment had to be tolerated by the patient according to their attending physician. All patients provided their written informed consent to participate in the study.

Objectives

Primary objectives were to investigate correlations between sleep quality, fatigue, and functional health status. Secondary objectives were to investigate correlations of sleep quality and daytime sleepiness, depression, anxiety, pain, and RLS.

Outcome variables

Primary outcome variables were sleep quality assessed with the Pittsburgh Sleep Quality Index (PSQI), fatigue assessed with the Modified Fatigue Impact Scale (MFIS), and functional health status assessed with the Short Form 36 (SF-36). Secondary outcome variables were daytime sleepiness measured with the Epworth Sleepiness Scale (ESS), depression and anxiety assessed with the Hospital Anxiety and Depression Scale (HADS), pain measured with the Hamburg Pain Adjective List (HSAL, Hamburger Schmerz Adjektiv Liste), and the severity of RLS assessed through the International RLS Study Group (IRLSSG) rating scale. Detailed information about the questionnaires is provided in the Additional file 1.

Statistical analyses

Statistical analyses were performed using SAS version 9.4 (SAS Institute Inc., Cary, NC). All analyses were exploratory. Continuous variables were described by sample statistics and categorical variables by frequency tables displaying the number of patients as well as percentages. The analyses were performed for the total population and stratified by baseline PSQI score (< 5, ≥ 5).

Correlations between the primary outcome variables and between sleep quality and the secondary outcome variables were calculated using Spearman rank correlation. Analyses were performed at baseline and all follow-up visits.

To further investigate the impact of potential confounders on the correlations, we also performed multivariable-adjusted regression analyses at baseline controlling for age, gender, EDSS score, and duration of disease.

In order to determine potential baseline predictors of poor sleep quality (PSQI≥5) at 12 and 24 months, we first performed univariate logistic regression for the dependent variable (PSQI< 5 vs. PSQI≥5). Second, we employed a stepwise selection procedure with an entry level of $p = 0.5$ and a stay level of $p = 0.1$. The following independent covariates were considered: gender (female, male), age (years), BMI (kg/m^2), type of MS (CIS, RRMS), baseline EDSS score (< 3, ≥ 3), baseline PSQI score (< 5, ≥ 5), MS duration (months), duration of interferon beta-1b treatment (< 3 months, ≥ 3 months), previous sleep disorder (no, yes), baseline ESS score, baseline HADS depression and anxiety scores (< 8, ≥ 8), and concomitant medication (no, yes) until initial visit.

For primary outcome variables, missing data were not imputed. Questionnaires were scored according to standard rules based on available instructions. For the regression models in secondary analyses, missing values in the questionnaire scores were either replaced by the mean or median of the available values (continuous data) or a separate category was created (categorical data).

In order to account for decreasing sample size, we performed sensitivity analyses among patients with available data at each visit.

Results

Patient disposition

From December 2012 to January 2015 a total of 139 patients were enrolled into the study, 128 patients were available for full analysis. A flow chart describing patient disposition is provided in Additional file 2. 45.5% of all patients completed the study. Of the patients who discontinued participation in the study, 35.3% were lost to follow up, 23.5% withdrew consent to participate in the study, 13.7% switched to another medication, and 27.5% discontinued study participation for other reasons.

Baseline characteristics

Baseline characteristics are summarized in Table 1. The median age of the sample was 41 years (range 19–70 years; mean 41.5; SD = 11.3), and 71.1% were female. 89.1% had RRMS, while 10.9% had CIS. The median duration of disease was 6.9 months (range 0.1–315.1 months). The median EDSS was 2 (range 0–5). Some differences in gender and disease duration were seen between the good and the poor sleepers.

Sleep quality

At the initial visit, the mean PSQI score was 7.31 (SD = 4.36; median 6; range 1–18). Among 128 patients (106 patients had evaluable PSQI questionnaires) 55.47% indicated poor sleep quality (Table 2, Additional file 3). The mean and median PSQI scores at the final visit were lower (mean 6.71; SD = 4.11; median 5; range 1–18), with 37.70% of 61 patients (41 patients with evaluable PSQI questionnaires) indicating poor sleep quality.

In the sensitivity analysis considering only patients with PSQI scores at all visits ($n = 28$), the mean PSQI score at baseline was 6.75 (SD = 3.95; median 5; range

1–14), and 57.14% of patients indicated poor sleep quality. At the final visit, the mean PSQI was 6.29 (SD = 3.61; median 5; range 1–16), and 53.57% of patients indicated poor sleep quality.

Health status course

At the initial visit, the mean MFIS score was 32.4 (SD = 20.3; median 34; range 0–76; Fig. 1). Poor sleepers had a higher MFIS score (mean 39.4; SD = 18.8; median 43; range 2–76) than good sleepers (mean 20.2; SD = 15.2; median 18; range 0–51). The differences between poor and good sleepers were apparent at each visit. The sensitivity analysis among participants with available data at each visit confirmed these findings.

Poor sleepers also performed worse than good sleepers in the mean SF-36 physical (PCS) and mental component scores (MCS; Fig. 1). These differences could be observed at each visit. In the sensitivity analysis, the differences between poor sleepers and good sleepers in the PCS were less pronounced, while the differences in the MCS were confirmed.

With respect to the ESS, HADS depression, and HADS anxiety scores, poor sleepers performed worse at each visit (Fig. 1).

The prevalence of RLS in the sample was low (4.48% [$n = 6$] at initial visit, 6.56% [$n = 4$] at final visit); all patients diagnosed with RLS were poor sleepers (Table 3). Likewise, the number of patients with reported chronic pain was low, hence the low number of HSAL scores (Table 3).

The MS Functional Composite was lower in poor sleepers throughout the study and the EDSS score was higher at most visits (Table 3).

Correlations of sleep quality and other comorbidities

There was a strong positive correlation between the PSQI and MFIS total scores at baseline and all follow-up visits, with correlation coefficients ranging from 0.62 to 0.71 (nominal $p < 0.0001$ at all time points; Table 4, Additional file 4). Moderate to strong positive correlations were also found between the PSQI and MFIS physical subscale ($r_s = 0.58–0.67$; nominal $p < 0.0001$ at all time points), MFIS cognitive subscale ($r_s = 0.56–0.67$; nominal $p < 0.0001$ at all time points), and MFIS psychological functioning subscale ($r_s = 0.56–0.65$; nominal $p < 0.0001$ at all time points; Table 4, Additional file 4).

Strong to moderate negative correlations at all visits were found between the PSQI total score and the SF-36 PCS ($r_s = -0.51–-0.63$; nominal $p < 0.0001$ at all time points) and the SF-36 MCS ($r_s = -0.47–-0.78$; nominal $p < 0.0001$ at all time points; Table 4, Additional file 4).

Weak to moderate positive correlations were found between the PSQI total score and ESS ($r_s = 0.27–0.55$; nominal p between 0.005 and < 0.0001), and between

Table 1 Baseline characteristics and scores

Characteristic	All Patients	Good sleepers (PSQI< 5)	Poor sleepers (PSQI≥5)
Age, years	$N = 128$	$N = 35$	$N = 71$
Mean (SD)	41.5 (11.3)	40.4 (11.8)	41.3 (10.7)
Median (range)	41.0 (19–70)	41.0 (19–61)	41.0 (19–65)
Gender, n (%)	$N = 128$	$N = 35$	$N = 71$
Women	91 (71.1)	21 (60.0)	53 (74.7)
Men	37 (28.9)	14 (40.0)	18 (25.4)
Diagnosis, n (%)	$N = 128$	$N = 35$	$N = 71$
RRMS	114 (89.1)	31 (88.6)	62 (87.3)
CIS	14 (10.9)	4 (11.4)	9 (12.7)
Duration of disease, months	$N = 113$	$N = 32$	$N = 61$
Mean (SD)	43.0 (71.6)	30.9 (63.8)	45.6 (74.3)
Median (range)	6.9 (0.1–315.1)	6.9 (0.3–262.3)	6.3 (0.1–315.1)
EDSS, median (range)	$N = 128$	$N = 35$	$N = 71$
	2.0 (0–5)	2.0 (0–5)	2.0 (0–5)
MFIS	$N = 122$	$N = 35$	$N = 71$
Mean (SD)	32.38 (20.33)	20.20 (15.24)	39.38 (18.78)
Median (range)	34.0 (0.0–76.0)	18.0 (0.0–51.0)	43.0 (2.0–76.0)
SF-36 physical component score	$N = 113$	$N = 33$	$N = 67$
Mean (SD)	44.56 (11.35)	50.86 (8.37)	41.80 (11.41)
Median (range)	46.53 (16.50–64.06)	53.00 (22.67–64.06)	41.21 (16.50–60.67)
SF-36 mental component score	$N = 113$	$N = 33$	$N = 67$
Mean (SD)	41.74 (13.28)	47.84 (9.98)	38.27 (13.31)
Median (range)	44.39 (12.44–63.82)	50.96 (22.76–63.82)	39.54 (12.44–59.53)
HADS-D	$N = 128$	$N = 35$	$N = 71$
HADS-D ≥ 8, n (%)	29 (22.66)	2 (5.71)	25 (35.21)
HADS-A	$N = 128$	$N = 35$	$N = 71$
HADS-A ≥ 8, n (%)	41 (32.03)	4 (11.43)	32 (45.07)
ESS	$N = 118$	$N = 35$	$N = 68$
Mean (SD)	8.03 (4.54)	6.69 (4.26)	8.88 (4.71)
Median (range)	8.0 (0.0–16.0)	6.0 (0.0–14.0)	9.0 (1.0–16.0)

Subgroups of good sleepers (PSQI< 5) and poor sleepers (PSQI≥5) do not add up to $N = 128$ (100%) due to missing PSQI baseline values
PSQI Pittsburgh Sleep Quality Index, *SD* standard deviation, *RRMS* relapsing-remitting multiple sclerosis, *CIS* clinically isolated syndrome, *EDSS* Expanded Disability Status Scale, *MFIS* Modified Fatigue Impact Scale, *SF-36* Short Form 36, *HADS* Hospital Anxiety and Depression Scale, *ESS* Epworth Sleepiness Scale

PSQI total score and HADS anxiety subscale (r_s = 0.51–0.56; nominal p between 0.0002 and < 0.0001; Table 4, Additional file 4). Moderate to strong positive correlations were found between the PSQI total score and HADS depression subscale (r_s = 0.44–0.60; nominal p between 0.0001 and < 0.0001; Table 4, Additional file 4).

The strengths of correlations among all primary and secondary outcome measures are visualized in Fig. 2.

Further investigations using multivariable-adjusted linear regression analyses controlling for age, gender, EDSS score, and duration of disease supported the significant relationships seen in the correlation analysis (Additional file 5). An impact of duration of disease on PSQI scores was seen

in most of these models. The influence of the questionnaire score was always the stronger one.

Predictors of poor sleep quality

In univariate logistic regression analysis, poor sleep quality (PSQI≥5) at the one-year follow-up was associated with higher BMI (odds ratio [OR] 1.122, 95% confidence interval [CI] 1.004–1.254), poor sleep quality at baseline (OR 6.270, 95% CI 2.211–17.784), baseline ESS scores (OR 1.200, 95% CI 1.066–1.351), depression at baseline (OR 4.833, 95% CI 1.001–23.344), and anxiety at baseline (OR 3.741, 95% CI 1.217–11.338). Poor sleep quality at the two-year follow-up was predicted by age (OR

Table 2 Course of sleep quality throughout the study

Patients	Baseline visit	6-month visit	12-month visit	18-month visit	24-month visit
All patients, N	128	109	96	65	61
Patients with evaluable questionnaires, N	106	90	82	51	41
PSQI mean (SD)	7.31 (4.36)	6.37 (3.99)	6.43 (4.03)	6.45 (4.48)	6.71 (4.11)
PSQI median (range)	6.0 (1.0–18.0)	5.5 (1.0–20.0)	5.0 (1.0–18.0)	5.0 (0.0–18.0)	5.0 (1.0–18.0)
Proportion of patients with PSQI≥5 (95% confidence interval)	55.47 (46.43–64.25)	46.79 (37.17–56.59)	50.00 (39.62–60.38)	49.23 (36.60–61.93)	37.70 (25.61–51.04)
Sensitivity analysis, N	28	28	28	28	28
PSQI mean (SD)	6.75 (3.95)	6.43 (4.26)	6.00 (3.22)	6.21 (4.07)	6.29 (3.61)
PSQI median (range)	5.0 (1.0–14.0)	4.0 (1.0–18.0)	5.5 (2.0–14.0)	5.0 (1.0–18.0)	5.0 (1.0–16.0)
Proportion of patients with PSQI≥5 (95% confidence interval)	57.14 (37.18–75.54)	46.43 (27.51–66.13)	57.14 (37.18–75.54)	64.29 (44.07–81.36)	53.57 (33.87–72.49)

PSQI Pittsburgh Sleep Quality Index, *SD* standard deviation

1.073, 95% CI 1.009–1.141), poor sleep quality at baseline (OR 4.500, 95% CI 1.06–19.111), and anxiety at baseline (OR 8.727, 95% CI 1.623–46.935).

In multivariate logistic regression using a stepwise selection procedure, baseline ESS values (OR 1.190, 95% CI 1.039–1.362) and poor sleep quality at baseline (OR 5.980, 95% CI 1.914–18.68) were identified as possible predictors for sleep quality at the one-year follow-up. No variable predicted sleep quality at the two-year follow-up.

Discussion

In the BETASLEEP study, more than half of the patients reported poor sleep quality (PSQI≥5) at baseline, while the proportion was only 37.7% (95% CI 25.61–51.04%) after two years. Poor sleep quality was correlated with fatigue, low functional health status, and high scores of daytime sleepiness, depression, and anxiety.

The proportion of poor sleepers reported at the beginning of our study (55.5%) is comparable to that reported in other studies in Germany [14, 15], confirming the high prevalence of poor sleep among patients with MS. In a prospective study by Kotterba et al. among 73 patients with RRMS or CIS, the proportion of poor sleepers was ~ 50% [14]. In a recent cross-sectional study by Rupprecht et al. among 2062 MS patients irrespective of disease course poor sleep quality was present in 54 to 60% of patients [15]. This proportion is higher than what was recently reported in the general population. A study among 9284 people from a German community sample showed poor sleep quality in 36% of participants [16]. The smaller proportion of poor sleepers at the end of our study compared to the beginning may be due to the decreasing number of participants with evaluable PSQI questionnaire results over the course of the study. On the other hand a stable course of disease during interferon beta-1b may reduce fears concerning the development of the disease and improve sleep quality.

The cross-sectional study by Rupprecht et al. [15] further found that depression (96%), anxiety (88%), and fatigue (45%) were the most common comorbidities. In our study, depression was only present in 15.4 to 22.7% and anxiety was only present in 25.0 to 34.9% of patients. HADS-D scores in our study ranged from 3.92 to 4.91, and HADS-A scores ranged from 4.72 to 6.28. A large study among 4516 MS patients from the UK [17] found higher values for HADS-D (7.73) and HADS-A (8.03). In a German study by Kleiter et al. [18], values for HADS-D (3.7) and HADS-A (5.3) were slightly lower than in our study. The low average EDSS values in our study could be one explanation for a lower prevalence of depression and anxiety.

The study by Rupprecht et al. [15] identified anxiety and fatigue as predictors of poor sleep, while medication showed no effect. Furthermore, in the study by Kotterba et al. [14], poor sleep and fatigue were correlated. Our study confirmed the correlation of poor sleep and fatigue, as well as the association of poor sleep and anxiety. Both fatigue and poor sleep quality have repeatedly been shown to negatively affect quality of life in MS patients [4, 19, 20]. In the present study, fatigue and poor sleep were also associated with reduced quality of life assessed with the SF-36.

In contrast to poor sleep, excessive daytime sleepiness was only reported by between 26.4 and 36.4% of our patients. This finding is consistent with previous findings showing presence of excessive daytime sleepiness in around a quarter of MS patients [14].

MS treatment may influence sleep quality. Available results on the effects of interferon beta-1b on sleep quality are mixed. Some studies report negative effects [19, 21], others beneficial [22] or no effect on sleep quality [6]. In animals, it was shown that interferon type I receptors affect the sleep wake cycle [23]. In order to minimize potential differences in medication effects, only patients who had been treated with interferon beta-1b (Betaferon®) for

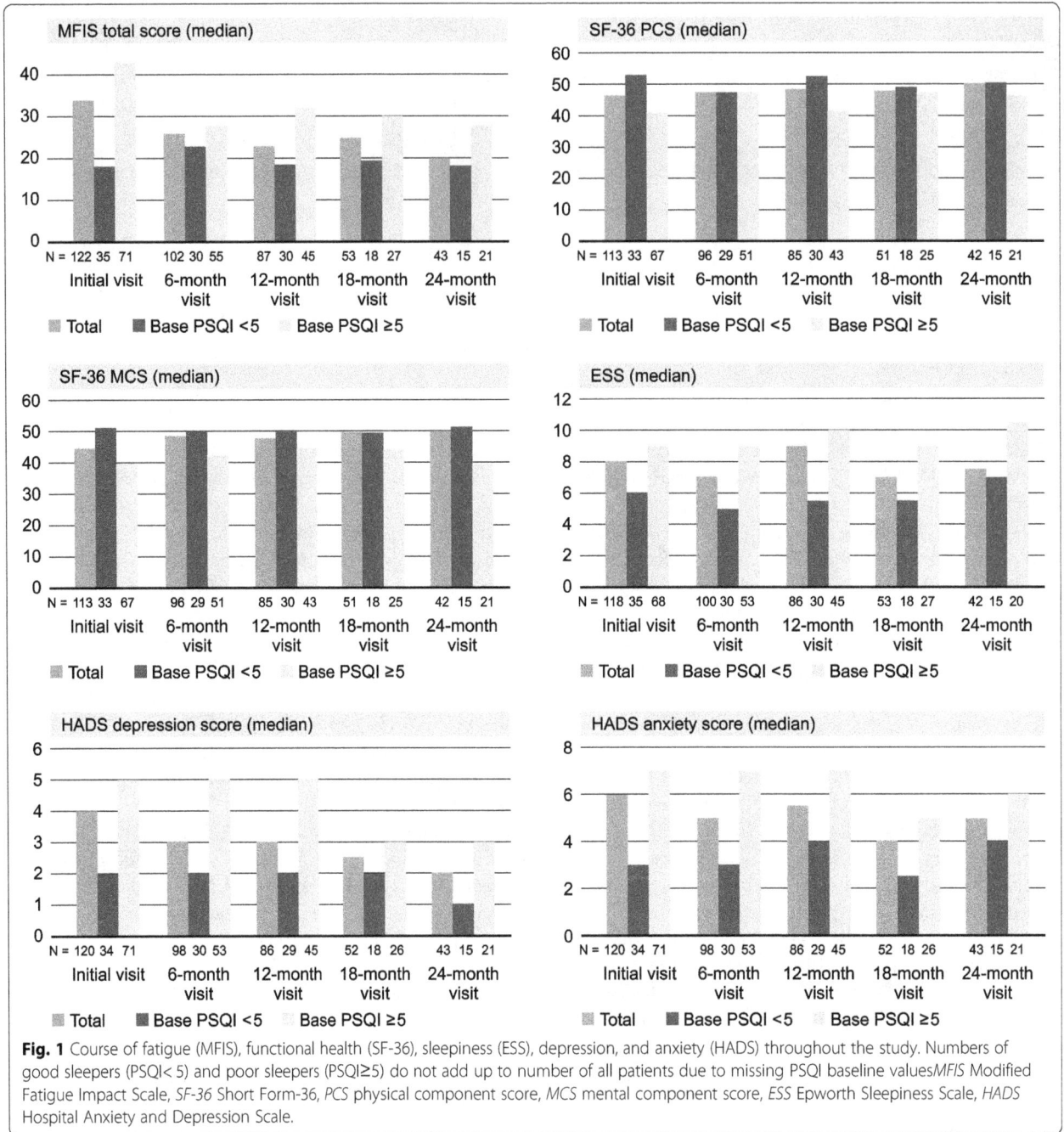

Fig. 1 Course of fatigue (MFIS), functional health (SF-36), sleepiness (ESS), depression, and anxiety (HADS) throughout the study. Numbers of good sleepers (PSQI< 5) and poor sleepers (PSQI≥5) do not add up to number of all patients due to missing PSQI baseline values*MFIS* Modified Fatigue Impact Scale, *SF-36* Short Form-36, *PCS* physical component score, *MCS* mental component score, *ESS* Epworth Sleepiness Scale, *HADS* Hospital Anxiety and Depression Scale.

less than six months and who had tolerated the treatment, were included in the study. Treatment tolerance was required in order to reduce the number of patients prematurely stopping the study.

In the present study, RLS was reported in 2.75 to 6.56% of patients. This proportion is much lower compared to other studies, where diagnosis of RLS was mostly based on questionnaires (prevalence of 14.4 to 57.5%; [2]) and standardized questionnaire-based interviews (prevalence of 32%; [18]). In contrast, in the present study, RLS was assessed by treating physicians based on their evaluation in routine clinical practice. When physicians diagnosed RLS in a patient, the severity was estimated with the IRLSSG. However, treating physicians might not have routinely asked for RLS symptoms. Thus, it is likely that RLS is underreported. The short duration of disease might have further contributed to the low prevalence of RLS in the present study. RLS increases with age in the general population and with disease duration and severity in MS (14). In the presented study patients are mildly impaired and in an early stage of the disease.

Table 3 Course of symptom severity, restless legs syndrome, and pain throughout the BETASLEEP study

Characteristic	Baseline visit			6-month visit			12-month visit			18-month visit			24-month visit		
	All Patients	Good sleepers (PSQI<5)	Poor sleepers (PSQI≥5)	All Patients	Good sleepers (PSQI<5)	Poor sleepers (PSQI≥5)	All Patients	Good sleepers (PSQI<5)	Poor sleepers (PSQI≥5)	All Patients	Good sleepers (PSQI<5)	Poor sleepers (PSQI≥5)	All Patients	Good sleepers (PSQI<5)	Poor sleepers (PSQI≥5)
EDSS	N=128	N=35	N=71	N=90	N=26	N=50	N=75	N=25	N=40	N=50	N=16	N=27	N=49	N=17	N=25
Median (range)	2.0 (0.0–5.0)	2.0 (0.0–5.0)	2.0 (0.0–5.0)	2.0 (0.0–6.5)	2.0 (0.0–4.0)	2.0 (0.0–6.5)	2.0 (0.0–6.5)	1.5 (0.0–4.5)	2.0 (0.0–6.5)	2.0 (0.0–6.5)	1.5 (0.0–4.5)	2.0 (0.0–6.5)	2.0 (0.0–5.0)	1.5 (0.0–5.0)	2.0 (0.0–5.0)
MSFC	N=93	N=26	N=55				N=54	N=18	N=31				N=31	N=8	N=17
Median (range)	0.11 (−3.46–1.49)	0.21 (−1.01–0.69)	0.08 (−3.46–1.49)				0.20 (−1.13–0.87)	0.26 (−0.76–0.87)	0.22 (−1.13–0.80)				0.17 (−1.52–0.99)	0.20 (−0.46–0.73)	0.17 (−1.52–0.99)
RLS, evaluable patients (N)	N=128	N=35	N=67	N=109	N=33	N=59	N=96	N=31	N=50	N=65	N=20	N=34	N=61	N=20	N=31
n (%)	5 (3.9)	0	4 (6.0)	3 (2.8)	0	2 (3.4)	4 (4.2)	0	2 (4.0)	1 (1.5)	0	1 (2.9)	2 (3.3)	0	2 (6.5)
HSAL	N=7	N=1	N=5	N=6	N=1	N=3	N=5	N=1	N=3	N=4	N=1	N=2	N=3	N=0	N=2
Median (range)	111.0 (18–193)	18.0 (18–18)	111.0 (38–193)	42.5 (0–151)	0.0 (0–0)	50.0 (6–133)	48.0 (0–89)	0.0 (0–0)	62.5 (48–77)	61.5 (0–109)	0.0 (0–0)	61.5 (30–93)	124.0 (26–137)	–	75.0 (26–124)

Numbers of good sleepers (PSQI<5) and poor sleepers (PSQI≥5) do not add up to number of all patients due to missing PSQI baseline values

PSQI Pittsburgh Sleep Quality Index, EDSS Expanded Disability Status Scale, RLS restless legs syndrome, MSFC Multiple Sclerosis Functional Composite, SD standard deviation, HSAL Hamburg Pain Adjective List

Table 4 Correlations between the primary and secondary outcome variables

	Baseline visit						12-month visit						24-month visit					
	PSQI (total score)			MFIS (total score)			PSQI (total score)			MFIS (total score)			PSQI (total score)			MFIS (total score)		
	N	r_s	p	N	r_s	p	N	r_s	p	N	r_s	p	N	r_s	p	N	r_s	p
PSQI (total score)		–	–	106	**0.62**	<.0001		–	–	82	**0.68**	<.0001				41	**0.66**	<.0001
MFIS(total score)	106	**0.62**	<.0001		–	–	82	**0.68**	<.0001		–	–	41	**0.66**	<.0001			
SF-36																		
Physical component score (PCS)	100	−0.54	<.0001	113	**−0.72**	<.0001	81	**−0.63**	<.0001	85	**−0.75**	<.0001	40	**−0.61**	<.0001	42	**−0.72**	<.0001
Mental component score (MCS)	100	−0.47	<.0001	113	**−0.68**	<.0001	81	−0.57	<.0001	85	**−0.81**	<.0001	40	**−0.78**	<.0001	42	**−0.78**	<.0001
ESS score	103	0.27	0.0049				82	0.55	<.0001				40	**0.49**	0.0011			
HADS anxiety	105	0.56	<.0001				81	0.51	<.0001				41	**0.53**	0.0002			
HADS depression	105	**0.60**	<.0001				81	0.44	<.0001				41	**0.55**	0.0001			
HSAL score	6	**0.93**	0.0045				5	**0.97**	0.0021				3	**1.00**	.			
IRLSSG score	4	**0.50**	0.5828				3	**0.50**	.				2	**1.00**	.			

Strong correlations are highlighted in **bold numbers**. *PSQI* Pittsburgh Sleep Quality Index, *MFIS* Modified Fatigue Impact Scale, *SF-36* Short Form-36, *ESS* Epworth Sleepiness Scale, *HADS* Hospital Anxiety and Depression Scale, *HSAL* Hamburg Pain Adjective List, *IRLSSG* International Restless Legs Symptom Study Group

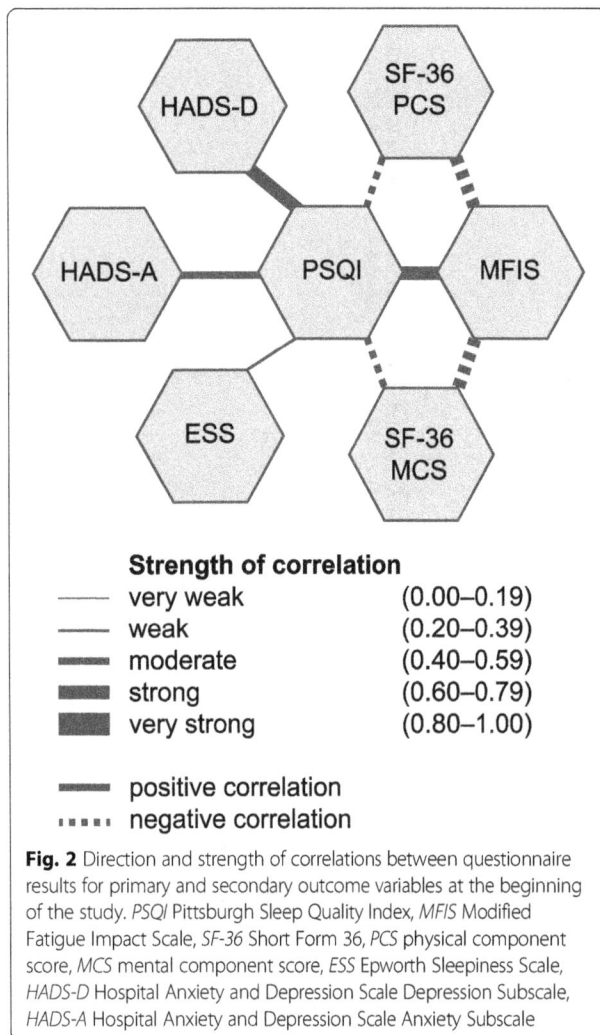

Strength of correlation

——	very weak	(0.00–0.19)
——	weak	(0.20–0.39)
▬▬	moderate	(0.40–0.59)
▬▬	strong	(0.60–0.79)
▬▬	very strong	(0.80–1.00)

▬▬	positive correlation
.....	negative correlation

Fig. 2 Direction and strength of correlations between questionnaire results for primary and secondary outcome variables at the beginning of the study. *PSQI* Pittsburgh Sleep Quality Index, *MFIS* Modified Fatigue Impact Scale, *SF-36* Short Form 36, *PCS* physical component score, *MCS* mental component score, *ESS* Epworth Sleepiness Scale, *HADS-D* Hospital Anxiety and Depression Scale Depression Subscale, *HADS-A* Hospital Anxiety and Depression Scale Anxiety Subscale

One of the advantages of our study is the prospective observational study design investigating sleep quality in German MS patients over two years, thus allowing a real-world picture to be drawn. Furthermore, key characteristics and results from questionnaires suggest that participants in the BETASLEEP study are comparable to other cohorts of patients with relapsing forms of MS with a similar functional health status [24] and a slightly lower level of depression and anxiety [17].

Limitations include the lack of a control group. The results therefore allow no conclusion regarding a possible treatment effect. However, the study was not designed to compare the effect of different medications on the course of sleep quality and fatigue, but rather to investigate sleep quality and fatigue under stable treatment conditions. The ideal situation would have been to prospectively investigate the natural course in untreated patients, which however is not possible due to ethical concerns. Further, obstructive sleep apnea was not excluded in patients. Given the observational study design reflecting real-world activities, such screening was not possible. Additional limitations include the low number of participants with RLS and chronic pain, precluding a reliable evaluation of the impact of these conditions on sleep quality and fatigue. Also, a considerable amount of patients was lost to follow-up. This might be due to the observational nature of the study, reflecting the real-world process in patient care. In addition, the patients were only mildly impaired and potentially observable changes may only occur over longer periods of time. Also we cannot draw any conclusion regarding the course of patients who are more severely affected. Finally, we used a forward selection procedure to identy potential predictors of poor sleep quality, which is prone

Sleep quality, daytime sleepiness, fatigue, and quality of life in patients with multiple sclerosis treated...

163

to type I error. Given that the performed analyses are exploratory we wanted to make sure that we do not miss a potential predictor. This could have been the case with backward stepwise selection, for example, which sometimes drops variables that would be significant when added to the final reduced model.

Conclusion

Taken together, our study confirms the high prevalence of poor sleep quality among patients with MS, which can also be seen in our cohort treated with interferon beta-1b over 2 years. Poor sleep quality was correlated with greater fatigue, lower functional health, and more depression and anxiety. The results highlight the importance of interventions targeted at improving sleep quality in patients with MS.

Additional files

Additional file 1: Additional information on questionnaires, training of investigators and data collection.

Additional file 2: Flow chart of patients enrolled into the BETASLEEP study.

Additional file 3: Sleep quality during the course of the BETASLEEP study.

Additional file 4: Correlations between primary and secondary outcome variables.

Additional file 5: Multivariable-adjusted linear regression analysis for the influence of health status questionnaires on PSQI controlling for age, gender, EDSS, and duration of disease at baseline.

Abbreviations

BMI: Body mass index; CI: Confidence interval; CIS: Clinically isolated syndrome; DMD: Disease modifying drug; EDSS: Expanded disability status scale; ESS: Epworth Sleepiness Scale; HADS: Hospital Anxiety and Depression Scale; HSAL: Hamburg Pain Adjective List; IRLSSG: International RLS Study Group; MCS: Mental component score; MFIS: Modified fatigue impact scale; MS: Multiple sclerosis; OR: Odds ratio; PCS: Physical component score; PSQI: Pittsburgh Sleep Quality Index; RLS: Restless legs syndrome; RRMS: Relapsing remitting multiple sclerosis; SD: Standard deviation

Acknowledgements

The authors wish to thank Sebastian Karl, medizinwelten-services GmbH, for his support in writing this paper.

Funding

The study was funded by Bayer Vital GmbH, Leverkusen, Germany. TN, MD, PB, TG, CN, and MS are former or current employees of Bayer and were involved in the design of the study and collection, analysis, and interpretation of data and in writing the manuscript as indicated in the section Authors' contributions.

Authors' contributions

SK, PB, TG, MS were responsible for the concept and design of the study. TN, MS were responsible for study coordination and conduct. CN, MS were responsible for the data analysis. SK, TN, CN, MD, MS interpreted the data. All authors contributed to and critically reviewed the manuscript during its development and approved the final version of the manuscript for submission.

Competing interests

SK received study grants from Bayer Vital GmbH and BiogenIdec, personal compensation as a speaker from Bayer Vital GmbH, BiogenIdec, UCB, Pfizer, and Novartis. TN, MD and MS are full-time employees of Bayer Vital GmbH. MS previously served as an associate editor to BMC Neurology. PB is a full-time employee of Bayer Consumer Care AG. TG is a former employee of Bayer Vital GmbH and currently a consultant to Bayer Vital GmbH. CN is a full-time employee of Bayer AG.

Author details

[1]Klinik für Geriatrie, Klinikum Leer gemeinnützige GmbH, Leer, Germany. [2]Bayer Vital GmbH, Leverkusen, Germany. [3]Bayer AG, Wuppertal, Germany. [4]Bayer Consumer Care AG, Basel, Switzerland.

References

1. Browne P, Chandraratna D, Angood C, Tremlett H, Baker C, Taylor BV, et al. Atlas of multiple sclerosis 2013: a growing global problem with widespread inequity. Neurology. 2014;83(11):1022–4.
2. Marrie RA, Reider N, Cohen J, Trojano M, Sorensen PS, Cutter G, et al. A systematic review of the incidence and prevalence of sleep disorders and seizure disorders in multiple sclerosis. Mult Scler. 2015;21(3):342–9. (Houndmills, Basingstoke, England)
3. Barun B. Pathophysiological background and clinical characteristics of sleep disorders in multiple sclerosis. Clin Neurol Neurosurg. 2013;115(1):S82–5.
4. Lobentanz IS, Asenbaum S, Vass K, Sauter C, Klosch G, Kollegger H, et al. Factors influencing quality of life in multiple sclerosis patients: disability, depressive mood, fatigue and sleep quality. Acta Neurol Scand. 2004; 110(1):6–13.
5. Fleming WE, Pollak CP. Sleep disorders in multiple sclerosis. Semin Neurol. 2005;25(1):64–8.
6. Neau JP, Paquereau J, Auche V, Mathis S, Godeneche G, Ciron J, et al. Sleep disorders and multiple sclerosis: a clinical and polysomnography study. Eur Neurol. 2012;68(1):8–15.
7. Cameron MH, Peterson V, Boudreau EA, Downs A, Lovera J, Kim E, et al. Fatigue is associated with poor sleep in people with multiple sclerosis and cognitive impairment. Mult Scler Int. 2014;2014:5.
8. Krupp LB, Serafin DJ, Christodoulou C. Multiple sclerosis-associated fatigue. Expert Rev Neurother. 2010;10(9):1437–47.
9. Veauthier C, Paul F. Sleep disorders in multiple sclerosis and their relationship to fatigue. Sleep Med. 2014;15(1):5–14.
10. Veauthier C, Radbruch H, Gaede G, Pfueller CF, Dorr J, Bellmann-Strobl J, et al. Fatigue in multiple sclerosis is closely related to sleep disorders: a polysomnographic cross-sectional study. Mult Scler. 2011;17(5):613–22. (Houndmills, Basingstoke, England)
11. Cote I, Trojan DA, Kaminska M, Cardoso M, Benedetti A, Weiss D, et al. Impact of sleep disorder treatment on fatigue in multiple sclerosis. Mult Scler. 2013;19(4):480–9. (Houndmills, Basingstoke, England)
12. Li Y, Munger KL, Batool-Anwar S, De Vito K, Ascherio A, Gao X. Association of multiple sclerosis with restless legs syndrome and other sleep disorders in women. Neurology. 2012;78(19):1500–6.
13. Lanza G, Ferri R, Bella R, Ferini-Strambi L. The impact of drugs for multiple sclerosis on sleep. Mult Scler. 2017;23(1):5–13. (Houndmills, Basingstoke, England)
14. Kotterba S, Schwenkreis P, Schölzel W, Haltenhof C. Fatigue and sleep problems in patients with relapsing-remitting multiple sclerosis (RRMS) under treatment with interferon β-1b. Klin Neurophysiol. 2016;47(03):136–41.
15. Rupprecht S, Witte OW, Schwab M, for the SLEEP-MS Study Group. SLEEP-MS: Prevalence of Sleep Disturbances, Fatigue, Anxiety and Depression in Multiple Sclerosis. Presentation at the 90 Congress of the German Society of Neurology. Leipzig; 2017.
16. Hinz A, Glaesmer H, Brahler E, Loffler M, Engel C, Enzenbach C, Hegerl U, Sander C. Sleep quality in the general population: psychometric properties of the Pittsburgh sleep quality index, derived from a German community sample of 9284 people. Sleep Med. 2017;30:57–63.
17. Jones KH, Jones PA, Middleton RM, Ford DV, Tuite-Dalton K, Lockhart-Jones H, et al. Physical disability, anxiety and depression in people with MS: an internet-based survey via the UK MS register. PLoS One. 2014;9(8):e104604.
18. Kleiter I, Lang M, Jeske J, Norenberg C, Stollfuss B, Schurks M. Adherence, satisfaction and functional health status among patients with multiple sclerosis using the BETACONNECT(R) autoinjector: a prospective observational cohort study. BMC Neurol. 2017;17(1):174.

19. Boe Lunde HM, Aae TF, Indrevag W, Aarseth J, Bjorvatn B, Myhr KM, et al. Poor sleep in patients with multiple sclerosis. PLoS One. 2012;7(11):e49996.

20. Amato MP, Ponziani G, Rossi F, Liedl CL, Stefanile C, Rossi L. Quality of life in multiple sclerosis: the impact of depression, fatigue and disability. Mult Scler. 2001;7(5):340–4. (Houndmills, Basingstoke, England)

21. Mendozzi L, Tronci F, Garegnani M, Pugnetti L. Sleep disturbance and fatigue in mild relapsing remitting multiple sclerosis patients on chronic immunomodulant therapy: an actigraphic study. Mult Scler J. 2009;16(2):238–47.

22. Pokryszko-Dragan A, Bilinska M, Gruszka E, Biel L, Kaminska K, Konieczna K. Sleep disturbances in patients with multiple sclerosis. Neurological Sci. 2013; 34(8):1291–6.

23. Bohnet SG, Traynor TR, Majde JA, Kacsoh B, Krueger JM. Mice deficient in the interferon type I receptor have reduced REM sleep and altered hypothalamic hypocretin, prolactin and 2',5'-oligoadenylate synthetase expression. Brain Res. 2004;1027(1–2):117–25.

24. Baumstarck K, Butzkueven H, Fernández O, Flachenecker P, Stecchi S, Idiman E, et al. Responsiveness of the multiple sclerosis international quality of life questionnaire to disability change: a longitudinal study. Health Qual Life Outcomes. 2013;11(1):127.

17

Performance in daily activities, cognitive impairment and perception in multiple sclerosis patients and their caregivers

G. Fenu*, M. Fronza, L. Lorefice, M. Arru, G. Coghe, J. Frau, M. G. Marrosu and E. Cocco

Abstract

Background: The relationship between cognitive assessment results in multiple sclerosis (MS) and performance in daily activities (DAs) remains unclear. Our study aimed to evaluate the relationship between cognitive functions (CF) measured by tests, performance in DAs, and the perception of CF in patients and their caregivers (CG) in MS.

Methods: The Brief International Cognitive Assessment for Multiple Sclerosis (BICAMS) battery was used to evaluate cognitive status. We created an ad hoc questionnaire (DaQ) to assess performance in DAs not requiring specific motor skills. We used the Multiple Sclerosis Neuropsychological Questionnaire (MSNQ) to measure each patient self-judgment and caregiver's perception of CF.

Results: Forty-nine patients and their caregivers were included in the study. Significant correlations were found between the BICAMS and the DaQ (Symbol Digit Modalities Test (SDMT): $r = -0.48$, $p < 0.001$; California Verbal Learning Test (CVLT): $r = -0.33$, $p = 0.01$; Brief Visual Memory Test (BVMT-R): $r = -0.42$; $p = 0.002$); patients self-judgment (SDMT: $r = -0.38$, $p = 0.004$; CVLT: $r = -0.26$, $p = 0.03$); caregiver perception of patient's CF (SDMT: $r = -0.52$, $p < 0.001$; CVLT: $r = -0.3$, $p = 0.01$; BVMT-R: $r = -0.42$, $p = 0.002$). The difference in perception between the patients and their caregivers was related to patient age ($p = 0.001$) and severity of cognitive impairment ($p = 0.03$).

Conclusions: Cognitive assessment results show a significant correlation with performance in daily activities and with patients and, especially, caregiver perception of cognitive impairment. These data support the importance of a routine evaluation of cognitive function in MS that includes an anamnestic evaluation of patients, and, when possible, consideration of the caregiver's point of view.

Keywords: Patients, Caregiver, Multiple sclerosis, Cognition, Daily activities, Perception, BICAMS, Neuropsychological assessment

Background

Multiple sclerosis is a chronic disease involving the central nervous system that is caused by a complex interplay between genetic and environmental factors [1–4]. In addition to motor involvement, other clinical manifestation significantly affects the quality of life of patients and their caregivers [5], including fatigue, pain, dysphagia, psychiatric disorders, and cognitive deficits [5–7].

In recent years, an increasing amount of attention has been paid to cognitive impairment in MS [8]. The availability of diagnostic tools such as the Brief International Cognitive Assessment for Multiple Sclerosis (BICAMS) [9], which can be used in daily clinical practice, has helped to better integrate cognitive function into patient monitoring and the evaluation of disability [10, 11].

MS patients with cognitive impairment experience more difficulty working and in social aspects of life, as well as in adherence to therapy and rehabilitative treatment [8, 12].

The correlation between neuropsychological test results and the actual ability of patient to complete tasks of daily life is a debatable issue [8, 12, 13].

Patients with impairment in cognitive function have greater difficulty carrying out tasks of daily life [13, 14].

* Correspondence: giuseppefenu@unica.it
Multiple Sclerosis Center, Binaghi Hospital, ATS Sardegna, Department of Medical Sciences and Public Health, University of Cagliari, via Is Guadazzonis, 2, 09126 Cagliari, Italy

Test results, as well as the perception of cognitive deficits by the patient and the caregiver, are affected by multiple factors [15]. Therefore, the role of mood disorders, current pharmacological treatments, and the severity of cognitive deficits have been assessed as possible determinants of subjective perception by the patient and family members regarding cognitive function [15].

Our study aimed to evaluate the relationship between cognitive functions, as measured by neuropsychological tests, performance in daily activities (DAs), and the perception of cognitive impairment in MS patients and their caregivers (CGs).

Methods

Subject inclusion and study design

Outpatients with a diagnosis of MS were recruited. For each patient just one caregiver was also included in the study.

Inclusion criteria: MS diagnosis according the 2010 revision of the Diagnostic Criteria [16]., age: 18–65 years; caregiver available to participate in the study. Exclusion criteria were: corticosteroid administration or relapse in the previous 30 days, major comorbidity, intake of drugs with activity on the central nervous system, physical disability that did not permit neuropsychological evaluation (i.e., blindness).The caregivers were classified on the basis of the relationship with the patients to confirm the consistency as a privileged informant.

Principal demographic and clinical features for patients included in the study, including sex, age at inclusion, years of education, age at disease onset, and disability (as evaluated by the EDSS scale [17]) were recorded. For the caregiver, we established the type of connection with the patients by classifying them as either partners or family (with their corresponding degree of kinship).

All included subjects signed informed consent form. Even if a significant percentage of included patients have cognitive impairment, the loss of the ability to express consent has been found in no case. In this case the subject would have been included in the study after acquiring the consent of the legal guardian.The study received approval from the local ethics committee.

Neuropsychological assessment

Cognitive function of all patients included in the study was evaluated using the Italian version of the BICAMS battery that implemented the normative values for the Italian population and corrections for sex, age, and years of education [18]. The BICAMS includes the Symbol Digit Modalities Test (SDMT) for evaluating the processing speed of information, the California Verbal Learning Test (CVLT-II) for evaluating verbal learning and memory, and the Brief Visual Memory Test-Revised

(BVMT-R) for evaluating visual learning and memory. According to the Italian Language validation procedure, the normative data have been established as it follows: raw test scores have been converted to scaled scores using the raw-to-scale-score conversions derived from the normative value. Multiple regression equations derived from the normative values have been applied to compute predicted scores for each patient on the basis of principal demographical features (sex, age, years of education). Predicted scores have been then subtracted from each patient's actual scores and the differences divided by the standard deviation of the normative values raw residuals for each measure. Finally, the values have been converted to T scores. The T score is standardised measurement of score. A t score is a type of standard score computed by multiplying a z-score by 10 and adding 50. Thus the T score, the average score is 50, and the standard deviation is 10, and the score shows how many standard deviations the result is from the mean. Result on each neuropsychological measure classified as either intact ($T > 35$) or impaired ($T \leq 35$). Patients showing at least one altered BICAMS test were classified as cognitive impaired. Patients showing no altered test were classified as cognitive preserved.

The perception of the patient's cognitive deficits was evaluated using the Multiple Sclerosis Neuropsychological Questionnaire patient version (pMSNQ) and caregiver version (cgMSNQ) [15] for the patient and their caregiver, respectively. In order to evaluate the magnitude of the difference in the perception of CI between patients and caregivers, a specific calculation (cgMSNQ - pMSNQ) was used.

Performance assessment of daily activities

We created an ad hoc questionnaire (DaQP) to evaluate performance in DAs that do not require specific motor skills (i.e., purchasing flight tickets via the Internet, sending an email, creating a shopping list).

Participants were asked to answer the following question:

"During the last year, how much difficulty did you have carrying out the following activities?"

Participants were asked to select an answer from the following options for each activity:

No difficulty
Some difficulties
Impossible to do it

Scores ranged from 12 (no difficulty carrying out activities) to 36 (impossible to do any of the activities). The full version of the questionnaire is shown in an Additional file 1.

To remove the effect of social context on DAs, we also tested the caregiver's performance using the DaQ

(DaQCG), and then subtracted the patient's score from that obtained by the caregivers to estimate the impact of MS on DAs (DaQP - DaQCG = cost of MS on DAs).

Depression and anxiety were evaluated using the Beck Depression Inventory [7] and Zung Scale [19, 20], respectively.

We also evaluated the patient's cognitive reserve using a previously validated tool, the Cognitive reserve index questionnaire (CRIQ) [21] as previous used in studies about cognition in MS [22].

Statistical analysis

All statistical analyses were performed using SPSS for Mac version 22.0 (SPSS Inc., Chicago, IL, USA).

Firstly, a descriptive analysis was performed summarising patients' demographic and clinical data as mean for quantitative variables and percentages for qualitative variables.

Pearson Test was used to assess correlation between continuous variable as score of BICAMS test and questionnaire results (MSNQp, MSNQcg, DaQP and DaQCG).

T-test was used to compare questionnaire results between the two groups (Cognitively impaired and cognitively preserved patients).

Finally, linear regression analyses were used to evaluate the possible relationship between the different perception of CI (patients/caregiver) and the clinical and demographical features. For all assays, statistical significance was set at $p < 0.05$.

Results

Forty-nine patients and their caregivers were included in the study. The demographic features of the patients included in the study are as follows: female sex: 37/49 (76.0%); mean age: 43.65 years (SD: 11.9); mean EDSS: 3.24 (SD: 2.06); mean disease duration: 12. years (SD: 7.82); mean years of education: 11.38 years (SD: 4.09); CI (at least one test with T-score < 35) was detected in 27/49 (55.1%) as reported in Table 1. Caregiver included as a follows: 29 partners (59.18%), 19 family caregivers (38.77%).

Pearson test showed a significant correlation between BICAMS tests T-scores (and the number of altered tests)

and both MSNQ versions, patients and caregivers. However the correlation was stronger between BICAMS results and cgMSNQ than pMSNQ as showed in Table 2.

Among the BICAMS tests, the strongest correlations were found between the SDMT T-score and the pMSNQ ($r = -3.81$, $p = 0.004$) and between the SDMT T-score and the cgMSNQ ($r = 0.52$, $p = 0.000$).

The caregiver's perception of cognitive deficit showed stronger correlations with the tests than the patient's perception. The correlation was stronger between the cgMSNQ for all three BICAMS tests (SDMT: $r = -0.52$, $p < 0.000$; CVLT: $r = -0.38$, p value = 0.012) than the pMSNQ, which was significantly correlated with the SDMT ($r = -0.38$, $p = 0.004$), and CVLT ($r = -0.26$, $p = 0.03$), but not with the BVMT-R.

Table 2 shows that the daily activity, assessed by DaQP, showed a significant correlation with the cognitive evaluation assessment, measured by the T score of SDMT, as well as the number of altered tests.

The difference in perception between caregivers and patients (cgMSNQ - pMSNQ) showed a significant correlation with number of altered BICAMS tests ($r = 0.40$, $p = 0.000$), age ($r = 0.50$, $p = 0.000$), and EDSS ($r = 0.38$, $p = 0.008$). Linear regression showed that the difference in perception between patients and caregivers depended mainly on age ($p = 0.006$) and the number of altered tests ($p = 0.03$) (Table 3).

The burden of cognitive impairment on DAs that do not require motor skills, as evaluated by the difference between DaQCG and DaQP, was significantly correlated with all BICAMS tests and with the number of altered BICAMS tests as reported in Table 2.

T-tests showed significant differences between cognitively impaired (CI) and cognitively preserved patients (not-CI) for the Cognitive Reserve Index Questionnaire, pMSNQ, cgMSNQ, and DaQ results. These results are presented in Table 4.

No correlations were found between anxiety and depression scores and the BICAMS results. However a strong correlation was found between Zung Score and pMSNG (r:0.581, p: 0.001) and also between Beck Score and pMSNQ (r: 0.543, p:0.001). No correlation was found between Zung and Beck scores and cgMSNQ.

Table 1 Demographic and clinical features of the study patients

	Patients ($n = 49$)
Age (years)	43.65 (S.D. 11.9)
Female sex	38 (76%)
EDSS	3.24 (S.D. 2.06)
Disease duration (years)	12.00 (S.D. 7.82)
Education (years)	11.38 (S.D. 4.09)
Cognitive impaired patients	37 (54%)

Discussion

Results of our study highlight the complexity of the relationship existing between perceived cognitive deficits and those observed through neuropsychological tools. Consistent with findings of previous studies [15,], we found the caregiver's perception to correlate more strongly with cognitive deficits than the patient's self-judgment, which had a less robust but still significant correlation with some objective parameters [23].

Table 2 Pearson Correlation Between the T-score in each BICAMS test, the number of altered tests, and the pMSNQ, cgMSNQ DaQP, DaQP-DaQCG scores

		T-score SDMT	T-score CVLT	T-score BVMT-R	Number of Altered Tests
pMSNQ	Correlation coefficient	−0.381	−0.269	−0.189	0.275
	P value	0.004	0.031	0.097	0.028
cgMSNQ	Correlation	−0.521	−0.338	−0.423	0.562
	P value	< 0.001	0.012	0.002	< 0.001
DaQP	Correlation	−0.487	−0.372	−0.395	0.477
	P value	< 0.001	0.004	0.002	< 0.001
DaQP - DaQCG	Correlation	0.358	0.461	0.256	−0.285
	P Value	0.010	0.001	0.049	0.032

One study [24] showed that the reliability of the caregiver version of the MSNQ was greater than the patient version, but we found the patient version of the MSNQ to also be significantly correlated with objective deficits.

These results support the importance to involve the caregiver in the anamnestic evaluation of cognitive deficit. In fact, the caregiver point of view may be a real expression of cognitive deficit more than patients' perception. This attitude is reflected in previous studies that concluded that self-judgment on cognitive function by patients with multiple sclerosis can be problematic and with a difficult interpretation. Several features as depression, and anxiety could play a role in this self-perception. [25–27]. In fact, also in our study self reported measures of cognitive functions are correlated to depression and anxiety.

In our study, the difference in the perception of cognitive deficiency reported by caregivers and patients correlated with the severity of cognitive deficiency, higher age, and disability. For these reasons, when evaluating patients with such characteristics, the caregiver's view of cognitive impairment should be evaluated with even greater attention.

Equally important is the use of specially developed instruments in the cognitive function anamnesis.

In our study, the BICAMS results were correlated with DAs, which is similar to the findings of a previous study

[13] that reported a strong correlation between the BICAMS test results and performance in daily activities (evaluated using computerized tools) in 41 MS patients.

Among the BICAMS tests, SDMT had the strongest correlation with DAs. These results confirm a role for the SDMT in the principle battery of tests used for MS neuropsychological assessment and as a possible screening test for MS. The correlation between assessment results and the ability in tasks in daily activities support the importance of a routinely cognitive function assessment in daily clinical practice. Moreover we found a significant difference in cognitive reserve score between preserved and impaired patients, as in previous study [22], also our data suggested that cognitive reserve could play a role in the complex interplay between structural damage and cognitive functions in multiple sclerosis.

Our study had several limitations. First, an Italian version of the MSNQ is not available.

The original version was translated by two Italian experts and then by a native English speaker. The translated MSNQ was then administered to 5 patients, 5 caregivers, and 5 healthy volunteers (not included in the study) to evaluate the presence of any difficulties in its ability to be understood.

However, a validation process is needed prior to MSNQ testing in a large Italian population. Despite these issues, we preferred using an instrument such as

Table 3 Linear regression showing the difference between cgMSNQ and pMSNQ as dependent variables, and age, EDSS, and the number of altered tests as dependent variables

Coefficients[a]								
Model		Unstandardized Coefficients		Standardized Coefficients	t	Sig.	95.0% Confidence Interval for B	
		B	Std. Error	Beta			Lower Bound	Upper Bound
1	(Constant)	−23,190	5809		−3.992	.000	−34.920	−11.459
	Age	.418	.144	.430	2.907	.006	.128	.708
	EDSS	.335	.847	.061	.395	.695	−1.377	2.046
	Number of Altered Tests	3.165	1.433	.293	2.208	.033	.270	6.060

Abbreviations: *pMSNQ* Patients version of the Multiple Sclerosis Neuropsychological Questionnaire, *cgMSNQ* Caregiver version of the Multiple Sclerosis Neuropsychological Questionnaire
[a] Dependent Variable: Difference between cgMSNQ and pMSNQ

Table 4 Independent samples t-test for evaluating the difference between cognitively impaired patients and cognitively preserved patients in the MSNQ, DaQP, and Cognitive Reserve Index Questionnaire scores

	Cognitively impaired patients	Cognitively preserved patients	P value (t-test)
pMSNQ	25.41(12.43)	16.83 (9.33)	0.008
cgMSNQ	26.64 (13.59)	12.55 (9.71)	< 0.001
DaQP	18.41 (6.99)	14.35 (4.32)	0.016
CRIq	85.43 (9.93)	98.89 (11.76)	< 0.001

Abbreviations: pMSNQ Patients version of the Multiple Sclerosis Neuropsychological Questionnaire, *cgMSNQ* Caregiver version of the Multiple Sclerosis Neuropsychological Questionnaire, *DaQP* ad hoc questionnaire to evaluating performance in daily activities of MS patients, *CRIq* Cognitive Reserve Index Questionnaire

the MSNQ, i.e., one specifically developed for the perception of cognitive deficiencies in MS by patients and caregivers, for the purpose of our study.

Likewise, for the evaluation of performance in DAs for both the patient and the caregiver, we did not find appropriate tools in the literature to allow us to adequately evaluate activities that require the involvement of cognitive function without the need for motor skills; thus, we built an ad hoc test. Activities could be an area of intervention without complications and additional costs.

Another limitation of the study is the use of a short evaluation battery such as BICAMS, an instrument widely used in everyday clinical practice. However, recent evidence highlighted a correlation with more extensive batteries [28].

Conclusions
In conclusion, although our findings require further study in order to be generalized, they offer several insights as to the perception of cognitive deficits in MS and the correlation between objective cognitive deficits and the actual impact on activities in daily life.

Abbreviations
BICAMS: Brief International Cognitive Assessment for Multiple Sclerosis; BVMT: Brief Visual Memory Test-Revised; CFs: Cognitive Functions; cgMSNQ: Multiple Sclerosis Neuropsychological Questionnaire- caregiver version; CGs: Caregivers; CI: Cognitive impairmet; CVLT: California Verbal Learning Test; DaQ: Daily Activities Questionnaire; DaQCG: Daily Activities Questionnaire- caregiver version; DaQP: Daily Activities Questionnaire-patient version; DAs: Daily Activities; MS: Multiple Sclerosis; pMSNQ: Multiple Sclerosis Neuropsychological Questionnaire-patient version; SDMT: Symbol Digit Modalities Test

Acknowledgements
The authors wish to thank the patients and their caregivers for their time and commitment to this research.

Funding
The author(s) received no financial support for the research, authorship, and/or publication of this article.

Authors' contributions
FG, LL participated in the design of the study and drafted the manuscript.

FM, AM carried out the neuropsychological evaluation and performed the statistical analysis and drafted the manuscript. FJ, CG revised the manuscript for important intellectual content and performed the statistical analysis. CE, MMG helped draft the manuscript and revise it critically for important intellectual content. All authors read and approved the final manuscript.

Competing interests
The author(s) declared no potential conflicts of interest with respect to the research, authorship,
and/or publication of this article.
Dr. Fenu is an editorial board member of BMC Neurology and received honoraria for consultancy from Novartis, Biogen and for speaking from Merck Serono and Teva.
Dr. Lorefice received speaker fee from Teva and serves on scientific advisory boards for Biogen.
Dr. Frau serves on scientific advisory boards for Biogen, received honoraria for speaking from Merck Serono and Teva.
Dr. Coghe and received speaker fee from Teva and Almirall.
Professor Cocco and Marrosu have received honoraria for consultancy or speaking from Bayer, Biogen, Novartis, Sanofi, Genzyme, Serono and Teva.
Dr. Fronza and Dr. Arru have nothing to disclose.

References
1. Steri M, Orrù V, Idda ML, Pitzalis M, Pala M, Zara I, Sidore C, Faà V, Floris M, Deiana M, Asunis I, Porcu E, Mulas A, Piras MG, Lobina M, Lai S, Marongiu M, Serra V, Marongiu M, Sole G, Busonero F, Maschio A, Cusano R, Cuccuru G, Deidda F, Poddie F, Farina G, Dei M, Virdis F, Olla S, Satta MA, Pani M, Delitala A, Cocco E, Frau J, Coghe G, Lorefice L, Fenu G, Ferrigno P, Ban M, Barizzone N, Leone M, Guerini FR, Piga M, Firinu D, Kockum I, Lima Bomfim I, Olsson T, Alfredsson L, Suarez A, Carreira PE, Castillo-Palma MJ, Marcus JH, Congia M, Angius A, Melis M, Gonzalez A, Alarcón Riquelme ME, da Silva BM, Marchini M, Danieli MG, Del Giacco S, Mathieu A, Pani A, Montgomery SB, Rosati G, Hillert J, Sawcer S, D'Alfonso S, Todd JA, Novembre J, Abecasis GR, Whalen MB, Marrosu MG, Meloni A, Sanna S, Gorospe M, Schlessinger D, Fiorillo E, Zoledziewska M, Cucca F. Overexpression of the cytokine BAFF and autoimmunity risk. N Engl J Med. 2017;376(17):1615–26.
2. Cocco E, Meloni A, Murru MR, et al. Vitamin D responsive elements within the HLA-DRB1 promoter region in Sardinian multiple sclerosis associated alleles. PLoS One. 2012;7(7):e41678.
3. Cocco E, Murru R, Costa G, Kumar A, Pieroni E, Melis C, Barberini L, Sardu C, Lorefice L, Fenu G, Frau J, Coghe G, Carboni N, Marrosu MG. Interaction between HLA-DRB1-DQB1 haplotypes in Sardinian multiple sclerosis population. PLoS One. 2013;8(4):e59790.
4. Thompson AJ, Baranzini SE, Geurts J, Hemmer B, Ciccarelli O. Multiple sclerosis. Lancet. 2018;391(10130):1622–36.
5. Lorefice L, Fenu G, Frau J, Coghe G, Marrosu MG, Cocco E. The impact of visible and invisible symptoms on employment status, work and social functioning in multiple sclerosis. Work. 2018;60(2):263–70.
6. Toosy A, Ciccarelli O, Thompson A. Symptomatic treatment and management of multiple sclerosis. Handb Clin Neurol. 2014;122:513–62.
7. Solaro C, Trabucco E, Signori A, Martinelli V, Radaelli M, Centonze D, Rossi S, Grasso MG, Clemenzi A, Bonavita S, D'Ambrosio A, Patti F, D'Amico E, Cruccu G, Truini A. Depressive symptoms correlate with disability and disease course in multiple sclerosis patients: an Italian multi-center study using the Beck depression inventory. PLoS One. 2016;11(9):e0160261.

8. Chiaravalloti ND, DeLuca J. Cognitive impairment in multiple sclerosis. Lancet Neurol. 2008;7(12):1139–51. https://doi.org/10.1016/S1474-4422(08)70259-X.

9. Langdon DW, Amato MP, Boringa J, Brochet B, Foley F, Fredrikson S, Hämäläinen P, Hartung HP, Krupp L, Penner IK, Reder AT, Benedict RH. Recommendations for arief international cognitive assessment for multiple sclerosis (BICAMS). Mult Scler. 2012;18(6):891–8.

10. Korakas N, Tsolaki M. Cognitive impairment in multiple sclerosis: a review of neuropsychological assessments. Cogn Behav Neurol. 2016;29(2):55–67.

11. Saccà F, Costabile T, Carotenuto A, Lanzillo R, Moccia M, Pane C, Russo CV, Barbarulo AM, Casertano S, Rossi F, Signoriello E, Lus G, Brescia Morra V. The EDSS integration with the brief international cognitive assessment for multiple sclerosis and orientation tests. Mult Scler. 2017;23(9):1289–96.

12. Langdon DW. Cognition in multiple sclerosis. Curr Opin Neurol. 2011;24(3): 244–9. https://doi.org/10.1097/WCO.0b013e328346a43b.Review.

13. Goverover Y, Chiaravalloti N, DeLuca J. Brief international cognitive assessment for multiple sclerosis (BICAMS) and performance of everyday life tasks: actual reality. Mult Scler. 2016;22(4):544–50.

14. Campbell J, Rashid W, Cercignani M, Langdon D. Cognitive impairment among patients with multiple sclerosis: associations with employment and quality of life. Postgrad Med J. 2017;93(1097):143–7.

15. Benedict RH, Munschauer F, Linn R, Miller C, Murphy E, Foley F, Jacobs L. Screening for multiple sclerosis cognitive impairment using a self-administered 15-item questionnaire. Mult Scler. 2003;9(1):95–101.

16. Polman CH, Reingold SC, Banwell B, Clanet M, Cohen JA, Filippi M, Fujihara K, Havrdova E, Hutchinson M, Kappos L, Lublin FD, Montalban X, O'Connor P, Sandberg-Wollheim M, Thompson AJ, Waubant E, Weinshenker B, Wolinsky JS. Diagnostic criteria for multiple sclerosis: 2010 revisions to the McDonald criteria. Ann Neurol. 2011;69(2):292–302.

17. Kurtzke JF. Rating neurologic impairment in multiple sclerosis: an expanded disability status scale (EDSS). Neurology. 1983;33(11):1444–52.

18. Goretti B, Niccolai C, Hakiki B, Sturchio A, Falautano M, Minacapelli E, Martinelli V, Incerti C, Nocentini U, Murgia M, Fenu G, Cocco E, Marrosu MG, Garofalo E, Ambra FI, Maddestra M, Consalvo M, Viterbo RG, Trojano M, Losignore NA, Pietrolongo E, Lugaresi A, Langdon D, Portaccio E, Amato MP. The brief international cognitive assessment for multiple sclerosis (BICAMS): normative values with gender, age and education corrections in the Italian population. BMC Neurol. 2014;14:171.

19. Zung WWK. The measurement of affects: depression and anxiety. Mod Probl Pharmacopsychiatry. 1974;7:170–88. https://doi.org/10.1159/000395075.

20. Dunstan DA, Scott N, Todd AK. Screening for anxiety and depression: reassessing the utility of the Zung scales. BMC Psychiatry. 2017;17(1):329. https://doi.org/10.1186/s12888-017-1489-6.

21. Nucci M, Mapelli D, Mondini S. Cognitive reserve index questionnaire (CRIq): a new instrument for measuring cognitive reserve. Aging Clin Exp Res. 2012; 24(3):218–26.

22. Fenu G, Lorefice L, Arru M, et al. Cognition in multiple sclerosis: between cognitive reserve and brain volume. J Neurol Sci. 2018;386:19–22.

23. Strober LB, Binder A, Nikelshpur OM, Chiaravalloti N, DeLuca J. The perceived deficits questionnaire: perception, deficit, or distress? Int J MS Care. 2016;18(4):183–90.

24. Benedict RH, Cox D, Thompson LL, Foley F, Weinstock-Guttman B, Munschauer F. Reliable screening for neuropsychological impairment in multiple sclerosis. Mult Scler. 2004;10(6):675–8.

25. Romero K, Shammi P, Feinstein A. Neurologists' accuracy in predicting cognitive impairment in multiple sclerosis. Mult Scler Relat Disord. 2015;4(4): 291–5. https://doi.org/10.1016/j.msard.2015.05.009 Epub 27 May 2015.

26. Julian L, Merluzzi NM, Mohr DC. The relationship among depression, subjective cognitive impairment, and neuropsychological performance in multiple sclerosis. Mult Scler. 2007;13(1):81–6.

27. Sundgren M, Maurex L, Wahlin Å, Piehl F, Brismar T. Cognitive impairment has a strong relation to nonsomatic symptoms of depression in relapsing-remitting multiple sclerosis. Arch Clin Neuropsychol. 2013;28(2):144–55. https://doi.org/10.1093/arclin/acs113 Epub 2013 Jan 4. PubMed PMID: 23291310.

28. Niccolai C, Portaccio E, Goretti B, Hakiki B, Giannini M, Pastò L, Righini I, Falautano M, Minacapelli E, Martinelli V, Incerti C, Nocentini U, Fenu G, Cocco E, Marrosu MG, Garofalo E, Ambra FI, Maddestra M, Consalvo M, Viterbo RG, Trojano M, Losignore NA, Zimatore GB, Pietrolongo E, Lugaresi A, Pippolo L, Roscio M, Ghezzi A, Castellano D, Stecchi S, Amato MP. A comparison of the brief international cognitive assessment for multiple sclerosis and the brief repeatable battery in multiple sclerosis patients. BMC Neurol. 2015;15:204.

18

A case of Alemtuzumab-induced neutropenia in multiple sclerosis in association with the expansion of large granular lymphocytes

A. G. Vakrakou[1*], D. Tzanetakos[1], S. Valsami[2], E. Grigoriou[3], K. Psarra[3], J. Tzartos[1], M. Anagnostouli[1], E. Andreadou[1], M. E. Evangelopoulos[1], G. Koutsis[1], C. Chrysovitsanou[1], E. Gialafos[1], A. Dimitrakopoulos[1], L. Stefanis[1] and C. Kilidireas[1]

Abstract

Background: Alemtuzumab has been demonstrated to reduce the risks of relapse and accumulation of sustained disability in Multiple Sclerosis (MS) patients compared to β-interferon. It acts against CD52, leading primarily to lymphopenia. Recent data have shown that mild neutropenia is observed in 16% of treated MS-patients whereas severe neutropenia occurred in 0.6%.

Case presentation: Herein, we present the case of a 34-year-old woman with relapsing-remitting MS, with a history of treatment with glatiramer acetate and natalizumab, who subsequently received Alemtuzumab (12 mg / 24 h × 5 days). 70-days after the last Alemtuzumab administration, the patient displayed neutropenia (500 neutrophils/μL) with virtual absence of B-cells (0.6% of total lymphocytes), low values of CD4-T-cells (6.6%) and predominance of CD8-T-cells (48%) and NK-cells (47%); while large granular lymphocytes (LGL) predominated in the blood-smear examination. Due to prolonged neutropenia (5-days) the patient was placed on low-dose corticosteroids leading to sustained remission.

Conclusion: This is the first case of a patient with relapsing-remitting MS with neutropenia two months post-Alemtuzumab, with simultaneous presence of LGL cells in the blood and a robust therapeutic response to prednisolone. We recommend testing with a complete blood count every 15 days in the first 3 months after the 1st Alemtuzumab administration and searching for large granular lymphocytes cell expansion on microscopic examination of the peripheral blood if neutropenia develops.

Keywords: Multiple sclerosis, Alemtuzumab, Neutropenia, Large granular cells

Background

Alemtuzumab is a humanized monoclonal antibody directed against CD52, a surface glycoprotein with poorly understood role, that mainly is expressed on lymphocytes (B and T cells) and to a lesser magnitude on monocytes, macrophages and eosinophil granulocytes [1]. Mature natural killer (NK) cells, plasma cells, neutrophil granulocytes (neutrophils have approximately 22% the

CD52 of lymphocytes), and most importantly, hematological stem cells show little or no expression of CD52 [2]. Alemtuzumab leads to depletion of CD52-positive cells through antibody-dependent cell-mediated cytolysis (ADCC) and complement-dependent cytolysis (CDC) [1, 3]. Recent data from the literature have shown that mild neutropenia is not a rare manifestation in Alemtuzumab-treated MS patients, as approximately 16% of patients developed Grade-I and II neutropenia, yet in unclear time point from drug initiation (Table 1) [4]. Nevertheless, severe neutropenia occurred only in 0.6% of patients (Table 1). Out of these patients, two developed agranulocytosis; one of them was treated with

* Correspondence: avakrakou@med.uoa.gr
[1]1st Department of Neurology, Medical School of Athens, National & Kapodistrian University, Aeginition Hospital, Athens, Greece
Full list of author information is available at the end of the article

Table 1 Studies showing the incidence and characteristics of neutropenia following alemtuzumab - based therapy in MS patients

Study	Treatment	No of patients	Incidence of neutropenia	Grade of neutropenia	Median time to neutropenia	Median duration of neutropenia	Treatment	Comments
Coles AJ et al., 2012 [16]	1rst year of infusion (24 mg/d)	1/161	0,60%	NA	NA	NA	NA	Febrile neutropenia
Willis et al, 2016 [9]	NA	1/100	1%	NA	Median time to development of acquired autoimmune manifestations was 995 days following first treatment.	NA	NA	None
Gaitán MI et al., 2017 [5]	1rst year of infusion (12 mg/d)	1	case report	IV	4 weeks	3 days	Granulocyte-stimulating factor (300 mg/day for 72 h)	Responsive to 1 cycle of G-SCF, but developed HSV-1 infection that needed advanced antibiotics
Gaitán MI et al., 2017 [5]	1rst year of infusion (12 mg/d)	1	case report	IV-III (two episodes)	6 and 8 weeks (two episodes)	3	Granulocyte-stimulating factor (300 mg/day for 72 h)	Responsive to 2 cycles of G-SCF. Febrile neutropenia andsinusitis that needed iv antibiotics
Baker D et al., 2017 [4]	1rst year of infusion (12 mg/d)	127/811	15,70%	I-II	NA	NA		Data from CARE-MS I and CARE-MS II.
Baker D et al., 2017 [4]	1rst year of infusion (12 mg/d)	5/811	0,60%	III-IV	NA	NA	2 patients developed agranulocytosis,the first teated with PLEX and the other with lenograstim	Data from CARE-MS I and CARE-MS II.
Baker D et al., 2017 [4]	2nd year of infusion	104/808	12,90%	I-II	NA	NA		Data from CARE-MS I and CARE-MS II.
Baker D et al., 2017 [4]	2nd year of infusion	12/808	1,50%	III-IV	NA	NA		Data from CARE-MS I and CARE-MS II.
Vakrakou. et al., 2018 [17]	1rst year of infusion (12 mg/d)	1	case report	III	9 weeks	9 days	Prezolon (25 mg for 3 days and 12,5 mg for another 3 days)	LGL cells predominated in peripheral blood
Galgani S et al., 2018 [6]	1rst year of infusion (12 mg/d)	1	Case report	III/IV	1 month	2 weeks	Resolved spontaneously	

Plasma Exchange (PLEX) and the other with leno-grastim [4]. Another study reported that two patients with Grade-III/IV neutropenia were successfully treated with Granulocyte-Colony Stimulating Factor (G-CSF) (Table 1) [5]. Recently, Galgani et al. published a case report of asymptomatic Grade-III neutropenia detected 1 month after first Alemtuzumab course with spontaneous resolution (Table 1) [6]. None of above studies has proposed a mechanism for Alemtuzumab-induced neutropenia. Herein, we present a patient with relapsing-remitting MS with severe neutropenia 2 months post-Alemtuzumab with simultaneous presence of large granular cells in the blood and a robust therapeutic response to prednis-olone treatment. We are the first to propose an immunological mechanism for Alemtuzumab-induced neutropenia that merits further investigation in the future.

Case presentation

A 34-year-old female, diagnosed with relapsing-remitting MS since the age of 26, suffered from 2008 to 2013 from recurrent attacks of optic neuritis that partially responded to corticosteroid treatment. The patient was initially treated with glatiramer acetate for 2 years, and then switched to natalizumab (NTM) treatment due to significant clinical relapses. John Cunningham virus seropositivity developed while the patient was receiving NTM intravenously and treatment was discontinued after 24 months. The patient subsequently switched to Alemtuzumab therapy (12 mg/day for 5 days). At the day prior to Alemtuzumab-initiation she had a white blood cell (WBC) count of 14,500/μL (absolute neutrophil count [ANC], 10,900/μL; lymphocytes, 2300/μL) (Additional file 1: Table S1). 9 weeks (Day 65) after the first Alemtuzumab induction therapy, during the standard follow-up, complete blood count revealed severe neutropenia (Grade III)

(WBC count, 2000/μL; ANC, 899/μL) (Additional file 1: Table S1), a finding that led to her hospitalization. We tested for the presence of an underlying infection/pathology.

At the onset of neutropenia and throughout its duration, clinical, serological and ultrasonic investigation did not reveal any underlying pathology (Additional file 1: Table S1). At the onset of neutropenia, peripheral blood smear analysis (May-Grünwald-Giemsa staining) revealed numerous large granular cells (LGL cells) (approximately 80–90%) that had variable numbers of randomly distributed azurophilic granules in their cytoplasm (Fig. 1). Neutrophils with apoptotic features were rare. To further verify the nature of LGL cells, immunophenotypic analysis of peripheral blood was performed by flow cytometry. Such analysis showed marked elevation in the percentage of a specific cell-subset that belongs to the NK lineage [CD3-CD(16 + 56+): 47%] (Additional file 1: Table S1). Moreover, the percentage of CD3 + CD8+ T cells was found elevated compared to the baseline levels (before Alemtuzumab initiation). Of notice, the fold increase of CD3 + CD8+ T over baseline values (fold increase: 1.5) was less than that of NK-cells (fold increase: 3.2).

At the 70th day post-Alemtuzumab initiation, neutropenia was further exacerbated (ANC = 500 /μL). The occurrence of sustained neutropenia for at least 5 days underscored the need for therapeutic intervention. The patient was placed on corticosteroids (prednisolone 25 mg for 3 days and subsequent dose tapering) and 3 days after, the values of WBC and ANC started to rise, reached normal levels (fourth day) and remained stable for 2 months (Fig. 2). Neutropenia resolution is stable for at least 1 year of follow up. Peripheral blood smear analysis showed that LGL cells were markedly reduced (approximately 50%) after prednisolone initiation and were further diminished 1 month later. Flow cytometry analysis showed that the percentage of NK cells

remained increased (48%), whereas the percentage of CD3 + CD8+ showed a significant reduction compared to their levels upon neutropenia development (27.3% versus 48%) (Additional file 1: Table S1). The constellation of neutropenia, along with normal hemoglobin and platelet counts, the expansion in the peripheral blood of LGL cells, in the absence of a common infection, and the responsiveness to corticosteroids were highly suggestive of an ensuing immune-mediated mechanism for Alemtuzumab-induced neutropenia.

During the phase of neutropenia, our patient was in disease remission, with moderate neurologic disability and an EDSS = 2 (pyramidal signs, mild ataxia). We did not perform MRI scanning during the short phase of neutropenia because there was no any disease exacerbation and our patient did not exhibit any new neurological signs. No signs of radiological disease activity were evident during alemtuzumab treatment and as shown in Additional file 2: Figure S1, the lesion size and signal intensity was slightly reduced after 6-months of therapy. Our patient responded well to alemtuzumab, exhibited disease stabilization and was thereof, she was placed in a follow up with neurological examination and assessment of her hematological profile every 1-month, for at least 1 year. Due to prolonged disease remission and the resolution of neutropenia we have not switched to another disease-modifying drug yet.

Discussion and conclusions

Herein, we present an interesting case of a MS patient who, 2 months following Alemtuzumab treatment, displayed neutropenia with essentially no B cells and very low levels of CD4 T cells; there was a predominance of CD8 T and NK cells, while LGL cells predominated in the blood smear examination. The exact mechanism of early neutropenia associated with Alemtuzumab treatment is a challenging issue. In our case of neutropenia, direct toxic effects of Alemtuzumab on neutrophils are

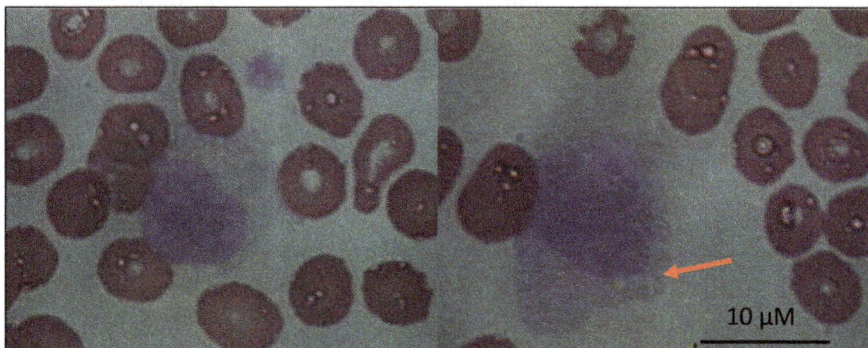

Fig. 1 Predominance of large granular lymphocytes in peripheral blood at the onset of Alemtuzumab-induced neutropenia. At the onset of neutropenia, peripheral blood smear analysis (Wright-Giemsa staining) revealed numerous large granular lymphocytes (LGL) (about 80–90%) that had azurophil granules in their cytoplasm (left image) and signs of cystic degeneration (right image, red arrow)

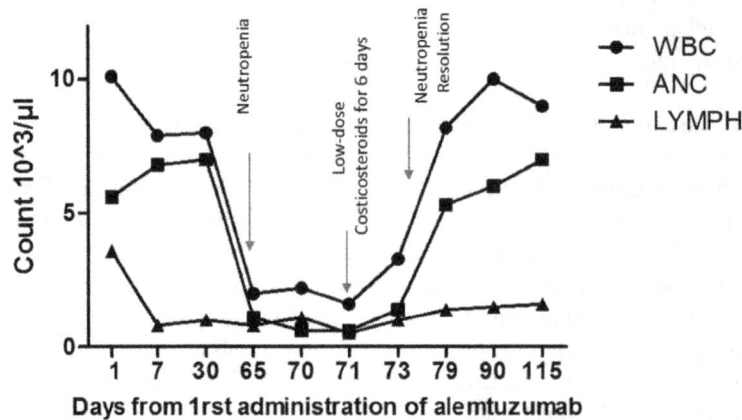

Fig. 2 Changes in blood count cells over time. Time points of neutropenia onset, therapeutic intervention and neutropenia resolution are indicated with red arrows. WBC; white blood cells, ANC; absolute neutrophil count, LYMPH; absolute lymphocyte count

unlikely. Consumption of complement constituents was not noted in the peripheral blood tests. The concept of autoimmune neutropenia, previously described in Alemtuzumab-treated MS patients (very rare), would seem an unlikely causative factor in our case, because such a manifestation would require a longer time interval from Alemtuzumab treatment [7]. Adverse events of Alemtuzumab treatment include infusion-related actions, infections, and secondary autoimmune disorders [8]. Neutropenia may also occur due to secondary autoimmunity after alemtuzumab [9]. The risk of developing secondary autoimmunity is greatest in the first 5 years of follow-up (mean time to development was 995 days following first treatment [9]. So, neutropenia is typically delayed and occurs after immune reconstitution [9]. The most intriguing feature of the present case concerns the expansion of the LGL cell population in the peripheral blood of this Alemtuzumab-treated MS patient. Immunophenotypic analysis showed that LGL cells are likely to be primarily NK and, to a lesser extent, CD8 T cells. Under healthy conditions, LGLs make up 5% to 15% of peripheral blood. LGL are characterized by elevated cytoplasmic:nuclear ratio and plenty azurophilic granules [10]. Initially, LGL were categorized in the lineage of natural killer (NK) cells. Nevertheless, it is now well-known that LGL comprise both cytotoxic T lymphocytes (CTL, CD3+) and NK cells (CD3-), both of which belong to the lymphoid lineage and act as principal mediators of cell-mediated cytotoxicity [10]. Polyclonal expansions of LGL have been observed in healthy elderly and are usually transient, after viral infections such as Epstein–Barr virus and cytomegalovirus, or associated with neoplasms and autoimmune disorders [11].

We suggest that LGL play an active role in the development of neutropenia in our case. Highly suggestive of the operation of an immune-mediated mechanism for the Alemtuzumab-induced neutropenia is the responsiveness

to corticosteroids. A short therapeutic protocol with low doses of prezolon led to a constant rise in neutrophil levels and to the normalization of white blood counts. This effect of corticosteroids was accompanied by a reduction in the levels of LGL in the peripheral blood and this effect was stable for at least of 1 month of close monitoring of our patient. Importantly, we performed immunophenotypic analysis of peripheral blood 1 month after the resolution of neutropenia. The percentage of NK cells remained increased, whereas the percentage of CD3 + CD8+ showed a significant reduction compared to their levels upon neutropenia development (Additional file 1: Table S1). This observation suggests that prednisolone treatment did not affect the survival of NK cells, but led to lympholysis of CD3 + CD8+ T cells and favored in overall the reconstitution of neutrophil numbers. This in turn suggests that such CD3 + CD8+ T cells were the main mediators of the neutropenic effect.

Our finding of neutropenia post-Alemtuzumab therapy in a setting of significant cytotoxic T cell-LGL proliferation is highly reminiscent of the potential role of the expanded LGL population in peripheral blood in the pathogenesis of Rituximab-induced neutropenia [12]. Late-onset neutropenia (LON) after rituximab was mainly reported in lymphoma-patients and occurred from 1 month up to 1 year after drug initiation. LGL phenotype has been shown to be associated with neutropenia through various mechanisms such as FAS\FAS ligand mediated neutrophil apoptosis, Fas\Fas ligand independent cytokine\chemokine-related myelosuppression and secretion of inflammatory mediators. Other proposed mechanisms include the presence of antineutrophil antibodies and the role of genetic polymorphisms in the immunoglobulin G (IgG) receptor FCγ RIIIA [13, 14]. An important recent study revealed that 6-months after alemtuzumab treatment CD56bright NK cells were expanded, albeit without alteration in their cytolytic function [15]. Of note, increased numbers of NK cells have also been observed in Hashimoto thyroiditis, which is considered to be a common autoimmune manifestation following alemtuzumab therapy. The exact mechanisms of autoimmunity following alemtuzumab therapy are not fully understood and immune reconstitution changes in cell repertoire could account for immune reactions against self. In this process, the role of CD56bright NK cells as well as cytotoxic CD8 T cells warrants further investigation.

In our patient, neutropenia was observed in a setting of normal hemoglobin level and platelet count (Additional file 1: Table S1), thus making the possibility of toxic (chemotherapy-related) or other (e.g. viral) underlying factors being responsible for our observations very remote. To our knowledge this if the first study to show the association of Alemtuzumab with LGL proliferation and neutropenia development. The exact triggering mechanism of LGL expansion is elusive until now. The present case indicates that clinicians should be aware of this particular side effect of Alemtuzumab, strongly implying the need of a close laboratory evaluation of patients after drug administration. Taken together, the results reported here challenge the currently published notion that severe Alemtuzumab-related neutropenia in the setting of MS should be treated with G-SCF. Considering the published data of the detrimental effect of G-SCF in MS disease evolution, we suggest prednisolone as an alternative therapeutic option. Therefore, we suggest complete blood count analysis every 15 days during the first 3 months following drug initiation and search for LGL cell expansion if neutropenia evolves. Moreover, we suggest early therapeutic intervention for Alemtuzumab-induced Grade-III neutropenia with low-dose corticosteroids.

Additional files

Additional file 1: Table S1. Table describing the hematological and serological profile of our patient with Alemtuzumab-induced neutropenia. Whole blood analysis, immunophenotypic analysis and serological analysis of parameters before, at the onset of neutropenia, throughout its duration and after neutropenia resolution.

Additional file 2: Figure S1. Brain MRI scanning for our patient before and after Alemtuzumab initiation. Brain MRI scanning revealed decline in lesion size and signal intensity 6-months after alemtuzumab initiation compared to baseline (2 months prior to alemtuzumab initiation).

Abbreviations

ADCC: Antibody-dependent cell-mediated cytolysis; ANC: Absolute neutrophil count; CDC: Complement-dependent cytolysis; CTL: Cytotoxic T lymphocytes; G-CSF: Granulocyte-Colony Stimulating Factor; LGL: Large granular lymphocytes; LON: Late onset neutropenia; MS: Multiple Sclerosis; NK: Natural killer cells; NTZ: Natalizumab; PLEX: Plasma exchange; RRMS: Relapsing remitting multiple sclerosis; WBC: White blood cells

Acknowledgements
The authors express their gratitude to the patient participating in the study.

Funding
No funding was obtained for the preparation of this case report.

Authors' contributions
VAG drafted the manuscript and reviewed the literature. VS performed the microscopic examination of the peripheral blood and took pictures. GE and PK performed flow cytometry in peripheral blood specimens and revised manuscript. TD and TJ analyzed the MRI, collected clinical data and revised the manuscript. AM, AE, EME, GE and KG contributed to obtaining and interpreting the clinical information and revised the manuscript. CC collected clinical data and revised manuscript. DA, AM, AE, and KC treated the case-patient at the Aeginition Hospital and critically revised the manuscript. SL, VS and KC participated in all parts of the review process and contributed to drafting of the article. VAG, SL, VS and KC provided substantial contributions to the conception or interpretation of data. All authors read and approved the final version of the manuscript and agreed to be accountable for all aspects of the work.

Competing interests
The authors declare that they have no competing interests.

Author details
[1]1st Department of Neurology, Medical School of Athens, National & Kapodistrian University, Aeginition Hospital, Athens, Greece. [2]Department of Blood Transfusion, Medical School of Athens, National & Kapodistrian University, Aretaieion Hospital, Athens, Greece. [3]Immunology and Histocompatibility Department, Evangelismos Hospital, Athens, Greece.

References
1. Ruck T, Bittner S, Wiendl H, Meuth SG. Alemtuzumab in multiple sclerosis: mechanism of action and beyond. Int J Mol Sci. 2015;16(7):16414–39.
2. Ambrose LR, Morel AS, Warrens AN. Neutrophils express CD52 and exhibit complement-mediated lysis in the presence of alemtuzumab. Blood. 2009; 114(14):3052–5.
3. Cohen JA, Coles AJ, Arnold DL, Confavreux C, Fox EJ, Hartung HP, et al. Alemtuzumab versus interferon beta 1a as first-line treatment for patients with relapsing-remitting multiple sclerosis: a randomised controlled phase 3 trial. Lancet (London England). 2012;380(9856):1819–28.
4. Baker D, Giovannoni G, Schmierer K. Marked neutropenia: significant but rare in people with multiple sclerosis after alemtuzumab treatment. Mult Scler Relat Disord. 2017;18:181–3.
5. Gaitan MI, Ysrraelit MC, Correale J. Neutropenia in patients with multiple sclerosis treated with Alemtuzumab. JAMA Neurol. 2017;74(9):1143–4.
6. Galgani S, Prosperini L, Haggiag S, Tortorella C, Gasperini C. Early transient asymptomatic neutropenia associated with alemtuzumab treatment in multiple sclerosis: a case report. J Neurol. 2018;265(9):2152–3.
7. Katsavos S, Coles A. Alemtuzumab as treatment for multiple sclerosis. Cold Spring Harb Perspect Med. 2018;8(10). https://doi.org/10.1101/cshperspect. a032029.
8. Sauer EM, Schliep S, Manger B, Lee DH, Linker RA. Microscopic polyangiitis after alemtuzumab treatment in relapsing-remitting MS. Neurol(R) Neuroimmunology Neuroinflammation. 2018;5(5):e488.
9. Willis MD, Harding KE, Pickersgill TP, Wardle M, Pearson OR, Scolding NJ, Robertson NP. Alemtuzumab for multiple sclerosis: long term follow-up in a multi-Centre cohort. Mult Scler (Houndmills, Basingstoke, England). 2016; 22(9):1215–23.
10. O'Malley DP. T-cell large granular leukemia and related proliferations. Am J Clin Pathol. 2007;127(6):850–9.
11. Zambello R, Teramo A, Gattazzo C, Semenzato G. Are T-LGL leukemia and NK-chronic Lymphoproliferative disorder really two distinct diseases? Transl Med @ UniSa. 2014;8:4–11.

12. Grant C, Wilson WH, Dunleavy K. Neutropenia associated with rituximab therapy. Curr Opin Hematol. 2011;18(1):49–54.

13. Wolach O, Bairey O, Lahav M. Late-onset neutropenia after rituximab treatment: case series and comprehensive review of the literature. Medicine. 2010;89(5):308–18.

14. Pontikoglou C, Kalpadakis C, Papadaki HA. Pathophysiologic mechanisms and management of neutropenia associated with large granular lymphocytic leukemia. Expert Rev Hematol. 2011;4(3):317–28.

15. Gross CC, Ahmetspahic D, Ruck T, Schulte-Mecklenbeck A, Schwarte K, Jorgens S, et al. Alemtuzumab treatment alters circulating innate immune cells in multiple sclerosis. Neurol(R) Neuroimmunology Neuroinflammation. 2016;3(6):e289.

16. Coles AJ, Twyman CL, Arnold DL, Cohen JA, Confavreux C, Fox EJ, Hartung HP, Havrdova E, Selmaj KW, Weiner HL, Miller T, Fisher E, Sandbrink R, Lake SL, Margolin DH, Oyuela P, Panzara MA, Compston DA; CARE-MS II investigators. Alemtuzumab for patients with relapsing multiple sclerosis after disease-modifying therapy: a randomised controlled phase 3 trial. Lancet. 2012;380(9856):1829–39.

17. Vakrakou AG, Tzanetakos D, Valsami S, Grigoriou E, Psarra K, Tzartos J, Anagnostouli M, Andreadou E, Evangelopoulos ME, Koutsis G, Chrysovitsanou C, Gialafos E, Dimitrakopoulos A, Stefanis L, Kilidireas C. A case of Alemtuzumab- induced neutropenia in multiple sclerosis in association with the expansion of large granular lymphocytes. BMC Neurology, 2018.

19

Structural MRI correlates of PASAT performance in multiple sclerosis

Jordi A. Matias-Guiu[1]*(iD), Ana Cortés-Martínez[1], Paloma Montero[1], Vanesa Pytel[1], Teresa Moreno-Ramos[1], Manuela Jorquera[2], Miguel Yus[2], Juan Arrazola[2] and Jorge Matías-Guiu[1]

Abstract

Background: The Paced Auditory Serial Addition Test (PASAT) is a useful cognitive test in patients with multiple sclerosis (MS), assessing sustained attention and information processing speed. However, the neural underpinnings of performance in the test are controversial. We aimed to study the neural basis of PASAT performance by using structural magnetic resonance imaging (MRI) in a series of 242 patients with MS.

Methods: PASAT (3-s) was administered together with a comprehensive neuropsychological battery. Global brain volumes and total T2-weighted lesion volumes were estimated. Voxel-based morphometry and lesion symptom mapping analyses were performed.

Results: Mean PASAT score was 42.98 ± 10.44; results indicated impairment in 75 cases (31.0%). PASAT score was correlated with several clusters involving the following regions: bilateral precuneus and posterior cingulate, bilateral caudate and putamen, and bilateral cerebellum. Voxel-based lesion symptom mapping showed no significant clusters. Region of interest–based analysis restricted to white matter regions revealed a correlation with the left cingulum, corpus callosum, bilateral corticospinal tracts, and right arcuate fasciculus. Correlations between PASAT scores and global volumes were weak.

Conclusion: PASAT score was associated with regional volumes of the posterior cingulate/precuneus and several subcortical structures, specifically the caudate, putamen, and cerebellum. This emphasises the role of both cortical and subcortical structures in cognitive functioning and information processing speed in patients with MS.

Keywords: Cognitive impairment, Multiple sclerosis, PASAT, Voxel-based lesion symptom mapping, Voxel-based morphometry

Background

The Paced Auditory Serial Addition Test (PASAT) is a useful cognitive tool with high sensitivity to sustained attention and information processing speed alterations [1]. It is one of the most frequently employed neuropsychological tests in patients with multiple sclerosis (MS), as it has been added to several widely used batteries in this setting, such as the Brief Repeatable Neuropsychological Battery (BRN-B), the Minimal Assessment of Cognitive Function in Multiple Sclerosis, and the Multiple Sclerosis Functional Composite scale [2–4].

In PASAT, patients have to add 60 pairs of digits by adding each digit to the immediately preceding one. Digits are usually presented every 3 s [1]. PASAT is considered to be a difficult and sometimes very stressful test, requiring a high level of concentration. However, it is highly sensitive to cognitive decline in patients with MS and has been found to be useful for evaluating information processing speed [5].

Although it is widely used for assessing MS, the neural basis of PASAT performance continues to be debated. Several previous articles have determined the correlation between PASAT performance and total brain volume and/or T2-weighted lesion volume [6]; but few studies have addressed the specific brain regions associated with the test. In this regard, Morgen et al. [7] correlated PASAT performance with atrophy of the prefrontal

* Correspondence: jordimatiasguiu@hotmail.com; jordi.matias-guiu@salud.madrid.org
[1]Department of Neurology, San Carlos Health Research Institute (IdISSC), Universidad Complutense de Madrid, C/ Profesor Martín Lagos s/n, 28040 Madrid, Spain
Full list of author information is available at the end of the article

cortex, precentral gyrus, superior parietal cortex and right cerebellum in a study of 19 patients with MS and 19 controls. Sbardella et al. [8] correlated PASAT performance with the orbitofrontal cortex, and white matter tracts located in the corpus callosum, internal capsule, thalamic radiations, and cerebral peduncles. In contrast, Nocentini et al. [9] found no significant correlations between PASAT performance and brain regions in a cohort of 18 patients with MS. And very recently, Riccitelli et al. [10] found correlations between PASAT performance and atrophy of grey matter nuclei and several fronto-temporo-occipital regions in a large cohort of 177 patients with MS.

Neuropsychological tests are standardised tools used to evaluate different cognitive functions, each of which has more or less specific neural underpinnings. Understanding the neural basis of a cognitive test may improve our interpretation of test results in clinical practice [11]. This is especially relevant in MS due to the multifocal nature of the disease, which constitutes a challenge in the interpretation of neuropsychological assessments; and in the particular case of PASAT, which probably involves several cognitive functions [5].

Our aim was to study the neural basis of PASAT performance in a large series of 242 patients with MS. We used structural magnetic resonance imaging (MRI) to estimate global brain volumes and performed a voxel-based morphometry and lesion symptom mapping analysis in order to identify the relationship between PASAT performance and global and regional brain atrophy and white matter lesions.

Methods
Study population and ethics
The study included patients meeting the revised McDonald criteria for MS [12]. We excluded patients with other causes of cognitive impairment besides MS, such as other neurological (e.g. stroke, brain tumour), medical (e.g. cancer, B_{12} vitamin deficiency), or psychiatric disorders (e.g. major depression, bipolar disorder, psychosis). Our hospital's Ethics Committee approved the research protocol; written consent was obtained from all participants.

Neuropsychological assessment
PASAT was administered according to the manual by a trained neuropsychologist. The stimulus was presented using an audiotape. Single digits were presented every 3 s. The total number of correct responses was recorded. Results were considered to represent impairment when the number of correct responses was > 1.5 standard deviations (SD) below the mean according to age- and education-adjusted normative data from our setting [13].

The patients were also examined using a comprehensive, co-normed battery assessing the main cognitive functions. This battery has been described elsewhere [14] and includes the following tests: forward and backward digit span, Corsi block-tapping test, Trail Making Test (TMT) parts A and B, Symbol Digit Modalities Test (written version) (SDMT), Boston Naming Test (BNT), Judgement of Line Orientation (JLO), Rey-Osterrieth Complex Figure (ROCF) (copy and recall at 3 and 30 min), Free and Cued Selective Reminding Test (FCSRT), verbal fluencies (animals and words beginning with "p", "m", and "r" in 1 min), Stroop Color Word Interference Test, and Tower of London-Drexel version (ToL) [15]. The Beck Depression Inventory and the Fatigue Severity Scale were also administered [16, 17].

MRI acquisition, preprocessing, and analysis
MRI was acquired using a 1.5 T scanner (Signa HDxt, GE Healthcare, Milwaukee, USA) including these sequences: a) T1-weighted 3D fast spoiled gradient-echo inversion recovery (repetition time [TR] 12 ms, echo time [TE] 2.3 ms, inversion time [TI] 400 ms; slice thickness 1 mm in 78 cases (32.2%) and 3 mm in 164 patients (67.8%); b) T2-weighted fluid-attenuated inversion recovery (FLAIR) (TR 9102 ms, TE 121 ms, TI 2260 ms; slice thickness 3 mm); c) T2-weighted double-echo fast spin-echo (FSE) (TR 2620 ms, TE 15/90 ms); d) T1-weighted post-contrast FSE sequence (TR 640 ms, TE 11.8 ms) following injection of gadoteric acid.

Image preprocessing and analysis were conducted using Statistical Parametric Mapping 8 (SPM8) (The Wellcome Trust Centre for Neuroimaging, Institute of Neurology, University College of London, UK) and the associated VBM8 and Lesion Segmentation Tool (LST) toolboxes [18]. LST is designed specifically for MS and performs a semi-automatic segmentation of T2-hyperintense white matter lesions using 3D-T1 and FLAIR sequences via a lesion-growth algorithm, in addition to lesion filling on T1-weighted images. Subsequently, 3D-T1 images were segmented into grey matter, white matter, and cerebrospinal fluid compartments, then normalised to the standard space of the Montreal Neurological Institute using the DARTEL template. Finally, images were smoothed at 8 mm full-width at half maximum. Preprocessing was performed blind to neuropsychological assessment data. Two expert neuroradiologists (MJ and MY) assessed the images and JAM-G conducted the statistical image analysis.

We calculated partial correlations between PASAT raw score and normalised brain volumes (white matter and grey matter fractions) and lesion burden, controlling for age, sex, and years of education. A multiple regression analysis was performed to estimate which brain regions were correlated with PASAT performance (raw score), using a voxel-based morphometry procedure with SPM8. Age, years of schooling, sex, protocol of 3D-T1 weighted acquisition, and total intracranial volume were included in the statistical model as nuisance covariates. In an additional analysis, depression was also added as a covariate. A false-discovery rate of $P < 0.05$ was considered statistically significant at cluster level. A minimum cluster size k = 100 was also used to avoid the multiple comparisons problem.

Normalised lesion maps of T2-hyperintense lesions detected in FLAIR sequences were smoothed at 8 mm full width at half maximum and then used to perform voxel- and region of interest (ROI)-based lesion symptom mapping. Voxel-based or ROI-based lesion symptom mapping is a method to analyse the relationship between localization of brain damage and a behaviour, which has been successfully used in cognitive neuroscience to advance in the identification of critical regions or networks for specific brain functions [19]. The "NiiStat" MATLAB® toolbox (9 October 2016 version) was used for these analyses [20]. The CAT atlas was used for the definition of white-matter ROIs [21]. Age, sex, and years of formal education were included as nuisance covariates. A minimum overlap of 15 subjects was considered, and 10,000 permutations were calculated to correct for multiple comparisons, using a P-value of < 0.05 as threshold.

Statistical analysis

Descriptive results are shown as frequencies (percentages), means ± SD, or medians (interquartile ranges), as appropriate. The chi-square and two-sample t tests were used for comparisons between 2 independent samples. Correlations between PASAT performance and other quantitative variables were calculated using Pearson's coefficient. A P-value of < 0.05 was considered statistically significant.

Statistical analysis was performed using the IBM® SPSS statistics package, version 20.0.

Results

Demographic, cognitive, and MRI variables

The 242 patients in the sample comprised 164 women (67.8%) and 78 men (32.2%) with a mean age of 45.35 ± 8.97 and 16.14 ± 2.89 years of schooling. According to clinical form of MS, 195 (80.6%) had relapsing-remitting, 30 (12.4%) secondary progressive, and 17 (7.0%) primary progressive MS. Median Expanded Disability Status Scale (EDSS) score was 2.0 (1–3.5).

Mean PASAT score was 42.98 ± 10.44 (range 16–60); scores were > 1.5 SD below the mean in 75 (31.0%) cases. There were no significant differences between patients with and without impairment in PASAT performance in terms of age (45.09 ± 9.1 vs 45.47 ± 8.93, $t = -0.303$, $P = 0.762$), EDSS score (2.48 ± 1.81 vs 2.35 ± 1.87, $t = 0.501$, $P = 0.617$), T2 lesion load (14.291 ± 16.992 vs 10.861 ± 12.440, $t = 1.57$,

$P = 0.118$), and normalised grey matter volume (0.42 ± 0.03 vs 0.42 ± 0.02, $t = 0.133$, $P = 0.894$). Level of schooling was slightly higher in the group with PASAT scores > 1.5 SD below the mean (16.95 ± 2.25 vs 15.77 ± 3.08, $t = 3.33$, $P = 0.001$).

PASAT performance was significantly correlated with most of the other cognitive tests. However, the size of the correlation was at least moderate ($r > 0.4$) with only the following tests: TMT-B ($r = -0.464$, $P < 0.0001$), SDMT ($r = 0.416$, $P < 0.0001$), Stroop part B ($r = 0.464$, $P < 0.0001$), Stroop part C ($r = 0.490$, $P < 0.0001$), semantic verbal fluency ($r = 0.408$, $P < 0.0001$), phonemic verbal fluency "p" and "m" words ($r = 0.444$, $P < 0.0001$; $r = 0.406$, $P < 0.0001$, respectively). Correlations with the other tests were as follows (all $P < 0.0001$): digit span forward ($r = 0.246$), digit span backward ($r = 0.310$), Corsi test forward ($r = 0.362$), Corsi test backward ($r = 0.367$), TMT-A ($r = -0.354$), Boston Naming Test ($r = 0.293$), ROCF copy accuracy ($r = 0.366$), ROCF memory at 3 min ($r = 0.296$), ROCF memory at 30 min ($r = 0.349$), FCSRT free recall 1 ($r = 0.250$), FCSRT total recall ($r = 0.238$), FCSRT delayed free recall ($r = 0.319$), FCSRT delayed total recall ($r = 0.273$), Stroop part A ($r = 0.384$), Tower of London correct moves ($r = 0.358$), and Judgement Line Orientation ($r = 0.349$). Regarding depression and fatigue, correlation with Beck Depression Inventory and Fatigue Severity Scale was $r = -0.233$ ($P < 0.0001$) and $r = -0.156$ ($P = 0.015$), respectively.

Correlation with MRI global measures

PASAT raw score correlated negatively with white matter lesion volume ($r = -0.186$, $P = 0.004$), and positively with grey matter volume ($r = 0.272$, $P < 0.0001$), white matter volume ($r = 0.244$, $P < 0.0001$), and total intracranial volume ($r = 0.250$, $P < 0.0001$). However, it was not correlated with normalised grey matter volume ($r = 0.026$, $P = 0.688$) or normalised white matter volume ($r = 0.118$, $P = 0.068$).

Voxel-based morphometry results: Multiple regression analysis

Voxel-based morphometry analysis showed that PASAT performance correlated with several clusters involving the following regions: bilateral precuneus and posterior cingulate, bilateral caudate and putamen, and bilateral anterior and posterior cerebellum (Table 1, Fig. 1). When controlling also depression scale as a covariate, results were very similar, showing an association of PASAT with several clusters involving precuneus/posterior cingulate, caudate/putamen, and cerebellum (Additional file 1).

Voxel- and ROI-based lesion symptom mapping

Voxel-based lesion symptom mapping did not show any significant clusters. ROI-based analysis restricted

Table 1 Voxel-based morphometry analysis. Multiple regression analysis showing correlations between PASAT and brain regions, using age, sex, years of education, and total intracranial volume as covariates. FDR corrected *p*-value < 0.05, k = 100

Brain region (Brodmann area)	MNI coordinates			T value	Z score	Cluster-level *p*-value (FWE corrected)	Peak-level *p*-value (FDR-corrected)	K (number of voxels)
	x	y	z					
Left and right precuneus and posterior cingulate [7, 31]	−4	−48	45	5.53	5.36	< 0.0001	0.003	5556
	4	−39	43	5.04	4.91		0.003	
	18	−64	16	4.39	4.30		0.007	
Right insula [13], caudate and putamen	34	2	−3	5.30	5.15	< 0.0001	0.003	3972
	40	−18	9	3.99	3.92		0.0014	
	18	16	−12	3.34	3.30		0.0046	
Right cerebellum (anterior and posterior lobes)	24	−57	−12	5.19	5.04	< 0.0001	0.003	2719
	24	−46	−12	5.02	4.89		0.003	
	39	−58	−14	3.87	3.81		0.018	
Left insula [13], caudate and putamen	−32	3	−3	4.70	4.59	< 0.0001	0.004	3548
	−27	14	1	4.24	4.16		0.009	
	−22	21	3	4.19	4.11		0.010	
Left cerebellum (anterior lobe)	−27	−49	−24	4.43	4.34	0.013	0.006	1375
Left thalamus	−2	−19	15	3.91	3.84	0.532	0.017	324

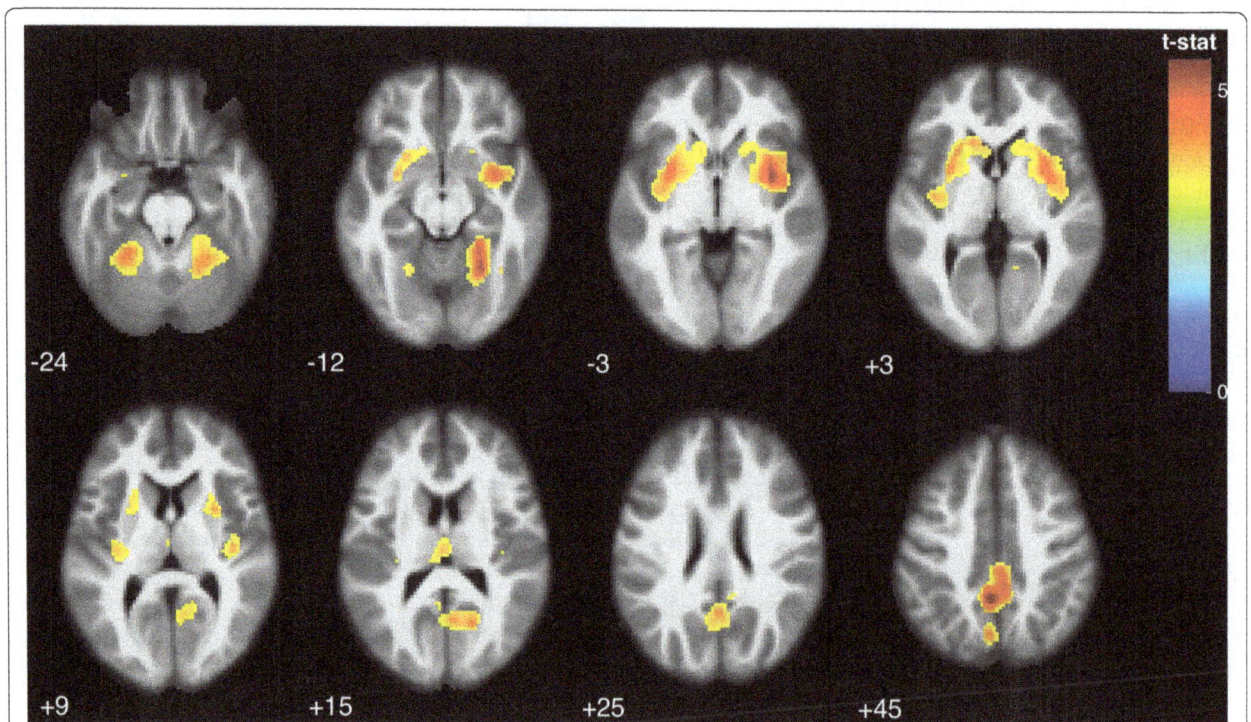

Fig. 1 Statistical parametric map showing brain regions positively correlated with PASAT performance (FDR *p* < 0.05, k = 100), rendered on MRI template with neurological orientation

to white matter regions showed five regions surviving the previously defined threshold: the left cingulum, corpus callosum, bilateral corticospinal tracts, and right arcuate fasciculus. When T2 total lesion volume was added to the statistical model as a regressor, no ROI reached statistical significance.

Discussion

In this study, we used voxel-based morphometry and lesion symptom mapping methods to explore MRI correlates of PASAT performance in MS. Poorer performance was correlated with atrophy of several brain regions including the posterior cingulate and precuneus, caudate, putamen, and cerebellum. Previous studies analysing correlation with brain atrophy at the regional level have found conflicting results (see Table 2 for a summary of these studies) [22–24]. However, these studies generally included relatively small samples. In contrast, a recent large study by Riccitelli et al. [10] found PASAT performance to be correlated with atrophy of the bilateral thalamus, caudate and putamen, the right anterior cingulate, right superior frontal gyrus, and the right precentral, left superior temporal, and right fusiform gyri. Our study also found a correlation with the basal ganglia, as well as with the cerebellum and, interestingly, with the posterior cingulate and precuneus. The posterior cingulate/precuneus is a central node within the default mode network, and functional MRI analysis has demonstrated posterior cingulate and precuneus atrophy to be a good predictor of default mode network dysfunction in patients with MS [25]. Furthermore, some of the regions observed by Riccitelli et al. also belong to the default mode network; and this network has been associated with PASAT performance in fMRI studies [10, 26].

In addition, we also observed a significant correlation between PASAT performance and 3 subcortical regions: caudate, putamen, and cerebellum. This emphasises the role of the basal ganglia and cerebellum in cognitive disorders in MS [27], and specifically in PASAT performance. The role of subcortical structures in cognitive disorders is increasingly recognised, with several structures participating in cognitive and behavioural functions through their connections with the cortex [28].

Table 2 Main studies evaluating the correlation between PASAT performance and MRI measures in multiple sclerosis

Author/year	Number of patients	MRI measures	Main results
Morgen et al., 2006 [7]	19 RRMS	T1	Correlation with bilateral prefrontal cortex, precentral gyrus, superior parietal cortex and right cerebellum
Dineen et al., 2009 [25]	37 MS	DTI (TBSS)	Correlation with fractional anisotropy in corpus callosum, parieto-occipital radiations of the forceps major, left cingulum, right inferior longitudinal fasciculus, left superior longitudinal fasciculus, and bilateral arcuate fasciculi
Sepulcre et al., 2009 [29]	54 MS	T2 (VLSM)	Correlation with bilateral parieto-frontal, centrum semiovale, temporo-occipital white matter, internal capsule, right pontomesencephalic tegmentum, right cerebellar peduncle, and right anterior cingulate
Van Hecke et al., 2010 [26]	20 MS	DTI	Correlation with fractional anisotropy in left inferior longitudinal fasciculus, forceps minor, internal and external capsule, corpus callosum, left cingulum, superior longitudinal fasciculus, and corona radiate
Nocentini et al., 2012 [9]	18 MS	T1	No significant correlations
Yu et al., 2012 [27]	37 RRMS	DTI	Correlation with reduced fractional anisotropy in sagittal striatum, posterior thalamic radiation, and external capsule
Sbardella et al., 2013 [8]	36 RRMS	T1 and DTI	Correlation with orbitofrontal cortex, and white matter tracts including the corpus callosum, internal capsule, posterior thalamic radiations, and cerebral peduncles
D'haeseleer et al., 2013 [30]	18 MS	Arterial spin labelling	Correlation between PASAT performance and cerebral blood flow in the left centrum semiovale
Baltruschat et al., 2015 [31]	17 RRMS	T1 and fMRI	No significant correlation between PASAT performance and functional connectivity in the MS group
Riccitelli et al., 2017 [10]	177 RRMS	T1 (VBM) and DTI (TBSS)	Correlation with atrophy of the bilateral thalamus, caudate and putamen, right anterior cingulate, right superior frontal gyrus, and right precentral, left superior temporal, and right fusiform gyri. Correlation with reduced fractional anisotropy and increased mean diffusivity in several white matter tracts
Present study	242 MS	T1 (VBM) and FLAIR (VLSM)	Correlation with bilateral precuneus and posterior cingulate, bilateral caudate and putamen, and bilateral anterior cerebellum

RRMS relapsing-remitting multiple sclerosis, *MS* multiple sclerosis, *DTI* diffusion tensor imaging, *TBSS* tract-based spatial statistics, *VLSM* voxel-based lesion symptom mapping; *fMRI* functional magnetic resonance imaging, *VBM* voxel-based morphometry, *FLAIR* fluid-attenuated inversion recovery

Lesion symptom mapping found several regions associated with poorer PASAT performance. In this regard, white matter lesions in the left cingulum, corpus callosum, corticospinal tract, and arcuate fasciculus were associated with poorer performance. These findings are similar to those of previous studies using diffusion tensor imaging (DTI), where multiple white matter tracts were associated with PASAT performance [8, 10, 29, 30]. Interestingly, whole-brain voxel-based analysis did not show any significant results, and ROI-based analyses lost statistical significance when total white matter lesion volume was included as a covariate in the statistical model. This may suggest that PASAT performance is influenced to a greater extent by the total lesion volume than by specific lesions in particular white matter regions and tracts. Analogously, previous studies using DTI have also found white matter impairment to have a secondary role in PASAT performance, in comparison to grey matter atrophy [10, 31].

Regarding whole-brain measures, our study found significant associations between PASAT performance and total white matter lesion volume, and raw grey and white matter volumes, but not normalised brain volumes. Although some correlations were statistically significant, the size of the correlation was small. This suggests a minor influence of these MRI measures in cognitive test performance, and statistical significance may be probably explained because of the large sample size included in this study. Previous studies have found conflicting results; a meta-analysis conducted in 2014 could not establish a definitive conclusion regarding the correlation between whole MRI findings and PASAT performance due to missing data and the heterogeneity of the studies [6]. Therefore, our findings, with a weak or non-significant correlation, support the search of brain regions as a better approach to explaining the pathophysiology of impaired PASAT performance and, thus, of impairment of the cognitive functions involved in the performance of this test in MS. However, the correlation between PASAT and global brain volumes could also be interpreted as a role of brain reserve in maintaining PASAT performance, as has been suggested previously [32].

In our study, PASAT results showed impairment in 31% of patients, a similar percentage to that found in previous studies [2, 10]. PASAT performance was correlated with most of tests of the neuropsychological battery examining several cognitive domains. This confirms the usefulness of PASAT as a general test in MS that may be applied as a neuropsychological screening test. However, the size of the correlation with most tests of memory, language, visuospatial functioning etc. was generally low. Conversely, PASAT was moderately correlated with several time-dependent neuropsychological tests, especially those associated to attention and executive functioning. Regarding fatigue and depression, the correlation with PASAT was low. This weak correlation suggests that fatigue and depression has a little influence in PASAT performance and, thus, impairment in this test is more related to cognitive issues than non-cognitive factors. Indeed, VBM analysis controlling for depression displayed the same brain regions associated to the PASAT performance.

PASAT involves several cognitive functions, including auditory perception and processing, speech production, mathematical abilities, working memory, several components of attention and concentration, processing capacity, and information processing speed [5, 33]. This suggests that PASAT, like almost all neuropsychological tests, should not be considered a measure of a single cognitive function (i.e. information processing speed) [5]. In the specific setting of MS, our results suggest that PASAT performance is associated with the status of several brain regions (posterior cingulate/precuneus, basal ganglia, and cerebellum), probably involved in the fronto-subcortical and default mode networks. White matter lesions may contribute to pathophysiology, but we could not find specific localisations associated with performance in the test. Overall, our findings support the status of PASAT as a test associated with information processing speed, among others cognitive functions. However, because correlation with other time-dependent neuropsychological tasks was moderate, information processing speed should not be regarded as a unitary concept. From this perspective, PASAT may be a measure of the efficiency of cognitive effort and concentration during a high-demand attentional task requiring the preservation of both cortical and subcortical structures; information processing speed may represent the level of efficiency that the patient achieves.

Our study has some limitations. Firstly, we included only 3D T1-weighted and FLAIR sequences, but not such other sequences of interest as DTI or fMRI. Thus, hypotheses about the brain networks involved in the execution of the test are speculative. Although we use findings from previous studies using these techniques, a multimodal MRI study of the same sample would be highly informative. Secondly, we included only patients who completed the PASAT, which may represent a selection bias. However, due to the large sample size and the clinical and demographic characteristics of the sample, we believe that our cohort of patients is representative of MS. Another interesting future point would be to examine the neural correlates of PASAT performance in each form of MS, in order to search potential differences between relapsing remitting and progressive variants [34]. Finally, our study has a cross-sectional design. Longitudinal studies may be of interest to better understand the dynamics of cognitive dysfunction in patients with MS.

Conclusions

Our study suggests that, on the one hand, the neural basis of PASAT performance involves the posterior cingulate/precuneus, probably associated with default mode network and participating in attention. On the other hand, the test is also correlated with several subcortical structures (particularly caudate, putamen, and cerebellum), which probably contribute to automation and behavioural adjustments during test performance. This emphasises the role of both cortical and subcortical structures in cognitive functioning and information processing speed in MS.

Abbreviations

BNT: Boston naming test; BRN-B: Brief repeatable neuropsychological battery; DTI: Diffusion tensor imaging; EDSS: Expanded disability status scale; FCSRT: Free and cued selective reminding test; fMRI: functional magnetic resonance imaging; JLO: Judgement of line orientation; MRI: Magnetic resonance imaging; MS: Multiple sclerosis; PASAT: Paced auditory serial addition test; ROCF: Rey-Osterrieth Complex Figure; ROI: Region of interest; SD: Standard deviation; SPM: Statistical parametric mapping; TMT: Trail making test; ToL: Tower of London-Drexel version

Acknowledgements

The authors thank the Spanish Society of Neurology's Research Operations Office for helping in the English language revision of this paper.

Funding

None

Authors' contributions

JAM-G: design of the study; statistical analysis; interpretation of data; writing of the manuscript; final approval of the manuscript. AC-M: data acquisition; statistical analysis; literature review; interpretation of data; writing of the manuscript; final approval of the manuscript. PM: data acquisition; literature review; interpretation of data; final approval of the manuscript. VP: data acquisition; design of the study; final approval of the manuscript. TMR: data acquisition; literature review; final approval of the manuscript. MY: data acquisition; study supervision; critical revision of manuscript for important intellectual content; final approval of the manuscript. MJ: data acquisition; literature review; final approval of the manuscript. JA: design of the study; data acquisition; final approval of the manuscript. JMG design of the study; study supervision; interpretation of data; critical revision of manuscript for important intellectual content; final approval of the manuscript.

Competing interests

The authors declare that they have no competing interest.

Author details

[1]Department of Neurology, San Carlos Health Research Institute (IdISSC), Universidad Complutense de Madrid, C/ Profesor Martín Lagos s/n, 28040 Madrid, Spain. [2]Department of Radiology, IdISSC, Universidad Complutense de Madrid, Madrid, Spain.

References

1. Gronwall DM. Paced auditory serial-addition task: a measure of recovery from concussion. Percept Mot Skills. 1977;44:367–73.
2. Rao SM, Leo GJ, Bernardin L, Unverzagt F. Cognitive dysfunction in multiple sclerosis. I. Frequency, patterns, and prediction. Neurology. 1991;41:685–91.
3. Benedict RH, Fischer JS, Archibald CJ, et al. Minimal neuropsychological assessment of MS patients: a consensus approach. Clin Neuropsychol. 2002; 16:381–97.
4. Cutter GR, Baier ML, Rudick RA, et al. Development of a multiple sclerosis functional composite as a clinical trial outcome measure. Brain. 1999;122: 871–82.
5. Tombaugh TN. A comprehensive review of the paced auditory serial addition test (PASAT). Arch Clin Neuropsychol. 2006;21:53–76.
6. Rao SM, Martin AL, Huelin R, et al. Correlations between MRI and information processing speed in MS: a meta-analysis. Mult Scler Int. 2014; 2014:975803.
7. Morgen K, Sammer G, Courtney SM, et al. Evidence for a direct association between cortical atrophy and cognitive impairment in relapsing-remitting MS. Neuroimage. 2006;30:891–8.
8. Sbardella E, Petsas N, Tona F, et al. Assessing the correlation between grey and white matter damage with motor and cognitive impairment in multiple sclerosis patients. PLoS One. 2013;8:e63250.
9. Nocentini U, Bozzali M, Spanò B, et al. Exploration of the relationships between regional grey matter atrophy and cognition in multiple sclerosis. Brain Imaging Behav. 2014;8:378–86.
10. Riccitelli GC, Pagani E, Rodegher M, et al. Imaging patterns of gray and white matter abnormalities associated with PASAT and SDMT performance in relapsing-remitting multiple sclerosis. Mult Scler. 2017. https://doi.org/10.1177/1352458517743091.
11. Matias-Guiu JA, Cabrera-Martín MN, Valles-Salgado M, et al. Neural basis of cognitive assessment in Alzheimer disease, amnestic mild cognitive impairment, and subjective memory complaints. Am J Geriatr Psychiatry. 2017;25:730–40.
12. Polman CH, Reingold SC, Banwell B, et al. Diagnostic criteria for multiple sclerosis: 2010 revisions to the McDonald criteria. Ann Neurol. 2012;69:292–302.
13. Sepulcre J, Vanotti S, Hernández R, et al. Cognitive impairment in patients with multiple sclerosis using the brief repeatable battery-neuropsychology test. Mult Scler. 2006;12:187–95.
14. Matias-Guiu JA, Cortés-Martínez A, Valles-Salgado M, et al. Functional components of cognitive impairment in multiple sclerosis: a cross-sectional investigation. Front Neurol. 2017;8:643.
15. Peña-Casanova J, Casals-Coll M, Quintana M, et al. Spanish normative studies in a young adult population (NEURONORMA young adults project): methods and characteristics of the sample. Neurologia. 2012;27:253–60.
16. Beck AT, Ward CH, Mendelson M, Mock J, Erbaugh J. An inventory for measuring depression. Arch Gen Psychiatry. 1961;4:561–71.
17. Krupp LB, LaRocca NG, Muir-Nash J, Steinberg AD. The fatigue severity scale. Application to patients with multiple sclerosis and systemic lupus erythematosus. Arch Neurol. 1989;46:1121–3.
18. Schmidt P, Gaster C, Arsic M, et al. An automated tool for detection of FLAIR-hyperintense white-matter lesions in multiple sclerosis. Neuroimage. 2012;59:3774–83.
19. Bates E, Wilson SM, Saygin AP, et al. Voxel-based lesion-symptom mapping. Nat Neurosci. 2003;6:448–50.
20. Rorden C, Karnath HO, Bonilha L. Improving lesion-symptom mapping. J Cogn Neurosci. 2007;19:1081–8.
21. Catani M, Thiebaut de Schotten M. A diffusion tensor imaging tractography atlas for virtual in vivo dissections. Cortex. 2008;44:1105–32.
22. Sepulcre J, Masdeu JC, Pastor MA, et al. Brain pathways of verbal working memory: a lesion-function correlation study. Neuroimage. 2009;47:773–8.
23. D'haeseleer M, Steen C, Hoogduin JM, et al. Performance on paced auditory serial addition test and cerebral blood flow in multiple sclerosis. Acta Neurol Scand. 2013;128:e26–9.
24. Baltruschat SA, Ventura-Campos N, Cruz-Gómez AJ, Belenguer A, Forn C. Gray matter atrophy is associated with functional connectivity reorganization during the paced auditory serial addition test (PASAT) execution in multiple sclerosis (MS). J Neuroradiol. 2015;42:141–9.
25. Louapre C, Perlbarg V, García-Lorenzo D, et al. Brain networks disconnection in early multiple sclerosis cognitive deficits: an anatomofunctional study. Hum Brain Mapp. 2014;35:4706–17.
26. Forn C, Belenguer A, Belloch V, Sanjuan A, Parcet MA, Avila C. Anatomical and functional differences between the paced auditory serial addition test and the symbol digit modalities test. J Clin Exp Neuropsychol. 2011;33:42–50.
27. Tobyne SM, Ochoa WM, Bireley JD, et al. Cognitive impairment and the regional distribution of cerebellar lesions in multiple sclerosis. Mult Scler. 2017. https://doi.org/10.1177/1352458517730132.

28. D'Ambrosio A, Hidalgo de la Cruz M, Valsasina P, et al. Structural
     connectivity-defined thalamic subregions have different functional
     connectivity abnormalities in multiple sclerosis patients: implications for
     clinical correlations. Hum Brain Mapp. 2017;38:6005–18.
29. Dineen RA, Vilisaar J, Hlinka J, et al. Disconnection as a mechanism for
     cognitive dysfunction in multiple sclerosis. Brain. 2009;132:239–49.
30. Van Hecke W, Nagels G, Leemans A, Vandervliet E, Sijbers J, Parizel PM.
     Correlation of cognitive dysfunction and diffusion tensor MRI measures in
     patients with mild and moderate multiple sclerosis. J Magn Reson Imaging.
     2010;31:1492–8.
31. Yu HJ, Christodoulou C, Bhise V, et al. Multiple white matter tract abnormalities
     underlie cognitive impairment in RRMS. Neuroimage. 2012;59:3713–22.
32. Sumowski JF, Rocca MA, Leavitt VM, et al. Brain reserve and cognitive
     reserve in multiple sclerosis: what you've got and how you use it.
     Neurology. 2013;80:2186–93.
33. Lockwood AH, Linn RT, Szymanski H, Coad ML, Wack DS. Mapping the
     neural systems that mediate the paced auditory serial addition task (PASAT).
     J Int Neuropsychol Soc. 2004;10:26–34.
34. Jonkman LE, Rosenthal DM, Sormani MP, et al. Gray matter correlates of
     cognitive performance differ between relasing-remitting and primary-
     progressive multiple sclerosis. PLoS One. 2015;10:e0129380.

Permissions

The contributors of this book come from diverse backgrounds, making this book a truly international effort. This book will bring forth new frontiers with its revolutionizing research information and detailed analysis of the nascent developments around the world.

We would like to thank all the contributing authors for lending their expertise to make the book truly unique. They have played a crucial role in the development of this book. Without their invaluable contributions this book wouldn't have been possible. They have made vital efforts to compile up to date information on the varied aspects of this subject to make this book a valuable addition to the collection of many professionals and students.

This book was conceptualized with the vision of imparting up-to-date information and advanced data in this field. To ensure the same, a matchless editorial board was set up. Every individual on the board went through rigorous rounds of assessment to prove their worth. After which they invested a large part of their time researching and compiling the most relevant data for our readers.

The editorial board has been involved in producing this book since its inception. They have spent rigorous hours researching and exploring the diverse topics which have resulted in the successful publishing of this book. They have passed on their knowledge of decades through this book. To expedite this challenging task, the publisher supported the team at every step. A small team of assistant editors was also appointed to further simplify the editing procedure and attain best results for the readers.

Apart from the editorial board, the designing team has also invested a significant amount of their time in understanding the subject and creating the most relevant covers. They scrutinized every image to scout for the most suitable representation of the subject and create an appropriate cover for the book.

The publishing team has been an ardent support to the editorial, designing and production team. Their endless efforts to recruit the best for this project, has resulted in the accomplishment of this book. They are a veteran in the field of academics and their pool of knowledge is as vast as their experience in printing. Their expertise and guidance has proved useful at every step. Their uncompromising quality standards have made this book an exceptional effort. Their encouragement from time to time has been an inspiration for everyone.

The publisher and the editorial board hope that this book will prove to be a valuable piece of knowledge for researchers, students, practitioners and scholars across the globe.

List of Contributors

Jessica Frau, Giuseppe Fenu, Giancarlo Coghe, Lorena Lorefice, Mauro Badas, Maria Giovanna Marrosu and Eleonora Cocco
Multiple Sclerosis Center Binaghi Hospital, Department of Medical Sciences and Public Health, University of Cagliari, via Is Guadazzonis 2, 09126 Cagliari, Italy

Alessio Signori
Department of Health Sciences, Section of Biostatistics, University of Genova, Via Pastore, 1, 16132 Genoa, Italy

Maria Antonietta Barracciu, Vincenzo Sechi and Federico Cabras
Unit of Radiology, Binaghi Hospital, ATS Sardegna, via Is Guadazzonis 2, 09126 Cagliari, Italy

Serkan Ozakbas, Pinar Yigit and Hatice Limoncu
Department of Neurology, Dokuz Eylul University, Izmir, Turkey

Bilge Piri Cinar
Department of Neurology, Samsun Training and Researce Hospital, Samsun, Turkey

Turhan Kahraman
School of Physical Therapy and Rehabilitation Department, İzmir Katip Celebi University, Izmir, Turkey

Görkem Kösehasanoğulları
Department of Neurology, Usak State Hospital, Usak, Turkey

Anat Achiron
Multiple Sclerosis Center, Sheba Medical Center, 52621 Tel-Hashomer, Israel

Hany Aref
Ain Shams University, Cairo, Egypt

Jihad Inshasi
Rashid Hospital and Dubai Medical College, Dubai, UAE

Mohamad Harb
Department in Monla Hospital, Tripoli, Lebanon

Raed Alroughani
Division of Neurology, Department of Medicine, Amiri Hospital, Sharq, Kuwait

Mahendra Bijarnia
Novartis Healthcare Pvt. Ltd., Hyderabad, India

Kathryn Cooke and Ozgur Yuksel
Novartis Pharma AG, Basel, Switzerland

Frank A. Hoffmann
Department of Neurology, Hospital Martha-Maria Halle-Dölau, Halle, Germany

Anastasiya Trenova
Department of Neurology, Medical University of Plovdiv, Plovdiv, Bulgaria

Miguel A. Llaneza
Neurology Department, Ferrol University Hospital, Ferrol, Spain

Johannes Fischer
Neurologische Praxis (NTDStudy-Group), Lappersdorf, Germany

Giacomo Lus
Multiple Sclerosi Center university of Campania L. Vanvitelli, Naples, Italy

Dorothea von Bredow
QuintilesIMS, IMS Health GmbH & Co. OHG, Munich, Germany

Núria Lara
QuintilesIMS, Barcelona, Spain

Elaine Lam
Novartis Pharmaceuticals Corporation, East Hanover, NJ, USA

Marlies Van Hoef and Rajesh Bakshi
Novartis Pharma AG, Fabrikstrasse 12-3.03.12, Postfach, CH-4002 Basel, Switzerland

Ingo Kleiter
St. Josef Hospital, University Hospital Bochum, Bochum, Germany
Marianne-Strauß-Klinik, Behandlungszentrum Kempfenhausen für Multiple Sklerose Kranke, Berg, Germany

Michael Lang
Joint Neurological Practice, Ulm, Germany

Judith Jeske
Neurological Practice, Wuppertal, Germany

Christiane Norenberg
Bayer AG, Wuppertal, Germany

Barbara Stollfuß and Markus Schürks
Bayer Vital GmbH, Leverkusen, Germany

D. Delgado, N. Cotterill, K. Inglis and D. Owen
Bristol Urological Institute, North Bristol NHS Trust, Southmead Hospital, Bristol BS10 5NB, UK

M. J. Drake
Bristol Urological Institute, North Bristol NHS Trust, Southmead Hospital, Bristol BS10 5NB, UK
School of Clinical Sciences, University of Bristol, Bristol, UK

D. Cottrell
Department of Neurology, North Bristol NHS Trust, Southmead Hospital, Bristol, UK

L. Canham
Department of Neurology, North Bristol NHS Trust, Southmead Hospital, Bristol, UK
School of Clinical Sciences, University of Bristol, Bristol, UK

P. White
University of West of England, Bristol, UK

Marcus J. Drake
School of Clinical Sciences, University of Bristol, Bristol, UK
Bristol Urological Institute, Southmead Hospital, Bristol BS10 5NB, UK

Nikki Cotterill, Debbie Delgado, Lyndsey Johnson and Mary C. Kisanga
Bristol Urological Institute, Southmead Hospital, Bristol BS10 5NB, UK

Luke Canham, Jenny Homewood, Kirsty Inglis, Denise Owen and David Cottrell
Neurology Department, Southmead Hospital, Bristol BS10 5NB, UK

Paul White
University of the West of England, Bristol, UK

Renxin Chu and Shahamat Tauhid
Laboratory for Neuroimaging Research, Brigham and Women's Hospital, Harvard Medical School, 60 Fenwood Rd, Mailbox 9002L, Boston, MA 02115, USA
Departments of Neurology, Brigham and Women's Hospital, Harvard Medical School, Boston, MA, USA

Rohit Bakshi
Laboratory for Neuroimaging Research, Brigham and Women's Hospital, Harvard Medical School, 60 Fenwood Rd, Mailbox 9002L, Boston, MA 02115, USA
Departments of Neurology, Brigham and Women's Hospital, Harvard Medical School, Boston, MA, USA
Radiology, Brigham and Women's Hospital, Harvard Medical School, Boston, MA, USA
Partners MS Center, Brigham and Women's Hospital, Harvard Medical School, Boston, MA, USA

Shelley Hurwitz
Department of Medicine, Brigham and Women's Hospital, Harvard Medical School, Boston, MA, USA

Nina Steinemann, Vladeta Ajdacic-Gross, Stephanie Rodgers, Milo Alan Puhan and Viktor von Wyl
Epidemiology, Biostatistics and Prevention Institute, University of Zurich, Hirschengraben 84, CH-8001 Zurich, Switzerland

Jens Kuhle
Neurological Policlinic, University Hospital Basel, Basel, Switzerland

Pasquale Calabrese
Department of Psychology, University of Basel, Basel, Switzerland

Jürg Kesselring
Rehabilitation Clinic Valens, Valens, Switzerland

Giulio Disanto
Department of Neurology, Regional Hospital Lugano (EOC), Lugano, Switzerland

Doron Merkler
Division of Clinical Pathology, Geneva University Hospital, Geneva, Switzerland

Caroline Pot
Department of Clinical Neuroscience, Centre hospitalier universitaire vaudois, Lausanne, Switzerland

Antoni Sicras-Mainar
Fundación Rediss (Red de Investigación en servicios Sanitarios), Barcelona, Spain

Elena Ruíz-Beato
Health Economics and Outcomes Research Unit, Roche Farma S.A., Madrid, Spain

Ruth Navarro-Artieda
Department of Medical Information, Hospital Universitari Germans Trias i Pujol, Badalona, Barcelona, Spain

Jorge Maurino
Medical Department, Roche Farma S.A., Madrid, Spain

Tjalf Ziemssen
Universitätsklinium Dresden, Fetscherstraße 74, 01307 Dresden, Germany

Christine Prosser, Jennifer Scarlet Haas and Sebastian Braun
Xcenda GmbH, Lange Laube 31, D-30159 Hannover, Germany

Andrew Lee and Ming-Yi Huang
Biogen, Cambridge, MA, USA

Pamela Landsman-Blumberg
Xcenda LLC, Palm Harbor, FL, USA

Angela Kempel, Erika Gleißner and Sarita Patel
Biogen GmbH, Carl-Zeiss-Ring 6, 85737 Ismaning, Germany

Spyros N. Deftereos, Dimitrios Sakellariou and Filippo DeLorenzo
Merck Hellas, 41-45 Kifisias av, 15123 Athens, Greece

Evangelos Koutlas
Neurology Department, Papageorgiou Hospital, Thessaloniki, Greece

Efrosini Koutsouraki and Nikolaos Vlaikidis
Neurology Department, Aristotle University of Thessaloniki, Thessaloniki, Greece

Athanassios Kyritsis
University of Ioannina Neurology Department, Ioannina, Greece

Panagiotis Papathanassopoulos
Neurology Department, University of Patras, Patras, Greece

Nikolaos Fakas
Neurology Department, 401 Army Hospital of Athens, Athens, Greece

Vaia Tsimourtou
Neurology Department, University of Thessaly, Larissa, Greece

Antonios Tavernarakis
Neurology Department, Evangelismos Hospital, Athens, Greece

Konstantinos Voumvourakis
B Neurology Department, University of Athens, Athens
Greece

Michalis Arvanitis
Private Practice, Athens, Greece

Maria Busch and Luise Krizek
Department of Neurology, University of Leipzig, Liebigstraße 20, 04103 Leipzig, Germany

Muriel Stoppe and Florian Then Bergh
Department of Neurology, University of Leipzig, Liebigstraße 20, 04103 Leipzig, Germany
Translational Centre for Regenerative Medicine, University of Leipzig, Liebigstraße 20, 04103 Leipzig, Germany

Robert Simpson, Frances S. Mair and Stewart W. Mercer
General Practice and Primary Care, Institute of Health and Wellbeing, University of Glasgow, House 1, 1 Horselethill Road, Glasgow, Scotland G12 9LX, UK

S. Michelle Driedger and Ryan Maier
Department of Community Health Sciences, Max Rady College of Medicine, Rady Faculty of Health Sciences, University of Manitoba, Winnipeg, MB, Canada

Ruth Ann Marrie
Departments of Internal Medicine and Community Health Sciences, Max Rady College of Medicine, Rady Faculty of Health Sciences, University of Manitoba, Winnipeg, MB, Canada

Melissa Brouwers
Department of Oncology, McMaster University, Hamilton, ON, Canada

Susan Coote and Sara Hayes
Department of Clinical Therapies, University of Limerick, Limerick, Ireland
Health Research Institute, University of Limerick, Limerick, Ireland

Aidan Larkin
Multiple Sclerosis Society of Ireland, Western office, Galway, Ireland

Marcin Uszynski
Department of Clinical Therapies, University of Limerick, Limerick, Ireland
Multiple Sclerosis Society of Ireland, Western office, Galway, Ireland

Matthew P. Herring
Health Research Institute, University of Limerick, Limerick, Ireland
Department of Physical Education and Sports Science, University of Limerick, Limerick, Ireland

Carl Scarrott
HRB Clinical Research Facility, National University of Ireland, Galway, Ireland
School of Mathematics and Statistics, University of Canterbury, Christchurch, New Zealand

John Newell
HRB Clinical Research Facility, National University of Ireland, Galway, Ireland
School of Mathematics, Statistics and Applied Mathematics, National University of Ireland, Galway, Ireland

Stephen Gallagher
Health Research Institute, University of Limerick, Limerick, Ireland
Department of Psychology, University of Limerick, Limerick, Ireland

Robert W Motl
Department of Physical Therapy, School of Health Professions, University of Alabama at Birmingham, Birmingham, USA

Sylvia Kotterba
Klinik für Geriatrie, Klinikum Leer gemeinnützige GmbH, Leer, Germany

Thomas Neusser, Thomas Glaser, Martin Dörner and Markus Schürks
Bayer Vital GmbH, Leverkusen, Germany

Christiane Norenberg
Bayer AG, Wuppertal, Germany

Patrick Bussfeld
Bayer Consumer Care AG, Basel, Switzerland

G. Fenu, M. Fronza, L. Lorefice, M. Arru, G. Coghe, J. Frau, M. G. Marrosu and E. Cocco
Multiple Sclerosis Center, Binaghi Hospital, ATS Sardegna, Department of Medical Sciences and Public Health, University of Cagliari, via Is Guadazzonis, 2, 09126 Cagliari, Italy

A. G. Vakrakou, D. Tzanetakos, J. Tzartos, M. Anagnostouli, E. Andreadou, M. E. Evangelopoulos, G. Koutsis, C. Chrysovitsanou, E. Gialafos, A. Dimitrakopoulos, L. Stefanis and C. Kilidireas
1st Department of Neurology, Medical School of Athens, National & Kapodistrian University, Aeginition Hospital, Athens, Greece

S. Valsami
Department of Blood Transfusion, Medical School of Athens, National & Kapodistrian University, Aretaieion Hospital, Athens, Greece

E. Grigoriou and K. Psarra
Immunology and Histocompatibility Department, Evangelismos Hospital, Athens, Greece

Jordi A. Matias-Guiu, Ana Cortés-Martínez, Paloma Montero, Vanesa Pytel, Teresa Moreno-Ramos and Jorge Matías-Guiu
Department of Neurology, San Carlos Health Research Institute (IdISSC), Universidad Complutense de Madrid, C/ Profesor Martín Lagos s/n, 28040 Madrid, Spain

Manuela Jorquera, Miguel Yus and Juan Arrazola
Department of Radiology, IdISSC, Universidad Complutense de Madrid, Madrid, Spain

Index

www.ingramcontent.com/pod-product-compliance
Lightning Source LLC
Chambersburg PA
CBHW082012190326
41458CB00010B/3163